Infant, Child and Adolescent Nutrition

Infant, Child and Adolescent Nutrition

A practical handbook

Judy More BSC DipNut&Diet RD RNutr
Paediatric Dietitian, Honorary Lecturer,
School of Health Professions,
University of Plymouth, Plymouth, UK

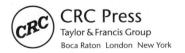
CRC Press
Taylor & Francis Group
Boca Raton London New York

CRC Press is an imprint of the
Taylor & Francis Group, an **informa** business

CRC Press
Taylor & Francis Group
6000 Broken Sound Parkway NW, Suite 300
Boca Raton, FL 33487-2742

© 2013 by Taylor & Francis Group, LLC
CRC Press is an imprint of Taylor & Francis Group, an Informa business

No claim to original U.S. Government works

Printed on acid-free paper
Version Date: 20121128

International Standard Book Number: 978-1-4441-1185-9 (Paperback)

Visit the Taylor & Francis Web site at
http://www.taylorandfrancis.com

and the CRC Press Web site at
http://www.crcpress.com

Contents

Preface

From conception through to adolescence, nutritional intake and status affect the health and wellbeing of children during their childhood and on into their adult years. Myths and confusion surrounding the topic of nutrition for children can compromise the health of some children. To combat this, evidence-based information has been compiled in this book to provide a comprehensive guide to the theory behind nutrition from preconception to adolescence.

Putting the theory into practice is another challenge that requires an understanding of how children's feeding skills develop, how children learn to like foods, how their attitudes to eating food change with age and why families and children choose the foods and drinks that they purchase and consume. These topics are explored in this text to help parents, carers, caterers, advisors and educators manage mealtime behaviour and provide suitable nutritious meals and snacks for children.

Health professionals working with children, be they paediatricians, general practitioners, nurses, health visitors, social workers, nursery nurses, school nurses, practice nurses, breast feeding counsellors, allied health professionals or dietitians, can use this text to find reliable nutritional information to pass on to parents and children. It is an essential reference for them and for students in all medical and social care courses.

Judy More

Section 1
Nutritional Requirements and Healthy Eating

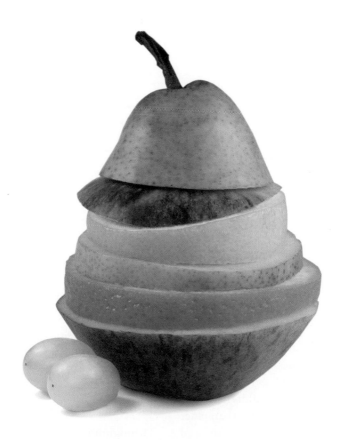

Nutritional Requirements

Summary

- Nutritional requirements increase as children grow and are theoretically defined for different age groups of children.

- Reference Nutrient Intakes (RNIs) are used to define the average daily amount of protein and each essential micronutrient that different age groups of children need.

- Energy requirements depend on weight and activity and are theoretically defined by Estimated Average Requirements (EARs) for each age group.

- There are no set fluid requirements for children over 1 year of age as the kidney functions well and can cope with varying amounts of fluid intake, however, dehydration should be avoided by offering 6–8 drinks per day.

- Different nutrients have different functions in the body and a combination of all the nutrients is required to maintain health and sustain growth and development.

Food and drinks provide water, energy and nutrients that are required for growth, development, health and a strong immune system to fight infection. A balanced, nutritious diet provides adequate amounts of water, energy and all the nutrients.

In general, energy and nutrient requirements increase with age as children grow, but to support rapid rates of growth in infancy there are some exceptions: calcium, iron and phosphorus requirements are higher in infancy than in subsequent years.

Water

Water makes up about 75 per cent of a newborn infant's body weight and about 70 per cent of that of a toddler. Throughout childhood this percentage slowly decreases to about 60 per cent of an adolescent. Infants and young children have a larger skin area in relation to their size than older children and can dehydrate very quickly, so need regular fluid intakes throughout the day.

Infant milk feeds are about 90 per cent water and a young infant's water intake can come entirely from milk feeds. Once solid food is introduced, some water will be obtained from food as well as drinks. Older children obtain about 60 per cent of their water intake from food and the remaining 40 per cent is from drinks.

Energy

Energy requirements in children must provide for (Wiskin *et al.* 2011):

- basal metabolic rate, which is around 60–70 per cent of energy expenditure

- physical activity, which varies considerably and can be up to 30–40 per cent of energy expenditure

- growth – the energy required varies throughout childhood as the rate of growth changes as described in Chapter 2.1.

Throughout childhood, energy requirements increase as weight increases and individual requirements vary specifically with activity levels and growth rate. Estimated average energy requirements for children are listed in Table 1.1.1. Inadequate energy intakes will reduce weight gain and if intakes are very low, growth and development can slow down. An excess energy intake will be stored on the child's body as excess fat, causing overweight or obesity.

Table 1.1.1 Estimated Average Requirement (EAR) of Energy for children in the UK (SACN, 2011)

| Age | Estimated Average Requirement for Energy | | | | |
| | Kilocalories/ Kg/day | Kilocalories/ day | | Megajoules/ day | |
		Males	Females	Males	Females
1-2 months*	96 (120)	526 (598)	478 (550)	2.2 (2.5)	2.0 (2.3)
3-4 months*	96	574 (622)	526 (598)	2.4 (2.6)	2.2 (2.5)
5-6 months*	72 (96)	598 (646)	550 (622)	2.5 (2.7)	2.3 (2.6)
7-12 months*	72	694 (742)	646 (670)	2.9 (3.1)	2.7 (2.8)
1 year		765	717	3.2	3.0
2 years		1004	932	4.2	3.9
3 years		1171	1076	4.9	4.5
4 years		1386	1291	5.8	5.4
5 years		1482	1362	6.2	5.7
6 years		1577	1482	6.6	6.2
7 years		1649	1530	6.9	6.4
8 years		1745	1625	7.3	6.8
9 years		1840	1721	7.7	7.2
10 years		2032	1936	8.5	8.1
11 years		2127	2032	8.9	8.5
12 years		2247	2103	9.4	8.8
13 years		2414	2223	10.1	9.3
14 years		2629	2342	11.0	9.8
15 years		2820	2390	11.8	10.0
16 years		2964	2414	12.4	10.1
17 years		3083	2462	12.9	10.3
18 years		3155	2462	13.2	10.3

*Figures are for breastfed infants 1–12 months. Where figures vary for formula fed infants, they are given in brackets.

1 megajoule = 1000 kilojoules

Energy intake is from foods and drinks, and is measured in either kilojoules or kilocalories. Energy is derived from the protein, fat, carbohydrate and alcohol in the foods. Differing amounts of energy are provided by each gram of these substances:

Protein	4 kcal/g (17 kJ/g)
Fat	9 kcal/g (37 kJ/g)
Carbohydrate	3.75 kcal/g (16 kJ/g)
Alcohol	7 kcal/g (29 kJ/g)

In a balanced diet for children over 12 months of age, the energy from each component is around:

Protein	15 per cent
Fat	35 per cent, including saturated fat providing up to 11 per cent total energy
Carbohydrate	50 per cent, including non-milk extrinsic sugars providing up to 11 per cent of total energy

For infants these percentages change as the diet changes from milk only, providing 8 per cent from protein, 47 per cent from fat and 45 per cent from carbohydrate towards the figures above as their intake of milk decreases and food increases.

Nutrients

Nutrients can be classified into two groups:

● macronutrients: protein, fat and carbohydrate
● micronutrients: vitamins and minerals.

Protein

Proteins are needed for building and maintaining all the cells in the body. During growth, vast numbers of new cells are created and extra protein is needed for this. Protein is made up of long chains of amino acids linked together. Some amino acids can be made by the human body (non-essential amino acids) but others cannot; these are called 'essential amino acids' and must be provided by food. All the essential amino acids needed are found in the protein in animal foods, such as milk, eggs, meat and fish. Proteins in plant-based foods contain some but not all of the essential amino acids. However, the combination of a starchy food, such as bread, pasta, potatoes or rice, together with pulses or nuts will provide all the essential amino acids together. Examples of this combination are baked beans on toast, rice and peas or a hummus (made from chickpeas) or peanut butter sandwich.

Carbohydrate

Carbohydrates provide energy and fibre. The energy comes from the starches and sugars. All carbohydrates are metabolised into glucose which is used by the cells for energy. The brain uses glucose for energy. Other cells can use glucose or fat.

Starch
Starches are long chains of sugar molecules that do not have a sweet taste.

Sugars
Sugars in food are either *monosaccharides*, e.g.

- glucose
- fructose – the main sugar in fruit

or *disaccharides*, e.g

- lactose – the sugar found in milk composed of glucose and galactose
- sucrose – white table sugar made from sugar cane or root vegetables composed of glucose and fructose
- maltose – the main sugar formed when starch breaks down composed of two glucose units.

Non-milk extrinsic sugars are the most harmful to teeth and include sucrose, fructose from processed fruit such as fruit juices and glucose and fructose in syrups.

Intrinsic sugars that are less harmful to teeth include lactose and fructose, when it is contained in raw unprocessed fruit as the cells of the fruit remain intact and the fructose is contained within each cell.

Fibre
Fibre is a term used for the particular types of carbohydrates that are not digested in the small intestine for absorption into the blood. They remain in the small intestines and pass right through to the large intestine and most are also excreted in the faeces. They help the digestive system to work properly, preventing constipation and diarrhoea.

Prebiotics
Prebiotics are the types of fibre that encourage the growth of beneficial bacteria in the intestine. Prebiotic fibre is found in fruits and vegetables, such as onions and leeks, garlic and bananas.

Fat

There are many different types of fat, all of which provide energy. Fat can be:

- saturated
- monounsaturated
- polyunsaturated
- complex, such as cholesterol.

The fat in foods is a mixture of all the types of fat but certain foods have more of one type than the others. Complex fats such as cholesterol account for a very small proportion of the fat in foods.

Saturated fat
About 60–70 per cent of the fat in meat, butter, cream, milk, cheese and palm oil is saturated fat. About 90 per cent of the fat in coconut oil is saturated. Processed commercial foods such as biscuits, cakes, pastries and ready meals also contain a lot of saturated fat in the form of hydrogenated fat. This is because hydrogenating unsaturated fats to change them into saturated fat extends the shelf-life of the foods; saturated fat is less likely go 'off' than unsaturated fats.

Trans fats
Trans fats are found naturally in milk and milk products and are not harmful, whereas the trans fats found in processed food are now known to raise cholesterol in the same way that an excess of saturated fat does.

Unsaturated fats – monounsaturated and polyunsaturated

Most vegetable oils, nuts and seeds contain more monounsaturated and polyunsaturated fat than saturated fat.

Essential fats: omega 3 and omega 6 fats

Two key groups of essential polyunsaturated fats that the body cannot make are omega 3 and omega 6 fats (Table 1.1.2). Plant foods provide these in a shorter chain form and the body converts them to a long-chain form to use in the cells in our body. Food from animal sources provides these essential fats directly in the long-chain form.

The long-chain form of omega 3 fat is particularly needed for the growing brain, the nervous system and for good vision. Infants can only make limited amounts of the long-chain form and rely on getting plenty of long-chain omega 3 in breast milk or infant formula as well as some oily fish during weaning. Children over 1 year of age should be able to make adequate amounts of the long-chain forms even if they eat a vegetarian diet without fish. Some research shows, however, that children who regularly eat oily fish a couple of times per week and have a good intake of omega 3 fat in the long-chain form are less likely to get asthma.

Balancing omega 3 and omega 6 fats in diets

The balance of these two groups of fats affects health. Up until about 50 years ago our diets had about equal quantities of these omega 3 and omega 6 fats, but nowadays we eat a much higher proportion of omega 6 fats and very little omega 3 fat. This change is thought to be one of the factors causing increased rates of allergy, asthma and hay fever in children.

Vitamins

Vitamins are chemicals that are needed for the proper functioning of the human body but cannot be made within the body. They are made by certain plants, animals or bacteria and thus the vitamins are acquired by eating those plant and animal foods. Certain bacteria in the gastrointestinal tract provide two of the vitamins – vitamin K and vitamin B12.

Vitamins A, D, E and K are fat-soluble vitamins and are found within the oils and fats in some foods. When an excess of these vitamins are eaten, reasonable amounts of them can be stored in the body. Vitamin C and the B vitamins are water-soluble and any excess amounts of them consumed are excreted in urine. The stores of these vitamins that are built up are much smaller and it is thus crucial to have a regular supply in the diet.

Table 1.1.2 Names and food sources of the various essential omega 3 and omega 6 fats

	Omega 3 fats	Omega 6 fats
Short-chain form – from plants		
Names	ALA (alpha-linolenic acid)	LA (linoleic acid)
Main food sources	Walnuts, linseeds, and their oils Rapeseed oil Olive oil and soya oil have smaller amounts	All nuts, seeds and vegetable oils
Long-chain form – from animal foods		
Names	EPA (eicosapentaenoic acid) DHA (docosahexaenoic acid)	GLA (gamma linolenic acid) AA (arachidonic acid)
Main food sources	Best source is oily fish[a] Other sources are red meat and egg yolks depending how the animals and chickens are fed[b]	Fish, meat and egg yolks

[a] Oily fish are: salmon, mackerel, trout, fresh tuna, sardines, pilchards and eel.

[b] Animals that have grazed on grass rather than been fed cereals have higher amounts of omega 3 in their meat. Egg yolks from chickens fed a special feed high in omega 3 fat will be a good source of omega 3 fats.

Vitamin A

Vitamin A comes in two forms: retinol in some animal foods (full-fat milk, butter, margarine, egg yolks and liver) and carotene in fruits and vegetables. Carotene is the orange colour in fruits and vegetables and it is also present in dark green vegetables such as spinach and broccoli.

Vitamin A is very important for growth and development as well as vision. As an antioxidant it is part of the immune system helping to prevent infections and illness. Young children do not always get enough vitamin A in their diet, which is why the Department of Health recommends a daily supplement for all under-fives. In the developing world, many children have impaired vision due to a deficiency of vitamin A. Fortunately this deficiency is not seen in the UK.

Excess vitamin A taken in the form of too many supplements could be a problem for children as excess amounts are stored in the body. Liver is very high in vitamin A now that animal feed is enriched with it. The Food Standards Agency recommends that children and adults should only consume liver once per week.

B vitamins

The B vitamins are thiamin, folic acid, niacin (nicotinamide), riboflavin, pyridoxine, biotin, pantothenic acid and vitamin B12. These are all important for growth and development of a healthy nervous system, and are needed to convert food into energy. Vitamin B12 and folate are important for preventing types of anaemia. Good sources of B vitamins include meat, milk products, fish, eggs, cereals, seeds and vegetables. Dark green vegetables, liver and pulses are high in folate.

Vitamin C

Vitamin C, also known as ascorbic acid, is essential for increasing the iron absorption from plant foods, protecting cells from damage and for maintaining blood vessels, cartilage, muscle and bone. Vitamin C is also involved in wound healing. A severe deficiency causes scurvy.

Vitamin D

Vitamin D is sometimes called the 'sunshine vitamin' as most is made in exposed skin when we are outside in daylight. The action of UV (ultraviolet) radiation of wavelength 290–310 nm converts 7-dehydrocholesterol to vitamin D3 (via its precursor). Skin synthesis is affected by many factors, including the following:

- Latitude: The intensity of the sunlight decreases with increasing distance from the equator. In the UK vitamin D is only made in the skin during the summer months from April to September. Hence in summer a store of vitamin D must be built up to last through the winter.
- Climate: Cloud cover decreases the intensity of the sunlight.
- Air pollution: This reduces the critical UV light waves available for skin synthesis.
- Skin type: Synthesis is higher in white populations than in darker pigmented skins of children of Asian, African and Middle Eastern origin.
- Lifestyle habits with regard to time spent outside or clothing. People who cover most of their skin when outside have limited synthesis and are more likely to be deficient in vitamin D.
- Sunscreen use, as sunscreens prevent skin synthesis. Although it is important not to let children's skin burn in the sunshine, it is also important for them to spend time outside everyday in summer in order to make plenty of vitamin D and build up a good store. Sunscreens should only be used to prevent sunburn when children are outside for extended periods in the middle of the day. If sunburn is unlikely then children should be encouraged to play outside without sunscreen.

Very few foods contain vitamin D – oily fish is the best source. In the UK, margarines, formula milks and some breakfast cereals are fortified with vitamin D. Meat and egg yolks contain tiny amounts.

The liver enzyme 25-hydroxylase converts endogenously synthesized vitamin D3 and diet-derived D2 and D3 to 25 hydroxyvitamin D. In the kidney, 25 hydroxyvitamin D can be converted to 1,25-dihydroxyvitamin D, the active hormone which has several roles in the body:

- the absorption of calcium from food and for depositing calcium and other minerals into bone to give it strength
- maintaining calcium levels in the blood – low levels of calcium can cause tetany and fitting which is seen in young infants who are deficient in vitamin D
- as a component of the immune system.

Many toddlers have low vitamin D levels and it has been reported that rickets, a disease that causes soft, misshapen bones, is on the increase in toddlers in the UK. Adolescents are also at risk of rickets. Children with dark skins are particularly at risk as they need longer in the sun to make enough vitamin D.

Because this vitamin is necessary to support the rapid rate of bone growth in the under-fives, a daily supplement is recommended for them. It used to be taken in cod liver oil but vitamin drops are now recommended (see pages 110, 136).

Vitamin E

Vitamin E is an important antioxidant that protects cell structures in the body. It is found in many foods such as vegetable oils, butter and margarines, meat, fish and eggs. Children usually have plenty of vitamin E in their food.

Vitamin K

Vitamin K is needed to ensure normal blood clotting and is provided mostly by the bacteria in the intestine. Green leafy vegetables are the best food source of vitamin K.

Minerals

Calcium is needed for the structure of healthy bones and teeth. It is also needed for many key functions in the body and the calcium in bone acts as a store so that there is always a ready supply enabling the muscles, including the heart, to contract and the nerves and cells to function as necessary. Milk, cheese and yogurt are the best sources. Soya beans are a reasonable source of calcium but soya milk needs to be fortified with extra calcium to provide the same amounts as cow's milk. White bread has been fortified with

calcium since the 1940s and tinned fish with bones such as sardines is another good source.

Copper is involved in energy and protein production. It is found in tiny amounts in all foods. Children usually get enough from their food.

Fluoride strengthens tooth enamel and makes it resistant to attack by the bacteria that cause tooth decay. The two main sources of fluoride are toothpaste and tap water. Teeth should be cleaned twice a day using a fluoride-containing toothpaste:

- up to the age of 3: a smear of toothpaste containing 1000 ppm of fluoride
- over the age of 3: a pea-sized amount of toothpaste containing 1350–1500 ppm of fluoride.

There are areas of the UK where tap water is fluoridated or the water naturally contains adequate levels of fluoride. However, there are large areas of the UK where water does not contain adequate fluoride. Dentists may recommend fluoride tablets or drops for children who are at high risk of dental disease. That is those who have:

- a family history of a high caries level
- medical conditions where treatment for dental caries should be avoided (e.g. bleeding disorders, cardiac problems)
- a mental or physical disability, which can make treatment for dental disease particularly difficult.

Advice from a dentist on giving supplements is crucial as too much fluoride can cause dental fluorosis – permanent brown spots on the teeth.

Iodine forms part of the hormone thyroxine which has several key roles in the body – converting food into energy and enabling growth and physical and mental development. Iodine deficiency is common in some areas of Europe but is rarely seen in children in the UK as British milk is a reasonable source of iodine. Fish, milk, yogurt and eggs are good sources.

Iron is part of the structure of haemoglobin, the chemical that carries oxygen to all the cells in the body via the blood. Oxygen is needed by cells to produce energy. Many under-fives and adolescents do not eat enough iron in their diet, and anaemia due to iron deficiency is fairly common among these two age groups in the UK. It causes tiredness, delayed growth and development and more illness as iron is also part of the immune system. Poor appetite is another consequence; this can create a vicious circle as less iron will be eaten by a child with a poor appetite. See page 147 for more information on iron-deficiency anaemia.

Iron in food is found in two forms:

● haem iron which is readily absorbed – good sources are red meat such as beef, lamb and pork, dark poultry meat such as chicken legs and thighs, and oily fish

● non-haem iron which is poorly absorbed unless vitamin C is present – good sources of non-haem iron are eggs, pulses, nuts, fortified breakfast cereals, dried fruit and some vegetables.

Magnesium is also involved in the process of converting food into energy as well as building bone and protein production. The best sources are wholegrain bread and breakfast cereals, milk and yogurt. Other good sources are meat, eggs, pulses and some vegetables.

Phosphorus forms the main structure of bones along with calcium. It is found in milk but unlike calcium it is also found in most other foods, so children usually have plenty in their food.

Potassium plays a key role in fluid balance, muscle contractions and proper nerve function. The best sources are milk, fruit, vegetables, cocoa and chocolate.

Selenium is an antioxidant and plays a role in the production of the thyroid hormone as well as energy production. The best sources for children are bread, meat, fish, eggs and other foods made from flour. Brazil nuts and cashew nuts are particularly rich.

The amount of selenium in the soil determines how much is in the food grown on that soil. Selenium levels in UK soil are on the low side compared to those in the United States where levels are higher.

Sodium plays a key role in fluid balance and maintaining blood pressure and is necessary to maintain growth in children. Sodium is found in several foods but the main source is in salt, which is used to preserve some foods and added to enhance flavour in most processed food. Too much salt can raise blood pressure in older children and adults, creating a higher risk of heart disease, but there is no evidence of harm in younger children. Children eating a lot of processed snack foods and ready meals, which all have added salt, may exceed the recommendations on salt/sodium intake published by the Scientific Advisory Committee on Nutrition (SACN) in 2003, as listed in Table 1.1.3.

Table 1.1.3 Salt/sodium intake recommendations

Age	Daily recommended maximum intake (SACN 2003)		Reference Nutrient Intake (Department of Health 1991)
	Salt (g/day)	Sodium (g/day)	Sodium (g/day)
0–3 months	1	0.4	0.21
4–6 months	1	0.4	0.28
7–9 months	1	0.4	0.32
10–12 months	1	0.4	0.35
1–3 years	2	0.8	0.5
4–6 years	3	1.2	0.7
7–10 years	5	2	1.3
11+ years	6	2.4	1.6

The SACN recommendations are not evidence based, are very difficult to achieve and are only slightly above the recommended intake expressed as the Reference Nutrient Intake.

Zinc helps wounds to heal and is part of the immune system. In children it is important for growth as it is part of two hormones – growth hormone and insulin. The best food sources are meat, fish, milk and eggs. Bread and breakfast cereals are also good sources.

Other Beneficial Components in Food

Phytochemicals

Phytochemicals are compounds that occur naturally in plants (phyto means 'plant' in Greek) and that have biological significance but are not established as essential nutrients. They include antioxidants, which are the brightly coloured pigments in plant foods – that is in fruits, vegetables, spices, herbs, nuts, cocoa beans and foods made from cereals. Tea and coffee also contain them. They are called a variety of names such as flavonoids, flavanols and isoflavones. Some of the commonly known phytochemicals are:

- lycopene in tomatoes
- quercetin in apples, onions, grapes and berries
- anthocyanins in berries.

There are thousands of these chemicals in plant foods, and research indicating that they may be protective against various cancers and cardiovascular disease has only been published in the last 30 or so years. Their mode of action in cancer prevention is by:

- increasing the body's ability to break down carcinogens
- acting as an antioxidant to mop up free radicals before they damage cells in the body
- enhancing the immune system
- altering hormones which are associated with the onset of cancer.

They help prevent cardiovascular disease by:

- decreasing blood cholesterol
- altering the profile of fats in the blood
- reducing the oxidation of fat present in arterial walls.

They have not been shown to be of critical importance for the day-to-day health of children, but during childhood it is important for children to learn to like the foods that contain them and to learn that eating fruit and vegetables at all meals is normal because of their likely disease prevention later in life.

Probiotics

Probiotics are bacteria in food that colonize the intestine and provide health benefits. Beneficial bacteria in the intestine help the intestine to function optimally and may help to prevent diarrhoea in children. Examples of beneficial bacteria are bifidobacteria and lactobacilli that are found in live yogurt.

Dietary Requirements

In general, the amount of energy and each nutrient that children need to stay healthy increases as they grow. In the UK energy and nutrient requirements have been set for different age groups of children in 1991 by the Committee on Medical Aspects of Food Policy (COMA). COMA was the forerunner of the current Scientific Advisory Committee on Nutrition (SACN) (www. sacn.gov.uk) (Department of Health 1991).

The relevant units used for dietary requirements are as follows:

- Reference Nutrient Intake (RNI) – the average daily amount of a nutrient that is considered to be enough to meet the requirements of 97 per cent of the population of each age group of children. This means only 3 in 100 children would require an amount higher than this. It is used as the daily recommendation for protein, vitamins and minerals.

- Estimated Average Requirement (EAR) is the daily mean/average requirement for each age group and would only be enough for 50 per cent of a population. It is used for energy requirements.

These recommended values vary somewhat from country to country.

RNIs for protein have been set for different age groups of children but an individual protein requirement can be calculated more specifically for individual infants and young children depending on their body weight (Table 1.1.4).

Table 1.1.4 UK Reference Nutrient Intakes for protein for children

Age	Protein RNI (g/day) Males	Females	Protein (g/kg body weight/day)
0–3 months	12.5	12.5	2.1
4–6 months	12.7	12.7	1.6
7–9 months	13.7	13.7	1.5
10–12 months	14.9	14.9	1.5
1–3 years	14.5	14.5	1.1
4–6 years	19.7	19.7	
7–10 years	28.3	28.3	
11–14 years	42.1	41.2	
15–18 years	55.2	45	

Micronutrient Requirements

UK Reference Nutrient Intakes for vitamins and minerals for children are listed in Tables 1.1.5 and 1.1.6.

For some of the micronutrients that are only required in very small amounts 'safe intakes' are set (Table 1.1.7).

Ensuring Adequate Energy and Nutrient Intakes

Children can store a certain amount of nutrients within their body and hence eating to meet the RNI for each nutrient each day is not necessary. An average daily intake over a few weeks is adequate.

Table 1.1.5 UK Reference Nutrient Intakes for vitamins for children

Age	Vitamin A (µg/day)	B Vitamins Thiamin (mg/day)	Riboflavin (mg/day)	Niacin (mg/day)	Vitamin B6 (mg/day)	Vitamin B12 (µg/day)	Folate (µg/day)	Vitamin C (mg/day)	Vitamin D (µg/day)
0–3 months	350	0.2	0.4	3	0.2	0.3	50	25	8.5
4–6 months	350	0.2	0.4	3	0.2	0.3	50	25	8.5
7–9 months	350	0.2	0.4	4	0.3	0.4	50	25	7
10–12 months	350	0.3	0.4	5	0.4	0.4	50	25	7
1–3 years	400	0.5	0.6	8	0.7	0.5	70	30	7
4–6 years	400	0.7	0.8	11	0.9	0.8	100	30	–
7–10 years	500	0.7	1.0	12	1.0	1.0	150	30	–
Males									
11–14 years	600	0.9	1.2	15	1.2	1.2	200	35	–
15–18 years	700	1.1	1.3	15	1.2	1.2	200	40	–
Females									
11–14 years	600	0.7	1.1	12	1.0	1.2	200	35	–
15–18 years	600	0.8	1.1	14	1.2	1.5	200	40	–

Table 1.1.6 UK Reference Nutrient Intakes for minerals for children

Age	Calcium mg/day	Chloride mg/day	Copper mg/day	Iodine µg/day	Iron mg/day	Magnesium mg/day	Phosphorus mg/day	Potassium mg/day	Sodium mg/day	Selenium µg/day	Zinc mg/day
0–3 months	525	320	0.2	50	1.7	55	400	800	210	10	4
4–6 months	525	400	0.3	60	4.3	60	400	850	280	13	4
7–9 months	525	500	0.3	60	7.8	75	400	700	320	10	5
10–12 months	525	500	0.3	60	7.8	80	400	700	350	10	5
1–3 years	350	800	0.4	70	6.9	85	270	800	500	15	5
4–6 years	450	1100	0.6	100	6.1	120	350	1100	700	20	6.5
7–10 years	550	1800	0.7	110	8.7	200	450	2000	1200	30	7
Males											
11–14 years	1000	2500	0.8	130	11.3	280	775	3100	1600	45	9
15–18 years	1000	2500	1.0	140	11.3	300	775	3500	1600	70	9.5
Females											
11–14 years	800	2500	0.8	130	14.8	280	625	3100	1600	45	9
15–18 years	800	2500	1.0	140	14.8	300	625	3500	1600	60	7

Table 1.1.7 Safe intakes for certain micronutrients

Nutrient		Safe intake
B vitamins	Pantothenic acid	3–7 mg/day
	Biotin	10–200 µg/day
Trace minerals	Chromium	0.104–1.976 µg/kg body weight/day
	Fluoride	0.12 mg/kg body weight/day
	Manganese	16.5 µg/kg body weight/day
	Molybdenum	0.480–1.440 µg/kg body weight/day

In general it is not necessary to calculate the nutrient intakes of children and compare them to the RNIs because foods can be grouped into food groups with all the foods in each food group providing a similar range of certain nutrients. By combining foods from each of the food groups in certain quantities each day all the nutrients needed will be automatically provided.

How to meet energy and nutrient requirements through food and drinks in a balanced nutritious diet is discussed in Chapter 1.2.

References and further reading

Department of Health (1991) *Report on Health and Social Subjects No. 41. Dietary Reference Values for Food Energy and Nutrients for the United Kingdom.* London: The Stationery Office.

Dietetic Department Great Ormond Street Hospital for Children NHS Trust (2009) *Nutritional Requirements for Children in Health and Disease*, 4th edn. London: Great Ormond Street Hospital Trust.

Scientific Advisory Committee on Nutrition (SACN) (2003) *Salt and Health.* London: The Stationery Office.

SACN (2011) *Dietary Reference Values for Energy.* London: The Stationery Office.

Wiskin AE, Davies JH, Wootton SA and Beatties RM (2011) Energy expenditure, nutrition and growth. *Archives of Disease in Childhood* **96**: 567–572.

Principles of a Balanced Nutritious Diet for Children over 1 Year

Summary

- Foods can be divided into five food groups based on the nutrients they contain, and an average daily combination of a number of servings from each food group provides nutritional adequacy.

- The food groups and number of servings children require are:

  - bread, rice, potatoes, pasta and other starchy foods – include at each meal and some snacks: 3–5 servings

  - fruit and vegetables – include at each meal and some snacks: about five servings

  - milk, cheese and yogurt – three servings per day

  - meat, fish, eggs, nuts and beans – two servings per day or three for vegetarians

- foods high in fat and foods high in sugar – small amounts that do not replace the other food groups.

- Sweet foods should be limited to four times per day.

- Between six and eight drinks should be offered each day.

- The number of average daily servings of each food group is the same throughout childhood from 12 months of age but portion sizes of food and drinks increase as children grow and their energy and nutrient requirements increase.

- Assessing the average number of daily servings from each food group can be used to help parents and children make changes to improve the nutritional adequacy of their diets.

Children can be assured of meeting the energy and nutrient intakes discussed in Chapter 1.1 by eating a combination of five food groups. The foods are grouped together according to the nutrients they contain and so all the foods within each food group provide a similar range of nutrients. The foods and the nutrients they contain along with the recommended number of average daily servings from each food group are set out in Table 1.2.1.

Food groups 1–4 provide most of the nutrients. Foods in group 5 provide fewer nutrients and are high in energy (calories). They can be included in small quantities but should not replace foods in groups 1–4.

In addition to the foods listed in Table 1.2.1 there are many foods that contribute to servings from more than one food group. For example, pizza provides a serving from three or four food groups depending on the ingredients used:

- Pizza base contains flour – providing a serving from food group 1.

- Cheese on top provides a serving from food group 3.

- If a meat is included it provides a serving from food group 4.

- If diced vegetables are included in the topping they provide a serving from food group 2.

Table 1.2.1 Food groups and recommended daily servings[a]

Food groups	Foods included	Main nutrients supplied	Recommendations			
			Infants 6–12 months	Toddlers and preschoolers 1–4 years	School children 5–18 years
Group 1: Bread, rice potatoes, pasta and other starchy foods	Bread, chapatti, breakfast cereals, rice, couscous, pasta, millet, potatoes, yam, and foods made with flour such as pizza bases, buns, pancakes	Carbohydrate B vitamins Fibre Some iron, zinc and calcium	3–4 servings a day	Serve at each meal and some snacks	Serve at each meal and some snacks
Group 2: Fruit and vegetables	Fresh, frozen, tinned and dried fruits and vegetables	Vitamin C Phytochemicals Fibre Carotenes	3–4 servings a day	Offer at each meal and some snacks – about 5 small servings a day	Serve at each meal and some snacks – aim for 5 servings a day
Group 3: Milk, cheese and yogurt	Breast milk, infant formulas, follow-on milks, cow's milk, goat's milk, yogurts, cheese, milk puddings, toddler milks, calcium-enriched soya milks, tofu	Calcium Protein Iodine Riboflavin	Demand feeds of breast milk or infant formula as main milk drink (decreases from about 1000 mls/day down to about 500 mls/day as food in take increases) Some yogurt and cheese	3 servings a day 1 serving is: – 120 mL milk drink – 1 pot yogurt (120 g) – a serving of cheese in a sandwich or on a pizza – a milk-based pudding – a serving of tofu	3 servings a day 1 serving is: – 150–250 mL milk drink – 1–2 pots yogurt (120 g) – a serving of cheese in a sandwich or on a pizza – a milk-based pudding – a serving of tofu
Group 4: Meat, fish, eggs, nuts and pulses	Meat, fish, eggs, nuts and pulses (lentils, dahl, chickpeas, hummus, kidney beans and other similar starchy beans)	Iron Protein Zinc Magnesium B vitamins Vitamin A Omega 3 long-chain fatty acids: EPA and DHA from oily fish	1–2 servings a day 2–3 for vegetarians	2 servings a day or 3 for vegetarians Fish should be offered twice per week and oily fish at least once per week[b]	2 servings a day or 3 for vegetarians Fish should be offered twice per week and oily fish at least once per week[b]

Group 5: Foods and drinks high in fat and/or sugar	Cream, butter, margarines, cooking and salad oils, mayonnaise, chocolate, confectionery, jam, honey, syrup, crisps and other high-fat savoury snacks, biscuits, cakes Fruit juices and sweetened drinks	Some foods provide: – vitamin E – omega 3 fatty acids: alpha-linolenic acid		In addition to but not instead of the other food groups	In addition to but not instead of the other food groups
Fluids	Drinks	Water Fluoride in areas with fluoridated tap water	Milk feeds and drinks of water offered with meals	6–8 drinks per day – each of 100–120 mL. More in hot weather or after extra physical activity	6–8 drinks per day – each of 150–250 mL. More in hot weather or after extra physical activity
Vitamin supplements			Vitamins A and D for breastfed infants and formula-fed infants drinking less than 500 mL formula milk/day	Vitamins A and D up to 5 years	Folic acid and vitamin D for adolescent girls who could become pregnant and during pregnancy

[a] Serving sizes of food and drinks will increase as children grow.

[b] Oily fish should be limited to two servings per week for girls and four servings per week for boys.

DHA, docosahexaenoic acid; EPA, eicosapentaenoic acid.

Drinks

Between six and eight drinks per day provide adequate fluid, although children may need more in very hot weather or after extra physical activity.

With the exception of water, drinks are also included in the five food group system. Milk and yogurt drinks are included in food group 3. Sweetened drinks and fruit juices are all included in food group 5 as they are high-sugar drinks that also contain acid which can cause dental decay if given frequently.

Water and milk are the safest drinks to offer between meals as they do not cause tooth erosion or increase the risk of dental decay. Up to three drinks per day can be milk but more than this can decrease the appetite for foods from the other food groups that contain iron.

Portion Sizes

Portion sizes of foods are discussed in the chapters for each age group in Sections 5 and 6. They increase as children grow and have higher energy and nutrient requirements. However, the recommended number of daily servings from each of the food groups is applicable for all children from 1 year of age.

It is not necessary for children to eat the exact Reference Nutrient Intakes (RNI) of each nutrient each day. Most nutrients are stored in the body and these stores will last them some time. Children may eat more of some nutrients on certain days and less on other days, depending on the foods offered and the quantities consumed. Over a period of two weeks or so, on a balanced diet with a reasonable variety of foods from each food group, children will be getting on average what they need.

The 'eatwell plate' is a visual representation developed for use in the UK describing how to combine the food groups on a daily basis (Figure 1.2.1). It has been devised for children over 5 years and adults. There is no UK visual representation of a combination of the five food groups for children under 5 years old.

This food group combination can be applied to whichever cultural diet families eat. The wider the variety of foods eaten within each food group the better the balance of nutrients provided. Most countries have developed their own visual

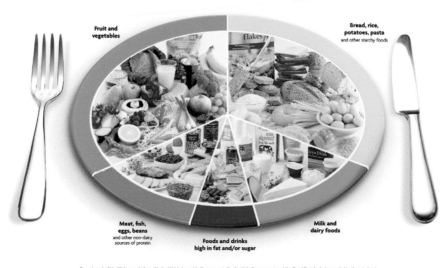

The eatwell plate

Use the eatwell plate to help you get the balance right. It shows how much of what you eat should come from each food group.

Fruit and vegetables

Bread, rice, potatoes, pasta and other starchy foods

Meat, fish, eggs, beans and other non-dairy sources of protein

Foods and drinks high in fat and/or sugar

Milk and dairy foods

Department of Health in association with the Welsh Assembly Government, the Scottish Government and the Food Standards Agency in Northern Ireland

Figure 1.2.1 The 'eatwell plate'. Copyright: Food Standards Agency

representation of how to combine food groups to provide a balanced nutritious diet according to the types of foods eaten. The principles are the same and the food groups vary very little from the UK 'eatwell plate'.

For example, in the United States 'MyPlate' is used (Figure 1.2.2), in Thailand the 'Nutrition Flag' (Figure 1.2.3) and in Singapore the food groups are displayed as a pyramid (Figure 1.2.4).

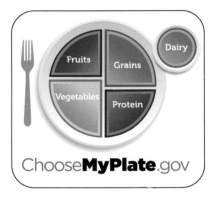

Figure 1.2.2 The US 'MyPlate'

Vegetarian and Vegan Diets

Vegetarianism can be divided into four main groups:

- partial vegetarian – red meat and offal are excluded
- lacto-ovo vegetarian – red meat, offal, poultry and fish are excluded but milk and eggs are eaten
- lacto-vegetarian – red meat, offal, poultry and fish and eggs are excluded but milk is included
- vegans – all animal products including eggs and cow's milk are excluded.

Vegetarian diets can provide a balanced, nutritious diet as long as they are well planned. Iron is the main nutrient at risk for children who do not eat meat as it is less well absorbed from plant-based foods than from meat and fish. Omega 3 fats may be low in diets that exclude all fish.

Nutritional requirements for growth and development can be achieved in the vegetarian diet by:

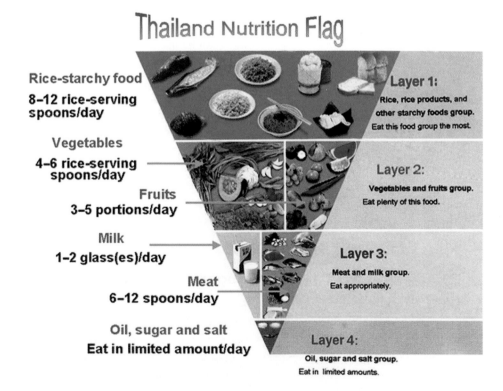

Figure 1.2.3 Thailand Nutrition Flag: 'Healthy Eating for Thais'

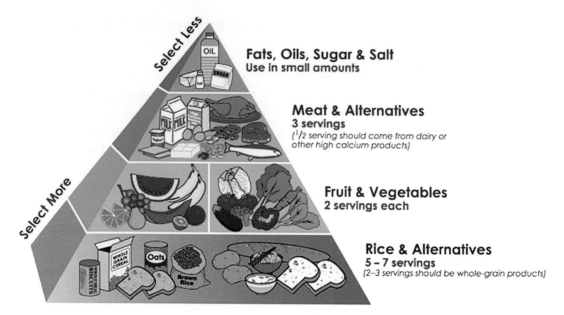

Fats, Oils, Sugar & Salt
Use in small amounts

Meat & Alternatives
3 servings
(¹/₂ serving should come from dairy or
other high calcium products)

Fruit & Vegetables
2 servings each

Rice & Alternatives
5 – 7 servings
(2–3 servings should be whole-grain products)

Select Less

Select More

Figure 1.2.4 Singapore healthy diet pyramid

- offering three servings/day of the vegetarian foods in food group 4 (i.e. eggs, nuts and pulses) and offering a food high in vitamin C at each meal to increase the iron absorbed from the plant-based foods
- including dried fruit often as it is a good source of iron
- including starchy foods from food group 1 in combination with nuts and pulses from food group 4 (e.g. as baked beans on toast, rice and dahl, rice and peas or peanut butter sandwich) as the amino acids in the protein of starchy foods complement the amino acids in the protein in nuts and pulses to provide together all the essential amino acids needed for growth
- offering breakfast cereals with added iron rather than those that are not fortified with iron
- increasing omega 3 fats from plant sources for those not eating fish by using rapeseed oil for cooking, walnut, soya or olive oil for dressings and chopped walnuts in place of other chopped nuts, or supplying a supplement of omega 3 fatty acids.

Vegan diets

Vegan diets are unlikely to provide adequate calcium, vitamin B12, omega 3 fats unless they are extremely well planned. A calcium-enriched soya milk can be used as a substitute for foods in food group 3. However, an extra supplement may be needed for the key 'at risk' nutrients, which are iron, zinc, calcium and vitamin B12. A vegan diet is not recommended for the under-fives (see Chapter 5.1).

Diets more restricted than a vegan diet, such as Zen macrobiotic, fruitarian or raw food diets, are not recommended for children as they cannot provide all the energy and nutrients for growth and development. A referral to social services and for a dietetic assessment are essential if parents reject this advice.

Sugar and Dental Health

Sugar has a place in all balanced nutritious diets, enhancing flavour and providing enjoyment from sweet tastes. As outlined in Chapter 1.1 sugar should be restricted to about 11 per cent of total energy intake and in practice this means that small amounts of sweet foods can be included at all meals and one snack, for example:

- breakfast – a breakfast cereal with added sugar or jam or honey on toast
- midday and evening meals – a second course or pudding that contains sugar
- one snack per day that contains sugar, such as biscuits, cake or bread/crackers/scone with jam or honey or another sweet spread.

Dental decay is caused by constant exposure to acid that is either contained in food and drink or produced by bacteria in the plaque on teeth as the bacteria break down the sugar present in food and drink. Acid is present in all drinks and fruit juices except water and milk.

When there is sufficient time between these acid attacks, saliva neutralizes any acid and the tooth enamel recovers its structure. Research has shown that by limiting sugar and sugar-containing foods to four times per day or less the risk of dental caries is reduced (Moynihan and Petersen 2004).

Sugars added to food come in a variety of forms and include: honey, sucrose, glucose, glucose syrup, maltose, dextrose, fructose, hydrolysed starch, corn or maize syrup, molasses, raw/brown sugar, treacle, golden syrup, Demerara and concentrated fruit juice.

Confectionery and chocolate are best eaten in small quantities at the end of a meal rather than in between meals.

All children should be registered with a dentist and have regular checkups.

Brushing teeth

Caries (decay) and gum disease can be avoided by twice daily brushing with a fluoride toothpaste (see Chapter 1.1) as it reduces the plaque coating teeth that contains the bacteria that convert sugar into acid.

A regime of brushing teeth last thing at night and one other time in the day should be encouraged, assisted and supervised by an adult until a child is at least 7 years old. Under-fives should be encouraged not to swallow the toothpaste but to spit it out and not to rinse the teeth with water after brushing.

Sugar-containing medicines

Children who require frequent and multiple medications are particularly at risk of dental decay if sweetened medicines are used. If a sugar-free alternative is not available, the medicine should be given at mealtimes if possible.

Salt

Salt is added to preserve some foods and to enhance flavour in others. Unfortunately, it is a very cheap flavour enhancer and has been used to excess in the food industry. The recommendations for restricting salt and sodium intake are list in Table 1.1.3 (page 8) but these recommendations are not evidence based and are very difficult to achieve. Furthermore, it is very difficult for families to estimate the intake of salt equivalent as some fresh foods naturally contain some sodium. Children will certainly not get ill or be harmed if they exceed these recommendations, but if they learn only to like salt-flavoured foods and develop a preference for them they may continue to eat mostly salt-flavoured foods as adults and are then at risk of raised blood pressure.

In practice, limiting salt intake to a reasonable intake in children means:

- including nutritious foods preserved with salt, such as bread, cheese, Marmite, ham, bacon and salamis as they also contain important nutrients
- not adding salt to food at the table
- using herbs and spices rather than extra salt to flavour food in cooking
- choosing tinned foods without added salt over those tinned with salt
- limiting the amount of processed foods offered as these usually have a higher salt content than home-cooked foods
- offering salty snack foods such as crisps and other packet snacks only occasionally.

Saturated Fat

Milk, cheese, yogurt, meat and eggs contain a mixture of fats, including saturated fat, but these foods should not be cut out of a children's diets as they are very nutritious foods. By limiting the foods high in fat in food group 5 to small quantities, the saturated fat content of children's food will be around 11 per cent total energy as recommended in Chapter 1.1. The foods to reduce are:

● crisps and similar packet snacks
● fried foods and pastry
● commercially prepared cakes and biscuits with a long shelflife.

Colours and Preservatives in Food and Drinks

The Food Standards Agency currently advises that the following colours should be avoided as research indicates they may affect children's behaviour:

● Tartrazine E102
● Ponceau 4R E124
● Sunset yellow E110
● Carmosine E122
● Quinoline yellow E104
● Allura red AC E129.

They also recommend avoidance of the preservative sodium benzoate E211.

Most manufacturers are working towards removing these substances from foods and replacing artificial colourings with natural food dyes.

Meals and Snack Routines

A planned routine of 3 meals and 2–3 nutritious planned snacks ensures children are not going for long periods of time without an energy boost from food, thus ensuring fairly even blood sugar levels throughout the day. When meals contain two courses of different foods they provide a wider range of foods and nutrients. The second course can be something simple like yogurt and fruit or it may be a nutritious pudding. Including a sweet second course after the savoury course makes the meal more of an occasion and more enjoyable for children. As discussed above, it can be included within the recommendations on limiting sugar intake.

Examples of nutritious puddings are those that contain one of more of the following ingredients: milk, flour, eggs, fruit, dried fruit, ground or chopped nuts. For example:

● yogurt with fruit
● fruit crumble with custard
● fruit pie with custard
● other fruit-based puddings such as apple Charlotte or summer pudding
● bread and butter pudding with dried fruit
● rice pudding served with fruit
● quick mixed milk puddings, such as Angel Delight, served with some fruit slices
● Bakewell tart served with fruit slices
● sponge cake with custard
● unsweetened tinned fruit with evaporated milk or ice cream
● jelly with fruit pieces
● fruit sponge cakes, such as apple sponge cake
● egg custard with fruit slices
● fruit salad with cream
● fresh fruit, such as strawberries, with cream
● fresh fruit with a biscuit or piece of cake or chocolate buttons.

Snacks

Children, particularly young children, may not be able to eat enough in just three meals to satisfy their nutrient requirements, so their snacks should include nutritious foods from food groups 1–4 to ensure adequate nutrient intakes.

Examples of nutritious snacks are:

- fresh fruit (dried fruit can be cariogenic (decay-causing) when eaten as a snack so it is not advised)
- vegetable sticks, such as carrot, cucumber, pepper, baby corn with dips based on yogurt, cream cheese or pulses such as hummus
- wholegrain breakfast cereals with milk
- cheese cubes and crackers/breadsticks or chapatti
- unsalted nuts (not whole nuts for children under 5 years)
- sandwiches, filled rolls and pitta breads
- French toast or toast with a range of spreads
- slices of pizza with a plain dough base that has not been fried
- yogurt and fromage frais
- crumpets, scones, pitta bread with a spread
- currant buns and teacakes
- pancakes, fruit muffins and plain biscuits
- home-made plain popcorn
- cakes containing dried fruit or vegetables or nuts (e.g. fruit cake and carrot cake).

Suitable drinks for meal and snack times include:

- still water
- milk (plain or flavoured)
- well-diluted pure fruit juice
- vegetable juices
- no added sugar (sugar-free) squashes – very dilute.

The best drinks to offer between meals and snacks are water and plain milk which do not have the same damaging effect on teeth as acidic and sugary drinks. Water has become a more popular drink in the UK in recent years but some parents never offer children water to drink as they do not drink water themselves and some think it is cruel to offer water in place of flavoured drinks.

Daily Meal Plans Combining the Five Food Groups

A variety of different eating plans, depending on a family routine, can provide a healthy eating regime with the desired combination of the food groups. There are two examples below. They both meet the principles of a balanced nutritious diet having:

- three meals
- two snacks
- six drinks
- two courses at each main meal
- bread, rice, potatoes, pasta and other starchy foods (group 1) at each meal
- fruit and vegetables (group 2) at each meal
- three servings of milk, cheese and yogurt (group 3)
- 2–3 servings of meat, fish, eggs, nuts or pulses (group 4)
- some high-fat high-sugar foods (group 5) included for flavour and enjoyment of meals
- sweet foods only offered a maximum of four times per day.

Example eating plan 1

In this example, breakfast is a quick meal based on cereal with fruit and milk – a quickly prepared breakfast that would suit a family that has little time in the morning. The midday meal might be served at nursery or school and the evening meal is a cooked meal that the family might eat together.

The three milk servings are taken at breakfast, mid-morning snack at nursery or school and for the evening meal pudding.

		Food groups included	Sample menu
Breakfast		Bread/rice/potatoes/pasta/starchy food	Breakfast cereal
		Milk/cheese/yogurt	Milk on cereal + ½ glass milk drink
		Fruit	Banana slices
		Drink	
Snack		Fruit	Apple slices
		Milk/cheese/yogurt	Cup of milk to drink
		Drink	
Midday meal	1st course	Meat/fish/eggs/nuts/pulses	Mini meatballs in a tomato and herb sauce
		Bread/rice/potatoes/pasta/starchy food	Pasta
		Vegetables	Broccoli florets
	2nd course	Foods high in fat and sugar	Apple crumble
		Fruit	With a small scoop of ice cream
	Drink	Drink	Water
Snack		Bread/rice/potatoes/pasta/starchy food	Crackers with Marmite
		Drink	Water to drink
Evening meal	1st course	Meat/fish/eggs/nuts/pulses	Fish and potato pie
		Bread/rice/potatoes/pasta/starchy food	Carrot and cucumber sticks
		Vegetables	
	2nd course	Milk/cheese/yogurt	Yogurt and ripe pear slices
		Fruit	A few chocolate squares or buttons
		Foods high in fat and sugar	
	Drink	Drink	Water

Example eating plan 2

In this example there is a more substantial breakfast that might suit a family that is not rushed in the morning, for example on a weekend day. The evening meal is a lighter meal with no food from the meat/fish/eggs/nuts/pulses group as there are already two servings from this group – one at breakfast and one at lunch.

		Food groups included	Sample menu
Breakfast		Bread/rice/potatoes/pasta/starchy food Meat/fish/eggs/nuts/pulses Fruit as drink	Scrambled egg with toast Diluted orange juice
Snack		Milk/cheese/yogurt	Glass milk 1 biscuit
Midday meal	1st course	Meat/fish/eggs/nuts/pulses Bread/rice/potatoes/pasta/starchy food Vegetable	Chicken curry and rice Green beans
	2nd course	Fruit Foods high in fat and sugar Milk/cheese/yogurt	Fruit sponge with custard
		Drink	Water
Snack		Fruit Bread/rice/potatoes/pasta/starchy food Drink	Grapes Rice cake Water
Evening meal	1st course	Bread/rice/potatoes/pasta/starchy food Milk/cheese/yogurt Vegetable	Cheese and tomato sandwiches
	2nd course	Foods high in fat and sugar Fruit	Jelly and peach slices
		Drink	Water

Activity

Plan a menu for one day using the appropriate number of servings from each food group for a child of 3–4 years and a child of 11–12 years. For each meal itemize the food and how it should be prepared.

Meal planner for a vegetarian diet

The following is a meal plan for a balanced vegetarian diet including the extra criteria:

- three servings of foods from food group 4: one at each meal
- a high-vitamin C food with each meal
- two courses at each main meal
- extra dried fruit and nuts to provide more iron.

	Day 1	Day 2	Day 3
Breakfast	Scrambled egg with toast and grilled tomatoes Milk to drink	Baked beans on toast Small glass diluted orange juice	Muesli with added ground almonds and dried fruit Milk on cereal and to drink
Midday meal	Chickpea curry with spinach and cauliflower Rice Bread and butter pudding with dried fruit	Lentil and parsnip soup with wheatgerm bread Yogurt and strawberries	Pasta with red kidney beans in bolognaise sauce Green beans Custard and sliced banana
Evening meal	Vegetable soup and peanut butter sandwiches Raspberries and cream	Tofu and vegetable stir fry with noodles Pear slices and a muffin	Pitta bread with hummus Red pepper and cucumber sticks Kiwi fruit with a mini Bakewell tart

Assessing Nutritional Adequacy Using the Five Food Groups

A child's diet can be assessed for adequate nutritional intake by comparing a record of what they have eaten with the principles of healthy eating.

How to assess the diet and help parents and children to improve a diet are discussed in Chapter 2.2.

Food group	Recommended number of daily age appropriate servings
1. Bread, rice, potatoes, pasta and other starchy foods	Included at each meal – and some snacks
2. Fruit and vegetables	Included at each meal – and some snacks
3. Milk, cheese and yogurt	3 servings per day
4. Meat, fish, eggs, nuts and beans	2–3 servings per day
5. Foods high in fat and foods high in sugar	Small amounts with meals Sweet foods limited to 4 times per day
Drinks	6–8 per day or 1 with each meal and snack
Vitamin supplements	Vitamins A and D daily for those under 5 years of age

References and further reading

Moynihan P and Petersen PE (2004) Diet, nutrition and the prevention of dental diseases. *Public Health Nutrition* 7(1A): 201–226.

Scientific Advisory Committee on Nutrition (SACN)/ Committee on Toxicity (COT) (2004) *Advice on Fish Consumption: Benefits and risks.* London: The Stationery Office.

Social and Cultural Influences on Food Choices

Summary

- Cultural and religious food traditions vary widely within the UK.

- Health professionals should not make assumptions about eating habits based on ethnic grouping or religion alone as traditions vary from family to family.

- Poverty and low income limits food choices and the ability to provide a healthy diet for children.

- Marketing and advertising influences children's food habits and requests for food.

- Parenting style affects the eating habits and foods consumed by children.

Throughout childhood, children tend to prefer to eat familiar foods. When given a choice of foods they will generally choose foods they have eaten before and enjoyed. They need to be motivated to try new foods. From the beginning of weaning onto solid foods children learn to like the foods their families choose to offer to them. Although adolescents may reject family foods, as young adults and parents, they are likely to revert to the eating habits they learned during their early childhood.

The very wide range of foods available within the UK today presents families with a huge choice of foods. Food choices are based on:

- availability
- cost and affordability, depending on socio-economic circumstances
- cultural and religious traditions
- family experience.

Poor food choices by families are key factors in the high rates of obesity, dental caries and iron-deficiency anaemia currently prevalent within the UK. Obesity in children is strongly associated with parental obesity and therefore family food habits.

Feeding practices are routed deeply in cultural and religious traditions. When health professionals understand why and how families make their food choices and engage in particular feeding practices they can give sensitive advice to help families improve their eating habits.

Cultural Food Traditions

Many different races have migrated to the UK, each bringing different cultural and religious traditions relating to food. Sharing food traditions and food restrictions can bind groups of people together and set groups apart from each other. This is seen in both religious and geographical food traditions.

Being fully aware of different food customs and practices is important but it is equally important that assumptions about a family's food habits are not made solely on the basis of their ethnic origin or religious grouping. There is enormous diversity in culture, traditions and food habits between and within different ethnic and religious groups and even within a family.

Migrant groups in the UK come from many different geographical areas. In the 2001 UK census the ethnic population was about 8 per cent of the general population or 4.6 million (Figure 1.3.1).

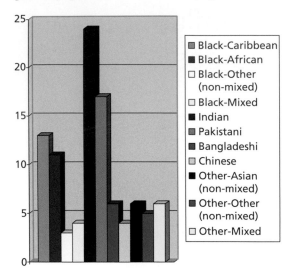

Figure 1.3.1 Distribution of total minority ethnic population by ethnic group in Great Britain in 2000. Data from www.statistics.gov.uk

On migrating to the UK, geographical groups tend to preserve their eating traditions (Table 1.3.1). This is seen particularly where larger groups have settled together and have a good source of traditional food through markets and local retailers. However, not all new migrants have access to their culturally acceptable foods – for example asylum seekers may be housed in areas where their traditional foods are unobtainable.

Western influences also affect traditional eating patterns of migrant groups to a considerable extent. Younger generations born in the UK generally move away from traditional dietary practices of their migrant parents and adopt the traditions of their friends and peers.

Activity 1

Visit a shop specializing in foods of one of the geographical regions below and make a list of 20 unfamiliar foods and then find out how they are used in the preparation of dishes for that ethnic group.

Table 1.3.1 Common traditional foods eaten by groups from different geographical regions that have migrated to the UK

Migration to the UK from	Traditional foods eaten
Caribbean Islands	Rice, sweet potatoes, yams, green bananas, plantain, dasheen, okra, cornmeal and coconut cream Beverages based on condensed milk with added sugar or honey Milk-based energy or malt drinks such as Nutriment, Nourishment, Supermalt, Mighty Malt
South Asia	Chapattis, parathas, puris, bhaura and naan are all types of bread made from wheat flour Spices Yogurt Fried snacks – samosas and pakoras
East Africa	Maize, millet, sorghum, matoke/cooking banana, cassava, sweet potato, yam
West Africa mainly Nigeria and Ghana	Cassava, green bananas, yam, plantain, ground rice, cornmeal, gari and kenkey Akra or black-eyed beans Ground nuts and seeds are often part of the meal Spices Tropical fruits
China	Balance of yin (coldness) and yang (hotness) is usually observed in meals Black beans Soy products such as tofu and soya milk Green leafy vegetables Cereals vary: in the north: wheat-based foods such as dumplings and noodles in the south: rice and foods made from rice flour such as noodles, cakes, vinegar

When ethnic groups do not have access to their traditional foods, they may need advice on how to choose a balanced, nutritious diet from the vast array of foods available in the UK. However, motivation to seek professional advice is low in many ethnic groups. Factors that influence the uptake of nutritional advice are complex. Those in the lower socio-economic groups are less likely to follow advice if they have a lower educational attainment or are affected by poverty.

A community worker, health professional or facilitator who is trusted and recognized and who speaks the language can improve the outcome of nutritional interventions (Stockley *et al.* 2009).

Activity 2

Make a list of the main barriers to healthy eating for the ethnic groups in your area.

Activity 3

Make a list of factors that reduce motivation of ethnic families to seek professional advice on healthy eating.

Religious Food Traditions

Within each religious grouping, families decide which food traditions to adopt. In some families one parent may observe certain food traditions while the other parent may not. Some common traditions are listed in Table 1.3.2.

Fasting

Most religions have a tradition of fasting (i.e. not eating any food or excluding certain foods) for particular periods of time (Table 1.3.3). Pregnant women and young children are usually exempt from fasting, however, some pregnant women may choose to observe these practices.

Religious festivals

Celebratory meals and specific foods are often eaten at festival times, as shown in Table 1.3.4. Dates of festivals are approximate as they are often based on lunar calendars.

Table 1.3.2 Common food traditions within religions

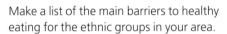

Religion	Food tradition
Buddhist and Jains	No meat or fish because of the belief of non-violence to all forms of life
Christian	Meat not eaten on Fridays
Jewish	No pork Only fish with fins or scales Milk and milk products not served with meat
Orthodox Jewish	Kosher meat and milk products
Hindu	No beef or beef products because cow is sacred Pork often avoided also as considered unclean Only fish with fins and scales Some are vegetarians
Muslim	No pork. Other meats are halal[a] No alcohol Hand and feet washing before meals
Rastafarian	Sometimes vegan or no pork or shellfish
Sikh	No pork and sometimes no beef Vegetarianism is common No alcohol

[a] Halal meat is from an animal that has been ritually slaughtered by being blessed and allowing the blood to drain – usually after the animal is stunned.

Table 1.3.3 Common fasting traditions within religions

Religion	Fasting tradition
Christian	Individual choices of certain foods not to be eaten during Lent – 40 days prior to Easter
Hindu and Sikh	Fasting between dawn and dusk on three festival days each year – the birthdays of Lord Shiva, Rama and Krishna. Degrees of further fasting are individual choice (e.g. fasting may be one or two days per week when only milk, yogurt, fruit, potatoes and nuts are eaten). More common in women than men
Jewish	24-hour fast over Yom Kippur Certain foods not eaten during Passover
Muslim	Fasting between dawn and dusk during the lunar month of Ramadan Pregnant women, the elderly and children under 12 years are exempt

Table 1.3.4 Religious festivals observed by different religions

Religion	Festival
Buddhist	Veska – birth enlightenment and death of Buddha – usually during May full moon
Christian	Easter – March/April Christmas – December
Hindu	Mahashrivatri – birthday of Lord Shiva – March Ram Navmi – birthday of Lord Rama – April Janmastami – birthday of Lord Krishna – late August Navaratri – nine nights October Holi – March Raksha Bandhan – August Diwali – Festival of Lights and New Year – October/November
Jewish	Rosh Hashana New Year – September/October Yom Kippur Day of Atonement – ten days later Passover – eight days in April
Muslim	Eid al-Fitr ('little Eid') – at the end of the Ramadan Eid al-Adah ('big Eid')
Sikh	Baissakha – New Year's day – April Diwali – Festival of Light – October/November Birth of Guru Nanak – November

Cultural variations in feeding practices

Cutlery

Some families use cutlery or chopsticks while others only use their hands; some only eat food with their right hand.

Eating environment

This may be a table, food on laps in front of the television, or eating while sitting on the floor. Some families always eat with the television on, others never with the television or distractions.

Self-feeding by infants and toddlers

Some families encourage self-feeding from the beginning of weaning, other parents prefer to take control of all the infant and toddler feeding and these children do not get the opportunity to learn to self-feed.

Mealtime routines

Some families do not eat around a planned daily routine of 3 meals and 2–3 snacks and allow grazing on food throughout the day.

Socio-economic factors influencing food choice

Nutritional content of diets and ill-health show a marked socio-economic gradient. National nutritional surveys and research (Gregory *et al.* 1995, Hinds and Gregory 1995, Gregory *et al.* 2000, North *et al.* 2000, Nelson *et al.* 2007) have shown that:

- poorer households have a less diverse diet and are less likely to experiment with new foods
- socio-demographic status of mothers influences the type of diet eaten during pregnancy and the foods fed to her children
- poverty and poor housing often have an effect on a mother's physical and emotional wellbeing and these in turn affect the choice of foods she makes for her children
- although there is no significant difference in energy intake between different socio-economic groups, the intakes of most vitamins and minerals in children is lower in lower socio-economic groups
- dental caries and iron-deficiency anaemia are both more common in under-fives in low-income households.

Costs that a low-income family might prioritize over buying food include:

- rent/housing
- heating and lighting
- gas and electricity bills
- clothes and shoes for children.

In 2003 a survey for the National Children's Home (2004) found that:

- $\frac{1}{5}$ of families didn't have enough money for food
- $\frac{2}{5}$ of families had only just enough money for food
- almost half of parents had gone short of food so the children had enough.

Food choices are limited in low-income families because:

- there may be no public transport links to large supermarkets where foods are cheaper than in smaller local shops
- families cannot take advantage of better value bulk buys as their fridge and cupboard storage is extremely limited or non-existent
- families are more likely to spend limited resources on cheap and filling foods that are less nutritious

- relatively inexpensive sweet foods are given as treats in place of more expensive treats such as toys and branded clothes and shoes
- the variety of fruit and vegetables available for purchase in small local shops may be limited and of poorer quality
- families are unlikely to purchase fruit and vegetables again if the children did not like them.

Government-funded schemes to support the nutritional intake of children in low-income families include:

- Healthy Start scheme
- free school milk for young children and subsidized milk for others
- free school meals.

Entitlement varies and is changed from time to time by governmental policy.

Healthy Start Scheme

This scheme is the latest version of a UK Government-funded scheme to give nutritional support to low-income families with pregnant women and children under 4 years (www.healthystart.nhs.uk). Eligibility to join the scheme depends on family income except for pregnant teenagers under 18 years who are all entitled to join irrespective of their financial circumstances.

Under the scheme low-income families and pregnant teenagers are entitled to:

- weekly vouchers to buy fruit, vegetables, milk and infant formula
- free vitamin supplements for pregnant and breastfeeding women and children under 4 years of age.

Activity 4

Make a list of factors that need to be addressed around food and nutrition in low-income families.

Social and Cultural Influences on Infant Feeding Choices

Factors affecting infant feeding practices adopted by families and how they follow the infant feeding recommendations include:

- socio-economic status
- parental age
- personality
- educational attainment of the mother
- infant's birth order
- consistency of advice from health professionals.

Breastfeeding vs. Formula Feeding

Although the health benefits of exclusive breastfeeding from birth until weaning for both infants and mothers are well documented, about 1 in 5 mothers in the UK do not initiate breastfeeding at birth and by 1 week of age less than half of infants are being exclusively breastfed. Breastfeeding rates are slowly increasing but for the past 80 years or so, infant formula milks (breast milk substitutes) have been widely available and have become accepted by many people as equivalent to breastfeeding. Formula feeding is often portrayed in the media as the socio-cultural norm and female breasts are associated with sexuality. As a result:

- many women are surrounded by family and friends who have not breastfed and have never seen a baby breastfeeding
- many mothers feel embarrassed breastfeeding in front of others both outside and within the home
- breastfeeding in public may be met with disapproval despite laws in both Scotland and England making it illegal not to allow breastfeeding in public places.

In addition:

- lack of appropriate staff training within health services leads to lack of knowledge, skills and confidence in health professionals and inappropriate practices and routines persist
- breastfeeding is not a priority in all maternity units and promotion is often left to advocates
- women may lack support to continue exclusive breastfeeding from health services and their social networks
- breastfeeding support services are frequently short-term initiatives rather than embedded in mainstream services.

Many women find breastfeeding challenging and give up earlier than they wish to. As shown in Figure 1.3.2, breastfeeding rates are higher among mothers:

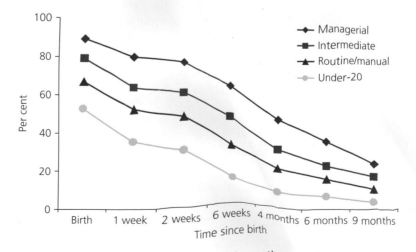

Figure 1.3.2 Duration of breastfeeding by mother's socio-economic group plus under-20s, 2005

- from higher occupational groups
- with highest educational levels
- aged 30 or over
- of first babies.

Some families are reluctant to change other infant feeding practices from those handed down by previous generations, and certain cultural practices are at variance with the Department of Health infant feeding guidelines and can compromise the nutritional intake of infants. Such practices include:

- women not taking vitamin D supplements during pregnancy and breastfeeding – particularly those at higher risk of low vitamin D levels (see page 65)
- giving water rather than colostrum to newborn babies as colostrum is seen as having a poor nutritional value or being unhealthy
- preference for formula feeding rather than breastfeeding because formula feeding is seen as a Western ideal and therefore assumed to be better for the baby
- herbal teas given during infancy as they are deemed to have health benefits
- boiled water and barley water given to infants as 'cooling' drinks to balance breast milk which is seen as a 'hot' food
- cow's milk introduced in place of formula milk before 12 months of age because it is cheaper than formula milks
- very early weaning before 4 months or late weaning after 6 months
- inappropriate weaning foods
- convenience and sweet foods that are low in iron given due to limited availability of halal or nutritious vegetarian savoury weaning foods
- little variety of weaning foods given (e.g. low-nutrient porridge given at all meals in the day)
- coercing infants to eat/drink to excess as a rapid weight gain or a 'bonny baby' is seen as an indicator of health and wellbeing.

Marketing and Media Influence on Food Choices

Eating behaviours and food choices can be strongly influenced by advertising, food packaging and presentation of food content.

Children are increasingly targeted with advertising and marketing. Large sums of money are spent targeting them with food advertising to build brand loyalty and persuade them to want a particular food product, starting from when they are toddlers. Marketing experts know that toddlers and children have considerable purchase influence and successfully negotiate purchases through 'nag factor' or 'pester power'. Requests are often for brand name products and food accounts for over half of total requests, with parents honouring these requests 50 per cent of the time (Story and French 2004). The most requested item is breakfast cereal, followed by snacks, drinks and toys.

Media messages about food are targeted at children through:

- television advertisements
- radio advertisements
- internet
- in-store displays
- child-friendly packaging, including familiar cartoon characters on the packaging.

Older children exposed to advertising chose advertised food products significantly more often than those who were not exposed (Story and French 2004).

Numerous studies have documented that children have little understanding of the persuasive intent of advertising. High-fat, high-sugar and low-fibre foods are regularly advertised on television and such advertisements often feature messages implying that these low-nutrient foods are beneficial. These implications, although not technically false may nonetheless confuse children and their parents about what makes a particular food a healthy choice.

Activity 5

Make a note of the foods advertised to children on television during several periods of children's television viewing time (e.g. 16:00–19:00) and calculate the percentages of nutritious and non-nutritious foods advertised.

Activity 6

List the negative effects that television viewing has on children's eating habits and health.

Influence of Family Feeding Practices and Parenting Skills

The mother is often the key decision-maker in feeding children, however, this is not so in all cultures and families. Other household members who may purchase the foods for the children and prepare and cook meals and snacks are:

- father
- maternal grandmother or grandfather
- paternal grandmother or grandfather
- most elderly member or members of the household
- older sibling who can speak English while other members of the household do not
- staff at the nursery the infant or young child attends
- babysitters
- child minders
- other carers.

Family meals

Eating together as a family in a relaxed and enjoyable way is an important social time in family life as well as a learning opportunity for children: they learn to eat different foods and improve their feeding skills.

Parents are very strong role models for young children, who learn by copying. When parents eat nutritious foods themselves and offer the same foods to their children, the children have the opportunity to learn to like those nutritious foods. Young children are less likely to try new foods that they have not seen other people eating.

However, eating together as a family has become less common due to:

- parents' long working hours and long commuting times
- shift work
- preference of parents not to eat with children.

With many young children eating separately from their parents, the concept of 'children's food' has developed. When young children are given control over what is served they tend to choose familiar foods, thereby narrowing down the range of foods they eat and forgoing the experience of a wider range of foods and the opportunity to learn to like the foods adults are eating.

Older children who consume more meals with their families have:

- better nutritional intakes (Gillman *et al.* 2000, Sweeting and West 2005)
- a lower risk of obesity (Taveras *et al.* 2005).

Videon and Manning (2003) found parental presence at the evening meal was associated with a higher consumption of fruits, vegetables, milk, yogurt and cheese, as well as less skipping of breakfast in adolescents.

Parenting styles

A parent or carer's role is to offer nutritious meals and snacks to young children in pleasant social environments but to allow each child to decide when they have had enough to eat, so that they develop an understanding of feeling hungry and eating to satisfy that feeling.

Parenting styles influence the range and type of foods that children are prepared to eat. A positive parenting style makes mealtimes enjoyable and improves nutritional intakes through a wider range of nutritious foods being eaten.

Rudolf (2009) has described four parenting styles that relate to responsiveness and control

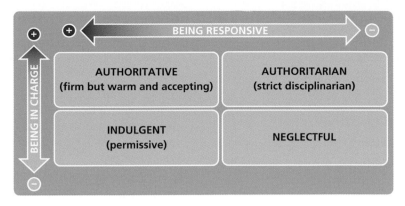

Figure 1.3.3 The model of parenting proposed by Mary Rudolf has four styles relating to responsiveness and control

(Figure 1.3.3). Positive parenting is being responsive to children's emotional and physical needs while being in charge and setting appropriate and clear boundaries. This is the *authoritative* style and parents using this style will buy a range of nutritious foods and encourage and prompt children to eat them while making allowances for their individual tastes and preferences. Children will be allowed to decide when they have had enough to eat.

The *authoritarian* parenting style takes control beyond any consideration of a child's needs, feelings or preferences. Parents may insist children eat certain foods and may resort to coercing and force-feeding. Children may be forced to finish all the food on their plates even when they have indicated they have had enough. Certain foods that the parent deems unsuitable may be denied altogether, making them very desirable in the child's mind.

The *indulgent* parenting style is responsive to the child's wishes and demands even when they are not in the child's best interests. This will include giving children full control over what food is to be served, thereby narrowing the range of foods they eat. In addition giving in to demands for frequent servings of sweet or high-fat foods which will provide less nutrients and excess calories. These children will also be at risk of dental caries.

A *neglectful* parenting style is where the parent is neither in charge nor responsive to the child. There may be no routine of meals and planned snacks and nutritious foods to maintain health and growth may not be offered.

Positive and negative feeding practices are described in Table 1.3.5.

Using food and drinks as rewards, treats or for comfort

The most desirable reward for young children is their parents' attention. However, sweet, energy-dense, low-nutrient foods are often used as a

Table 1.3.5 Positive and negative feeding practices by parents and carers

Positive feeding practices	Negative feeding practices
Praising when food is eaten	Coercion or coaxing children to eat healthy foods
Taking away uneaten food without comment	Coercion or coaxing children to eat more when they indicate they have had enough
Parents eating with children and eating the foods they want the young children to eat	Offering alternatives or rewards to encourage more food to be eaten
Pleasant interaction with young children during the mealtime	Encouraging children to finish up everything on their plate
Offering appropriate portion sizes	

substitute for this and given outside of meal and planned snack times to:

- show love and affection
- receive affection from the child
- comfort them
- reward for good behaviour
- bribe young children to modify their behaviour
- bribe young children to eat a food or meal they are refusing.

Encouraging such foods to be regarded as desirable is not compliant with teaching healthy eating.

Advantages of a meal and snack routine

Routines help young children to feel secure. A feeding routine of 3 meals and 2–3 planned nutritious snacks throughout the day:

- prevents grazing on less nutritious food throughout the day
- prevents young children becoming over hungry or thirsty by going too long between eating occasions
- avoids attempts to feed young children when they are ready to sleep and too tired to eat
- prevents toddlers not being hungry at meal times because they have just eaten snacks or had large sweet drinks just before the meal.

Activity 7

Make a list of factors to consider before giving advice to families.

Activity 8

Make a list of how parents can encourage healthy eating in their young children.

Activity 9

Make a list of non-food rewards that could be offered to a child.

Activity 10

Make a list of the disadvantages of not eating together as a family.

References and further reading

Ashton D (2004) Food advertising and childhood obesity. *Journal of the Royal Society of Medicine* **97**(2): 51–52.

Birch LL and Davison KK (2001) Family environmental factors influencing the developing behavioural controls of food intake and childhood overweight. *Pediatrics Clinics of North America* **48**(4): 893–907.

Blake CE (2008) Individual differences in the conceptualization of food across eating contexts. *Food Quality and Preference* **19**(1): 62–70.

Boyland EJ, Harrold JA, Kirkham TC, *et al.* (2011) Food commercials increase preference for energy-dense foods, particularly in children who watch more television. *Pediatrics* **128**(1): e93–e100.

Burgess-Champoux TL, Larson N, Neumark-Sztainer D, Hannan PJ and Story M (2009) Are family meal patterns associated with overall diet quality during the transition from early to middle adolescence. *Journal of Nutrition Education and Behavior* **41**(2): 79–86.

Daly A, MacDonald A and Booth IW (1998) Diet and disadvantage: observations on infant feeding from an inner city. *Journal of Human Nutrition and Dietetics* **11**: 381–389.

Faith MS, Scanlon KS, Birch LL, Francis LA and Sherry B (2004) Parent-child feeding strategies and their relationships to child eating and weight status. *Obesity Research* **12**(11): 1711–1722.

Fisher JO and Birch LL (1999) Restricting access to palatable foods affects children's behavioural response, food selection, and intake. *American Journal of Clinical Nutrition* **69**: 1264–1272.

Gillman MW, Rifas-Shiman SL, Frazier AL, *et al.* (2000) Family dinner and diet quality among older children and adolescents. *Archives of Family Medicine* **93**(3): 235–240.

Gregory JR, Collins DL, Davies PSW, Hughes JM and Clarke PC (1995) *National Diet and Nutrition Survey: Children aged 1½ and 4½ years*, Volume 1. Report of the Diet and Nutrition Survey. London: HMSO.

Gregory J, Lowe S, Bates CJ, *et al.* (2000) *National Diet and Nutrition Survey: Young people aged 4–18 years*. London: The Stationery Office.

Hare-Bruun H, Nielsen BM, Kristensen PL, Møller NC, Togo P and Heitmann BL (2011) Television viewing, food preferences, and food habits among children: a prospective epidemiological study. *BMC Public Health* **11**: 311.

Harrison K and Marske AL (2005) Nutritional content of foods advertised during the television programs children watch most. *American Journal of Public Health* **95**(9): 1568–1574.

Hastings G and Rayner M (2003a) *Review of Research on the Effects of Food Promotion to Children*. London: Food Standards Agency.

Hastings G and Rayner M (2003b) *Does Food Promotion Influence Children? A systematic review of the evidence*. London: Food Standards Agency.

Hinds K and Gregory JR (1995) *National Diet and Nutrition Survey: Children aged $1\frac{1}{2}$ to $4\frac{1}{2}$ years*, Volume 2. Report of the Dental Survey. London: HMSO.

Hughes SO, Shewchuk RM, Baskin ML, Nicklas TA and Qu H (2008) Indulgent feeding style and children's weight status in preschool. *Journal of Developmental and Behavioral Pediatrics* **29**(5): 403–410.

Jastran M, Bisogni CA, Sobal J, Blake C and Devine CM (2009) Eating routines: embedded, value based, modifiable, and reflective. *Appetite* **52**(1): 127–136.

National Children's Home (NCH) (2004) *Going Hungry: The struggle to eat healthily on a low income*. London: NCH.

Nelson M, Erens R, Bates B, Church S and Boshier T (2007) *Low Income Diet and Nutrition Survey*, Volume 2: *Food consumption and nutrient intakes*. London: The Stationery Office.

Netto G, Bhopal R, Lederle N, Khatoon J and Jackson A (2010) How can health promotion interventions be adapted for minority ethnic communities? Five principles for guiding the development of behavioural interventions. *Health Promotion International* **25**(2): 248–257.

North K, Emmett P, Noble S and the ALSPAC Study Team (2000) Types of drinks consumed by infants at 4 and 8 months of age: sociodemographic variations. *Journal of Human Nutrition and Dietetics* **13**: 71–82.

O'Connor TM, Hughes SO, Watson KB, *et al.* (2010) Parenting practices are associated with fruit and vegetable consumption in pre-school children. *Public Health Nutrition* **13**(1): 91–101.

Rudolf M (2009) *Tackling Obesity through the Healthy Child Programme. A Framework for Action*. Leeds: University of Leeds.

Sarwar T (2002) Infant feeding practices of Pakistani mothers in England and Pakistan. *Journal of Human Nutrition and Dietetics* **15**: 419–428.

Sharma S and Cruickshank JK (2001) Cultural differences in assessing dietary intake and providing relevant dietary information to British African-Caribbean populations. *Journal of Human Nutrition and Dietetics* **14**: 449–456.

Stockley L and Associates (2009) *Review of Dietary Intervention Models for Black and Minority Ethnic Groups*. Cardiff: The Food Standards Agency Wales.

Story M and French S (2004) Food advertising and marketing directed at children and adolescents in the US. *International Journal of Behavioral Nutrition and Physical Activity* **1**: 3.

Sweeting H and West P (2005) Dietary habits and children's family lives. *Journal of Human Nutrition and Dietetics* **18**: 93–97.

Taveras EM, Rifas-Shiman SL, Berkey CS, *et al.* (2005) Family dinner and adolescent overweight. *Obesity Research* **13**(5): 900–906.

Videon TM and Manning CK (2003) Influences on adolescent eating patterns: the importance of family meals. *Journal of Adolescent Health* **32**(5): 365–373.

Resources

The Ishmali Nutrition Centre – a guide to traditional foods of African, Central and South Asian, and Middle Eastern origin (**www.theismaili.org/nutrition**)

Healthy Start Scheme (**www.healthystart.org.uk**)

Working with homeless people (**www.qni.org.uk/for_nurses/opening_doors/homeless_health_initiative/resource_pack**)

World Health Organization's 2010 Recommendations on marketing foods and beverages to children (**www.who.int/dietphysicalactivity/marketing-food-to-children/en/index.html**)

Section 2
Assessment of Growth and Nutritional Intake

2.1 Measuring and Assessing Growth

2.2 Assessing Nutritional Intake

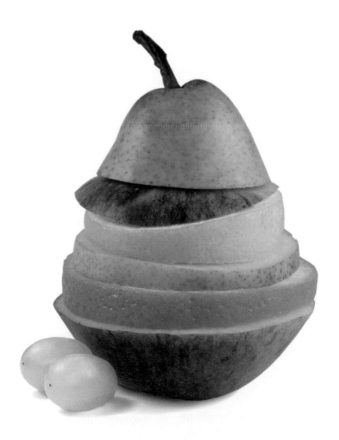

Measuring and Assessing Growth

Summary

- Measuring growth is key to monitoring the nutritional, endocrine, emotional and physical health of children.

- Growth assessment requires training to take accurate measurements using calibrated equipment and to plot and interpret growth and body mass index (BMI) charts.

- Growth charts describe how big or heavy healthy children are expected to be at any age.

- Infants and children normally grow parallel to centile lines on growth charts although some variation is normal due to illness in infancy, cyclical growth and varying ages of the pubertal growth spurt.

- Frequent measurements are not necessary in normal healthy infants and children and can cause unnecessary stress and concern.

Measuring growth is a key tool in monitoring normal development and is used as part of a nutritional assessment. When energy intake from food and drinks is adequate, weight gain will be within normal parameters. Normal growth measurements can reassure health professionals and parents while variations from expected growth can be an important indicator in diagnosing obesity, growth faltering, endocrine disorders, emotional neglect and other medical conditions. Growth rates vary throughout childhood and knowledge of how and why they vary is important for interpreting growth measurements.

Anthropometric Measures

The most common measurements taken to assess growth are:

- weight (Figure 2.1.1c)
- length for children under 2 years and height for children over 2 years (Figure 2.1.1a and 2.1.1d)
- head circumference measured around the widest part of the head (Figure 2.1.1b).

Additional measures can be used:

- waist circumference – a measure of the amount of fat stored centrally
- mid upper arm circumference (MUAC) – used to screen for malnutrition in under-fives in the developing world. A MUAC <11 cm in infants 2–6 months and MUAC <11.5 cm in children 6 months to 5 years is used as one indicator of severe malnutrition
- skinfold thicknesses – not regularly used but can be a useful measure when weight is inaccurate because of fluid retention such as oedema or ascites.

Growth Rates Throughout Childhood

Prenatal growth is the most rapid phase of growth in children. Growth rate slowly declines during infancy and early childhood until during the primary school years when children grow at a fairly steady rate of about 5–6 cm/year. This declines to about 4–5 cm/ year just prior to the pubertal growth spurt, during

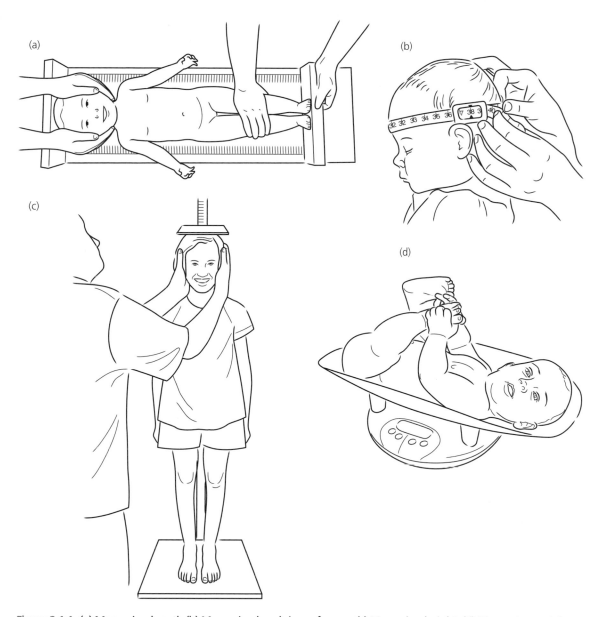

Figure 2.1.1 (a) Measuring length (b) Measuring head circumference (c) Measuring height (d) Measuring weight of an infant. You would measure the weight of older children this way!

which the growth rate increases rapidly for a period of about 3 years (Tables 2.1.1 and 2.1.2).

Biological drivers of growth

The regulation of growth is a complex process and the key drivers change as age increases. The main drivers (Table 2.1.3) are:

● nutrition

● hormones

● growth factors such as insulin-like growth factor 1 (IGF-I), insulin-like growth factor 2 (IGF-II), epidermal growth factor (EGF), fibroblast growth factor (FGF) and transforming growth factor (TGF).

The influence of hormonal and growth factors will be largely under genetic control, hence the tendency for children's growth patterns to relate to their parent's stature.

Table 2.1.1 Average growth rates at different ages

Age/developmental stage	Weight gain (kg/year)	Height increase (cm/year)
Infant	6.6	25
1–2 years	2.5	12
3 years–puberty	2	5–6
Female adolescent growth spurt	3.9	8 (6–10)
Male adolescent growth spurt	3.7	9 (6–13)

Table 2.1.2 Pubertal growth spurt statistics

	Girls	Boys
Average age of peak growth rate	12 years	14 years
Mean total gain in height over the 3-year growth spurt	20–25 cm	25–30 cm
Average final height	1.63 m	1.78 m

Table 2.1.3 Main drivers of growth at different ages

Age	Main drivers of growth in length or height
Prenatal	Maternal nutrition, IGF-1, IGF-2, EGF, FGF, TGF, insulin
Infancy 0–12 months	Nutrition, growth hormone, IGF-1
Childhood	Growth hormone, IGF-1, thyroxine
Puberty	Growth hormone, IGF-1, sex steroids: testosterone in boys and oestrogen in girls

Assessing Growth and Body Mass Index on Centile Charts

Children's growth is assessed by plotting successive accurate measurements of weight and length/height on centile charts that describe weight for age and length/height for age, respectively. Accurate measurements must be taken on calibrated scales. Staff taking measurements, and plotting and interpreting growth charts should undertake training for this purpose. Practical training is usually done on the job with more experienced staff but online resources are available and are listed at the end of this chapter.

Body mass index (BMI) is a measure of thinness and fatness and is calculated by dividing the weight in kilograms by the square of the height in metres:

$$BMI = \frac{Weight\ in\ kg}{(Height\ in\ m)^2}$$

For example a young child weighing 13.2 kg and measuring 91 cm or 0.91 m will have a BMI of $13.2/(0.91)^2 = 15.9$. This figure should then be plotted on the BMI-for-age centile chart.

Recommendations for measuring children

Frequency of measuring infants and children

As a minimum, infants should be weighed at (NICE 2008):

- birth
- 5 and 10 days, as part of an overall assessment of feeding
- 6–8-week check
- times of routine immunizations at 2, 3 and 4 months and 12–13 months.

If there is concern, children should be weighed and measured as part of monitoring; however, weights measured too closely together are often misleading and can cause stress and concern. A full or empty bladder can make a significant difference to the weight of an infant. Weighing more frequently than:

- once a month up to 6 months of age
- once every 2 months from 6 to 12 months of age
- once every 3 months over the age of 1 year

is not necessary in healthy children.

Length is not normally measured during infancy as it is hard to measure accurately and weight is an adequate indication of growth during the first year.

Head circumference is usually measured within 24 hours of birth and at the 6–8-week check; thereafter only if there are neurodevelopmental concerns.

Clothing

Infants and children up to 2 years should be weighed naked, without a nappy. Thereafter they can be weighed in underwear or very light clothing without shoes or socks.

Supine (lying on the back) length is measured up until 2 years and without clothing or a nappy as this can distort the hips and make the measurement inaccurate. Standing height is measured after 2 years of age and children can wear clothing but should remove shoes and socks. Any head wear such as topknots must also be removed.

Measuring equipment

Only class III clinical electronic scales in metric setting should be used to weigh children. These should be maintained and calibrated annually, in line with medical devices standards EC Directive 90/384 EEC.

Most equipment for measuring length and height is self-calibrating or should be adjusted with a standard measure.

Tapes for measuring head, waist, hip or limb circumferences should be made of a narrow, non-stretchable material such as paper or plastic.

Growth charts

Growth charts have been constructed by measuring a large number of healthy children at varying ages. Centile lines are then constructed showing the normal distribution of weight/height/head circumference measurements at each age. The 50th centile line is the median of the measurements for that age. Fifty per cent of children will have measurements below that line and the other 50 per cent will be above that line. The other centile lines are constructed using standard deviations from the median. The 25th and 75th centile lines are 2/3 standard deviation from the median. Twenty-five per cent of children's measurements will be below the 25th centile line and 75 per cent of children's measurements will be above that centile line.

The 2nd and 98th centiles are two standard deviations (or two z scores) above and below the median.

In the UK, two sources of data for construction of the recommended reference charts are used (Table 2.1.4):

- The UK 90 reference data is from a large number of measurements of children living in the UK during the 1980s and up to 1990. These charts describe the average growth of children at this time before the epidemic of childhood obesity began. They are considered a reference for normal growth in the UK.

- The World Health Organization data WHO Child Growth Standards were developed using data collected in the WHO Multicentre Growth Reference Study, which was a community-based, multi-country project conducted in Brazil, Ghana, India, Norway, Oman and the United States. In each of the six countries a sample of breastfed infants from non-smoking, non-deprived mothers were measured longitudinally. Growth was found to be similar in all six countries and growth charts using the data describe the optimal growth 0–4 years for all children from different ethnic groups.

Table 2.1.4 Data sources for different age groups

Age group	Source of data
Preterm infants	UK 90 reference data
Term infants at birth	UK 90 reference data
2 weeks to 4 years of age	WHO data collected in the WHO Multicentre Growth Reference Study
5–18 years	UK 90 reference data

Growth charts recommended for use in the UK

The growth charts in the UK have nine centile lines: 0.4th, 2nd, 9th, 25th, 50th, 75th, 91st, 98th and 99.6th (Table 2.1.5). Each type comes in one version for boys and one for girls as boys and girls have slightly different growth patterns. The correct term for the area between the centile lines is 'centile space'.

Table 2.1.5 Growth charts recommended for use in the UK

Charts	Use for
Neonatal and Infant Close Monitoring Chart (NICM) – boys and girls	1) births before 32 weeks gestation 2) unwell neonates born after 32 weeks 3) term infants with significant growth and weight faltering
UK–WHO Growth Chart 0–4 years – boys and girls (see Figure 2.1.2)	Healthy preterm infants born after 32 weeks gestation Term infants Young children 1–4 years
4–18 years Growth and BMI Chart – boys and girls	Children 5–18 years

These charts all come in two formats:

● A4 which are used mainly in clinical notes

● A5 for use in the Personal Child Health Record (Growth charts for boys 0–4 years and 2–18 years, and girls 0–4 years and 2–18 years are given in Appendix 2 p. 232–239)

The PCHR, also known as the 'Red Book', is used in the UK to record the health and development of a child. It is given to parents/carers following the birth of every child (Figure 2.1.2).

BMI centile charts are used for assessing if children aged over 2 years are underweight, normal weight for height, overweight or obese.

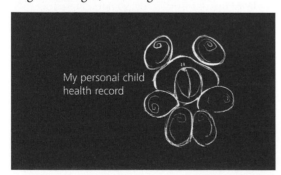

Figure 2.1.2 Personal Child Health Record used in the UK – also called 'Red Book'

Any other growth charts for normal children are now considered out of date by the Royal College of Paediatrics and Child Health (Wright *et al.* 2002, 2010). However, there are specialized growth charts for children with:

● Down syndrome

● Turner syndrome

● homozygous sickle cell disease.

All recommended charts are produced and printed by Harlow Printing Ltd and can be ordered from them (www.healthforallchildren.co.uk).

Plotting on growth charts

Charts should be plotted in pencil with a dot. Pencil is used because mistakes in plotting are often made and can be corrected more easily if plotted in pencil. The dots should not be joined up with a line, nor emphasized with a circle around them.

Age correction for preterm babies

The measurements of preterm babies should be age-corrected when plotting for:

● 1 year for infants born 32–36 weeks gestation

● 2 years for infants born before 32 weeks gestation.

Age correction adjusts the plot of a measurement to account for the number of weeks a baby was born early. The number of weeks early is equal to 40 weeks minus the gestational age at birth. Hence a baby born at 31 weeks gestation will have been born 9 weeks (40–31 = 9) early and his or her age since birth should be reduced by 9 weeks when plotting measurements taken up until the age of 2 years.

Normal Growth Patterns

The weight and length/height of infants and children are expected to increase along, or parallel to, the centile lines. However, growth is not usually regular so some small variation over about a centile space is usually seen in normal growth patterns. Growth anywhere between the 2nd and 98th centile lines is considered normal. Growth between the 0.4th and 2nd centile and between the 98th and 99.6th is usually normal and should be interpreted considering the ethnic origin and stature of parents.

Infants and young children may lose weight when they are ill and not eating well but normally regain the weight within a few weeks once they are well and their appetite has returned.

Weight loss after birth

Infants normally lose weight after birth and then regain their birthweight by 7–10 days. The weight loss is mainly due to a net fluid loss in the first 2–3 days. A weight loss of up to 10 per cent of birthweight is considered normal: more than 10 per cent needs careful assessment to ensure feeding is effective and such infants should be carefully monitored until they have regained their birthweight.

Because of the variability of this weight loss and gain, there are no centile lines between birth and 2 weeks of age on the growth charts for 0–4 years. However, weights measured at this time should be plotted on the chart and compared with birthweight.

Birthweight centile does not always predict the weight centile later in infancy

The birth weight reflects fetal growth, which is dependent on prenatal nutrition and also any growth restriction or acceleration within the womb. For example, intrauterine growth restriction may occur if the mother is very small in stature, or growth acceleration may occur in fetuses of mothers with diabetes, possibly due to extra insulin produced in response to the hyperglycaemia of the mother and consequently a high glucose level in cord blood.

Within the first 6–8 weeks infants may cross centiles up or down, usually towards the 50th centile, to compensate for either slow or rapid fetal growth.

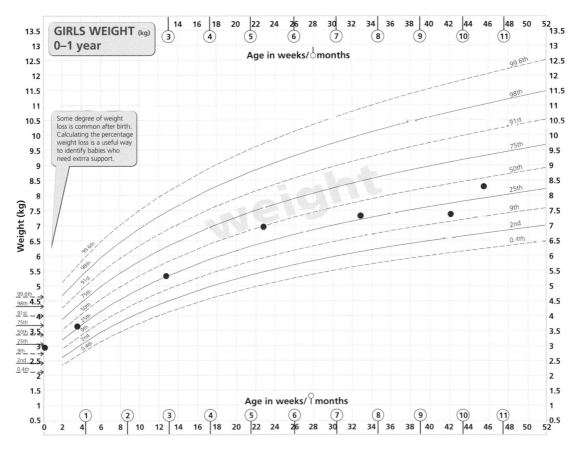

Figure 2.1.3 Normal growth in an infant girl on an A5 format growth chart

Weight gain in infancy

From about 6 to 8 weeks of age infants usually follow along a weight centile line or space but there will normally be some variation above and below it (see Figure 2.1.3).

Following length centiles in the first 2 years

Some catch-up or catch-down in length centile is usually seen in the first 2 years to compensate for any constraints in intrauterine growth. By 3 years there is good correlation between the height centile and the final height centile to be reached following the pubertal growth spurt.

BMI and body fat differences in girls and boys

BMI varies throughout childhood and this variation is slightly different between boys and girls. Hence there are gender-specific BMI-for-age centile charts. BMI increases during infancy, decreases between 1 and 5/6 years and then slowly increases throughout the rest of childhood.

The body fat content is similar in boys and girls at 5 and 7 years old but thereafter begins to increase

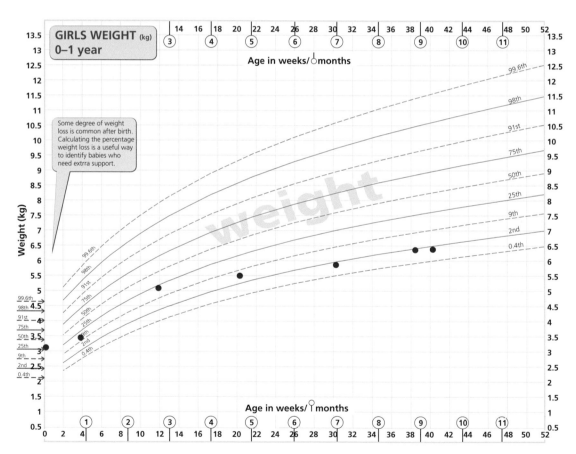

Figure 2.1.4 Faltering growth in an infant girl showing weight falling through 2 centile spaces. Measurements after 6-8 weeks show a fall across two centile spaces.

along with BMI, with girls gaining fat at a slightly higher rate than boys. This increase in BMI is termed the adiposity rebound. The timing of it is a crucial marker and intervention point for childhood obesity.

Crossing centiles during adolescence

The pubertal growth spurt occurs at different ages in children but the growth charts describe an average growth spurt at the average age of the pubertal growth spurt. Children who go through their pubertal growth spurt at a younger or older age than the average age will therefore cross centile lines on the chart. This needs to be taken into consideration when assessing height and weight gain around this time. See Chapter 6.2, page 173.

Abnormal Growth

Poor growth or extremely rapid growth may be the first indication of an underlying medical condition that requires further investigation. Faltering growth is defined as weight or height falling through 2 centile spaces after allowing for adjustments up or down on the centile charts in the first 6–8 weeks (see Figure 2.1.4). Rapid growth is defined as crossing centiles upwards on the weight or height centile charts. Rapid weight gain is a risk factor for obesity.

Referral to a paediatrician should be considered if:

- weight or height is noted, for the first time, to be below the 0.4th centile
- weight or length/height falls through 2 centile spaces and increasing energy intake from food is not successful in restoring normal growth velocity
- BMI centile is below the 2nd centile.

Height crossing more than one centile space upwards in children over 3 years of age and before puberty may be an indication of excess growth hormone but a referral needs careful consideration as the accuracy of height measurements is often poor. In addition, early puberty is becoming more common.

In children over 2 years, a BMI that is over the 91st centile is considered overweight and a BMI over the 98th centile is considered obese. Families of these children may need to make lifestyle changes to reduce the rate of weight gain in the child (see Chapter 7.2).

Acknowledgements

Thanks are due to Professor Mehul Dattani, London Centre for Paediatric Endocrinology, University College London and Professor Tim Cole, MRC Centre of Epidemiology for Child Health, University College London.

References and further reading

Department of Health (2011) *National Child Measurement Programme.* **www.dh.gov.uk/en/Publichealth/Obesity/DH_073787** (accessed 28 July 2011).

Elliman D and Hall DMB (2006) *Health for All Children*, revised 4th edn. Oxford: Oxford University Press.

Fayter D, Nixon I, Hartley S, *et al.* (2008) Effectiveness and cost-effectiveness of height screening programmes during the primary school years: a systematic review. *Archives of Disease in Childhood* **93**: 278–284.

NICE (National Institute for Health and Clinical Excellence) (2008) *Public Health Guidance 11. Improving the nutrition of pregnant and breastfeeding mothers and children in low-income households.* March 2008. London: NICE.

Tasker R, McClure R and Acerini C (2008) *Oxford Handbook of Paediatrics.* Oxford: Oxford University Press.

Wiskin AE, Davies JH, Wootton SA and Beattie RM (2011) Energy expenditure, nutrition and growth. *Archives of Disease in Childhood* **96**: 567–572.

Wright CM, Booth IW, Buckler JM, *et al.* (2002) Growth reference charts for use in the United Kingdom. *Archives of Disease in Childhood* **86**: 11–14.

Wright CM, Williams AF, Elliman D, *et al.* (2010) Using the new UK–WHO growth charts. *British Medical Journal* **340**: c1140.

Resources

Growth charts and BMI charts can be ordered from: **www.healthforallchildren.co.uk**

Growth charts and online training exercises in plotting and interpreting growth charts (**www.rcpch.ac.uk/growthcharts**)

Self-learning programme: Module 8 Growth and Nutrition (**www.e-lfh.org.uk/healthychild**)

Assessing Nutritional Intake

Summary

- Dietary intake can be assessed by:

  - estimating or weighing food consumed over one or more days and recording this in a food diary or

  - completing a 24-hour recall of all food and drink consumed, or a food frequency questionnaire (FFQ).

- A recorded food diary can be used to assess energy and nutritional adequacy by either comparison with the principles of healthy eating or by using dietary analysis software containing a database of foods, energy and nutrients.

- Parents and older children can be taught how to assess food and drink intake using the principles of healthy eating and they can use this to make changes to improve the nutritional adequacy of the diet.

- Nutritional analysis of the diets of large populations of children (e.g. Avon Longitudinal Study of Parents and Children; ALSPAC) have been used to find associations between dietary intakes and later health outcomes. The adequacy of the diet is assessed by comparison with Dietary Reference Values (DRV).

As discussed in Chapter 1.1, a child's diet is considered nutritionally adequate if the nutrient content of the foods, drinks and any supplements consumed meet:

- the Reference Nutrient Intakes (RNIs) for each of the nutrients and

- the Estimated Average Requirement (EAR) for energy for that child's age and activity level.

In Chapter 1.2 the principles of healthy eating are discussed, and individual diets can be assessed against those principles.

To be able to assess the nutritional adequacy of an individual child's diet you need to know:

- what the child has consumed or normally consumes in terms of food, drinks and supplements

- the energy and nutrient content of those foods, drinks and supplements

- the age, gender and physical activity of the child.

Assessing the recent or usual dietary intake can be done by either taking a dietary history or weighing the food and drink offered to a child over a set period of time.

Taking a dietary history is usually done in one of the following ways:

- Food and drink diary: A carer or the child records the food and drinks consumed over one or several days – ideally including a mixture of weekdays and weekend days.

- 24-hour recall: The child, parents or carers are asked to remember what the child has eaten in the last 24 hours or on the previous day.

- Food frequency questionnaire: The child or parent or carer reports how often and in what quantity a range of different foods are generally eaten.

Alternatively the second method entails weighing both the food and drinks offered to the child over a set period of time. After each eating episode the food and drinks that the child did not consume must also be weighed. The difference in weights of each food or drink item will be what the child has consumed.

There are advantages and disadvantages to each method:

- Recording a dietary diary may not be done accurately and there may be some underreporting of certain foods and overreporting of other foods. This method can be enhanced by a subsequent interview to clarify any anomalies and also to check the validity and accuracy of measurement of any quantities.

- Food frequency questionnaires (FFQ) are less expensive to administer and are therefore used more extensively in large-scale epidemiological studies investigating the relationship between diet and health outcomes. The key point about an FFQ is that it records the type of food eaten and the frequency of consumption. They reflect what the interviewee estimates that they eat but may not be accurate. They also have a use in checking the dietary intake of specific nutrients. In young children they may be used to estimate iron intake by asking how often specific foods with significant iron content are eaten.

- Weighing food and drinks is considered the best estimate of dietary intake but it is time consuming for whoever has to weigh the food and drinks and that person must be trained to do it accurately. Weighing each food and drink will disrupt the normal flow of meal and snack patterns in the household and consequently may also influence which foods and drinks are offered to the child. Hence the results may not reflect what the child would have eaten had there been no interference to the normal routine. A certain amount of the food and drinks offered to infants and young children may be spilt or regurgitated so a weighed intake for this age group may be less accurate than in older age groups.

Assessing Nutritional Adequacy of a Child's Diet with a Recorded Food Intake

For assessing individual diets a recorded food diary is a very useful method. Parents of younger children or older children themselves are asked to complete a food diary such as that shown in Figure 2.2.1.

Daily food and drinks diary					
DATE:					
Time	Location	All food and drinks offered	Quantity or weight eaten	Time taken	Who else was also eating
7:30	Kitchen table	Bowl Cheerios with full fat milk + 1 tsp sugar 1 slice toast with butter and jam	All milk left All toast eaten	10 minutes	Sister and mother
10:30	School playground	200mL carton apple juice 2 cereal bars	All	15 minutes	Friends
12:00	School canteen	5 tbsp pasta 3 tbsp meat sauce 6 carrot sticks 3 cauliflower florets Bowl apple crumble and custard glass of water	½ pasta and meat sauce no carrots or cauliflower All dessert ½ water	20 minutes	Friends

Figure 2.2.1 A daily food and drinks diary

A professional trained in assessing dietary intake (e.g. a dietitian) can use this information to assess the nutritional adequacy by one of two methods:

- assessment against the principles of healthy eating using the number of daily servings and portion sizes of the five food groups
- computer software to compare the dietary intake of energy and each nutrient against the RNIs for each nutrient and EAR for energy.

Assessing nutritional adequacy using the five food groups

This assessment method is simple and older children and parents can be taught to do it themselves. If the number of servings from the five food groups (as described in Table 1.2.1, pages 14–15) is followed then the child can be assumed to be consuming an adequate intake of nutrients.

Food group	Recommended number of daily age-appropriate servings
1. Bread, rice, potatoes, pasta and other starchy foods	Included at each meal – and some snacks
2. Fruit and vegetables	Included at each meal – and some snacks
3. Milk, cheese and yogurt	3 servings per day
4. Meat, fish, eggs, nuts and beans	2–3 servings per day
5. Foods high in fat and foods high in sugar	Very small amounts with meals Sweet foods limited to 4 times per day
Drinks	6–8 per day or 1 with each meal and snack
Vitamin supplements	Vitamins A and D daily for those under five years of age

A chart such as in Figure 2.2.2 can be used for the assessment of foods from a record of a 24-hour intake. All the food and drinks consumed over a 24-hour period are listed in the left-hand column. A mark is made in the food group columns when a

Date:	Name :					
All food and drinks		**Food groups**				**Fluid**
	Bread, rice, potato, pasta, other starchy food	Fruit & veg	Milk, cheese, yogurt	Meat, fish, eggs, nuts, pulses	Foods high in fat &/or sugar	Drinks
TOTALS :						
RECOMMENDED :	3–5 At each meal and some snacks	5 At each meal and some snacks	3	2–3	Some high-fat foods	6–8 cups

Figure 2.2.2 Food chart for 24-hour intake

food or drink contributes to a serving from that food group. Whether a mark of 1, 2 or ½ is put in depends on the quantity consumed and the appropriate portion size for the child's age.

For example, the food diary could report that the child had eaten the food shown in Figure 2.2.3.

For breakfast a '1' would be marked in the 'Bread, rice, potato, pasta, other starchy food' column for the bowl of breakfast cereal. Then a '1' in the 'Milk, cheese and yogurt' column for the cup of milk that would have been poured onto the breakfast cereal. If the child leaves half of the milk in the bowl then this could be reduced to a '½'. A '1' in the 'Fruit and vegetable' column would be for the blueberries that were added to the cereal.

The rest of the day's intake would be assessed and marked in the same way. Finally the '1's and '½'s in each food group column would be added up then recorded in the row for totals. A comparison can then be made of these figures to the daily recommendations.

An assessment of the intake in Figure 2.2.3 would be shown as in Figure 2.2.4.

Breakfast	Breakfast cereal with milk Blueberries Pure fruit juice diluted with water
Mid-morning snack	Apple slices Cup milk
Lunch	Mini meatballs Pasta Broccoli florets Apple crumble with ice cream Pure fruit juice diluted with water
Afternoon snack	Crackers with Marmite and cheese cubes Water to drink
Evening meal	Fish and potato pie Carrot and cucumber sticks Plain yogurt mixed with strawberries and sugar Water

Figure 2.2.3 Example food intake recorded

All food and drinks	Food groups					Fluid
	Bread, rice, potato, pasta, other starchy food	Fruit & veg	Milk, cheese, yogurt	Meat, fish, eggs, nuts, pulses	Foods high in fat &/or sugar	Drinks
Breakfast:						
Breakfast cereal	1					
Milk on cereal			½			
Blueberries		1				
Pure fruit juice diluted with water					1	1
Mid-morning snack:						
Apple slices		1				
Cup milk to drink			1			1
Lunch:						
Mini meatballs				1		
Pasta	1					
Cauliflower florets		1				
Apple crumble		1			1	
Ice cream					1	
Pure fruit juice diluted with water					1	1
Mid-afternoon snack:						
Crackers with Marmite and cheese cubes	1		1			
Water to drink						1

(Continued)

All food and drinks	Food groups					Fluid
	Bread, rice, potato, pasta, other starchy food	Fruit & veg	Milk, cheese, yogurt	Meat, fish, eggs, nuts, pulses	Foods high in fat &/or sugar	Drinks
Evening meal:						
Fish and potato pie	1			1		
Carrot and cucumber sticks		1				
Plain yogurt mixed with			1			
strawberries and sugar		1			1	
Water to drink						1
Extra drinks of water						2
TOTALS :	4	6	3½	2	5	7
RECOMMENDED :	3–5 At each meal and some snacks	5 At each meal and some snacks	3	2–3	Some high-fat foods	6–8 cups

Figure 2.2.4 Completed assessment of example intake

All food and drinks	Food groups					Fluid
	Bread, rice, potato, pasta, other starchy food	Fruit & veg	Milk, cheese, yogurt	Meat, fish, eggs, nuts, pulses	Foods high in fat &/or sugar	Drinks
Breakfast:						
Cornflakes and milk	1		½			
Orange Squash to drink					1	1
At nursery:						
Pieces fruit and milk to drink		1	1			1
Lunch:						
Jam sandwich and cake	1				3	
Milk to drink			1			1
Afternoon:						
1 packet Wotsits					1	
Carton of fruit juice drink					1	1
Evening meal:						
Fish fingers and chips	1			1	1	
Chocolate biscuit					1	
Milk to drink			1			1
Before bed:						
Full bottle of milk			2			2
TOTALS :	3	1	5½	1	8	7
RECOMMENDED :	3–5 At each meal and some snacks	5 At each meal and some snacks	3	2–3	Some high-fat foods	6–8 cups

Figure 2.2.5 Ellie's food and drinks in one day

Case Study

Ellie is now 2 years 9 months and goes to nursery in the morning. She still has a sleep after lunch and her mother is concerned that she eats very poorly at lunchtime. She usually gives her bread and jam just to make sure she has had something. There are no problems with her growth and her mother was asked to write down everything Ellie had eaten the day before: 'Breakfast: cornflakes and milk, orange squash to drink. Milk to drink and fruit at breaktime at nursery. Lunch: jam sandwich and cake. A packet of Wotsits and a carton of a fruit juice drink in the afternoon with her older brother on the way home from school. Fish fingers with chips for tea, milk and a chocalate biscuit for pudding. A bottle of milk on going to bed.'

Ellie's food and drinks in one day are thus as shown in Figure 2.2.5.

Ellie is getting enough calories to keep growing for the time being. She is probably tired when she comes home from her busy morning at nursery which is why she is not eating well at lunchtime. After her afternoon sleep she is hungry and eats well but is given the same snack as her brother, which is not nutritious enough to replace the nutrients she has not had at lunch.

The combination of the food groups is very poor and by comparing the totals to the recommendations you can see she has too much milk and a lot of foods that are high in fat and sugar and not enough foods from the other food groups. Consequently Ellie's diet will be low in iron and other minerals. If she continues to eat like this she would become deficient in iron and might get iron-deficiency anaemia.

As the rest of the family do not eat fruit and vegetables Ellie is not being offered

→

them at home. The only fruit she is having is that which is given for a snack at nursery.

There are several changes that Ellie's mother can make to improve Ellie's diet:

- cut out the bottle of milk before bed as soon as possible
- change the lunch to a more nutritious sandwich, for example she could try a peanut butter and jam sandwich
- change the afternoon snack to a more nutritious snack such as carrot sticks with breadsticks which are crunchy like the Wotsits. She could also add in some pieces of cold meat such as ham or cooked chicken to make up for the small lunch that is being eaten.

The whole family needs to begin eating more fruit and vegetables so that they are offered at each meal. As this change will take some time Ellie could be given diluted pure fruit juice in place of fruit juice drink that will only contain about 5 per cent fruit juice – the rest will be sugar and colouring. The pure fruit juice will provide a few more nutrients from fruit that squash does not contain.

If Ellie's mother is able to make these changes then eventually her one day's intake would be as shown in Figure 2.2.6.

Activity 1

Make a recorded intake of all the food and drinks you have over the next three days and analyse it for nutritional adequacy using the method above.

A one-day record of a child's intake may not be indicative of his or her average intake. Young children will often eat well some days and not so well on other days. The eating pattern Monday to

All food and drinks	Food groups					Fluid
	Bread, rice, potato, pasta, other starchy food	Fruit & veg	Milk, cheese, yogurt	Meat, fish, eggs, nuts, pulses	Foods high in fat &/or sugar	Drinks
Breakfast:						
Cornflakes and milk	1		½			
Diluted fruit juice to drink					1	1
At nursery:						
Pieces fruit and milk to drink		1	1			1
Lunch:						
Jam and peanut butter sandwich	1			1	1	
Fruit pieces		1				
Milk to drink			1			1
Afternoon:						
Carrot sticks and breadsticks	1	1				
Chunks of cold chicken				1		
Diluted fruit juice					1	1
Evening meal:						
Fish fingers and chips with peas	1	1		1	1	
Chocolate biscuit and fruit pieces		1			1	
Milk to drink			1			1
Before bed/during the day						
Extra water to drink						1
TOTALS :	4	5	3½	3	5	6
RECOMMENDED :	3–5 At each meal and some snacks	5 At each meal and some snacks	3	2–3	Some high-fat foods	6–8 cups

Figure 2.2.6 If Ellie's mother is able to make these changes then eventually her one day's intake would look like this

Friday may be quite different to the days on the weekend. Days a child goes to nursery, a child minder or school might be quite different to days when he or she stays at home. Birthday party days will also be quite different. Assessing a child's intake over several days or a week is therefore preferable to an assessment of just one day.

Total servings from each food group each day can be added together and then divided by 7 to give an average for this food group for the week (Figure 2.2.7).

In this example, the combination of the food groups over the week is good enough. The average for each food group is very close to the recommendation.

When the combination of the food groups over the week is not ideal then advice can be given by deciding which food groups the child is not having

	Food groups					Fluid
	Bread, rice, potato, pasta, other starchy food	Fruit & veg	Milk, cheese, yogurt	Meat, fish, eggs, nuts, pulses	Foods high in fat &/or sugar	Drinks
Sunday	5	5	3	2	2	6
Monday	6	4	4	1	3	8
Tuesday	4	6	2	2	2	5
Wednesday	5	3	1	2	4	6
Thursday	3	3	3	3	2	7
Friday	6	4	3	2	1	6
Saturday – went to a birthday party	4	2	3	1	5	9
Totals for the week:	33	27	19	13	19	47
Average for the week	4.7	3.8	2.7	1.9	2.7	6.7
RECOMMENDED :	3–5 At each meal and some snacks	5 At each meal and some snacks	3	2–3	Some high-fat foods	6–8 cups

Figure 2.2.7 Average for each food group for the week

enough of and providing ideas of ways to increase his/her intake of this food group by substituting this food group for another food group he may be having too much of.

Using computer software

There are computer software programmes that calculate the energy and nutrient content of a dietary intake. The adequacy of the diet is assessed by comparison with estimated average energy requirement and RNIs of each nutrient. Several companies sell computer software packages to do this. However, the analysis obtained is only as accurate as:

● the nutrient content of the food database that is in the software – the foods in the database may not match exactly the food that has been bought or prepared

● the accuracy of the diet history taken of the exact quantities that the child has consumed

● the accuracy with which the food and drinks consumed by a child are entered into the software.

Such software can also be used to assess the nutrient contents of menus and individual recipes.

Nutritional Assessments for Epidemiological Data

In the past, weighing food over a four-day period was the method used in national dietary surveys of children in the UK (Gregory et al. 1995, 2000) but it was a very expensive way to collect nationally representative data. The current national nutritional data collection is a rolling programme of dietary assessment and uses a four-day food diary recorded by the family and is followed up by an interview to clarify quantities consumed by the family member who is in the study.

Case Study

The food diary record method was used in the Avon Longitudinal Study of Parents and Children (ALSPAC). The data collected has been used in many scientific publications relating health outcomes to dietary intakes in children. Three-day diet records were recorded by parents of a cohort of over 14 000 children, all born in the early 1990s in Avon. A diet record booklet was sent to the parents just prior to them making a clinic visit to have their child weighed and measured at various ages from 4 months to 18 years. The parents were asked to describe everything their child was offered in household measures and to record leftover foods/drinks.

The diary was checked through in an interview with the parents by a nutrition fieldworker to improve accuracy. The fieldworker allocated food weights according to the parental description of the portion size using guideline measures for the various foods. For manufactured foods, parents provided packet weights when available. The full details of the methods used and the nutrient and food intakes of the children are described in various papers (Emmett *et al.* 2002, Cowin and Emmett 2007).

Biochemical Measures Used for Nutritional Assessment

Nutrient intake can be measured using biomarkers.

- Doubly-labelled water is used to measure energy expenditure which can be used to validate energy intake from a recorded food diary.

- A 24-hour urine collection can be measured for sodium, potassium and nitrogen content. Total nitrogen is a measure of protein intake.

- Blood levels of certain nutrients indicate an adequate or inadequate intake (e.g. plasma levels of vitamin C, beta-carotene, folate and vitamin D).

Activity 2

Ask the parents of a child to fill in a three-day recorded intake and then analyse it in terms of the five food groups.

References and further reading

Cowin I and Emmett P (2007) Diet in a group of 18-month-old children in South West England, and comparison with the results of a national survey. *Journal of Human Nutrition and Dietetics* **20**: 254–267.

Department of Health (2011) *National Diet and Nutrition Survey: Headline results from Years 1 and 2 (combined) of the rolling programme 2008/9–2009/10.* **www.dh.gov.uk/en/Publicationsandstatistics/Publications/PublicationsStatistics/DH_128166** (accessed April 2012).

Emmett P, Rogers I, Symes C and the ALSPAC Study Team (2002) Food and nutrient intakes of a population sample of 3-year-old children in the South West of England in 1996. *Public Health Nutrition* **5**: 55–64.

Gregory JR, Collins DL, Davies PSW, Hughes JM and Clarke PC (1995) *National Diet and Nutrition Survey: Children aged 1½ and 4½ years*, Volume 1. Report of the Diet and Nutrition Survey. London: HMSO.

Gregory J, Lowe S, Bates CJ, *et al.* (2000) *National Diet and Nutrition Survey: Young people aged 4–18 years.* London: The Stationery Office.

Resources

Software packages available in the UK for dietary analysis:

CompEat – Dietary Analysis Software (**www.compeat.co.uk**)

Dietplan6 (**www.foresoft.co.uk**)

Section 3
Prenatal Nutrition

3.1 Preconception and Fertility

3.2 Pregnancy

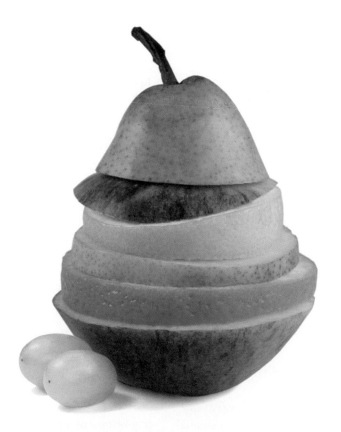

Preconception and Fertility

Summary

- Maternal nutritional status at conception affects fetal growth and development and has implications for postnatal health.

- About 50 per cent of pregnancies are unplanned and fetal health and birth outcomes are disadvantaged in a poorly nourished mother.

- Both men and women planning conception should follow a balanced nutritious diet and aim for an ideal body mass index (BMI) of 18.5–25 kg/m^2.

- Ideally, overweight and obese women should aim to reduce their weight to this ideal BMI at least four months prior to conception.

- Women planning a pregnancy should take folic acid and vitamin D supplements and avoid the same foods that should be avoided in pregnancy.

- Nutritional factors can affect fertility in both males and females.

The nutritional status of both parents can affect fertility and the chance of conception. Furthermore, maternal nutritional status, in particular at the time of conception, is an important determinant of fetal growth and development and lays the foundations of the child's future health.

Mothers with a history of poor nutrition before conception may have low nutrient stores and, consequently, the fetus may have reduced access to the nutrients needed for growth and development, particularly in the early stages of gestation. This is particularly important for mothers whose nutritional intake is compromised by nausea and vomiting in the first three months.

Women most at risk of poor nutritional status at conception are those who:

- eat a poor or unbalanced diet (this includes many teenagers)

- are trying to lose weight on very low-calorie diets that may be deficient in essential nutrients

- have had several closely spaced pregnancies.

Nutritional Advice Preconception

If pregnancies are planned, nutritional status preconception can be improved. However, only about 50 per cent of pregnancies in the UK are planned, with higher income, better educated and older women more likely to plan than low-income, young and poorly educated women. Good nutritional status in all women of childbearing age is therefore an ideal.

Those planning a pregnancy should follow a balanced nutritious diet as detailed for pregnancy in Chapter 3.2. In addition, women should take daily supplements of:

- 400 μg folic acid and

- 10 μg (400 IU) vitamin D.

A higher dose of 5 mg folic acid/day is recommended for women with:

- spina bifida

- a history of a previous child with a neural tube defect

- diabetes.

This high-dose folic acid preparation is available on prescription only.

Preconception, women should also avoid or limit certain foods and drinks as is advised for pregnant women (see Chapter 3.2, page 71).

Optimizing Body Weight

Women with a BMI above 27 should be encouraged to lose weight prior to conception. Excess maternal body weight combined with the weight of the baby can lead to problems during the course of the pregnancy. Overweight pregnant women are at increased risk of complications such as high blood pressure, gestational diabetes and preterm delivery. They are also more likely to have a low-birthweight baby.

The National Institute for Health and Clinical Excellence (NICE) recommends that women with a BMI over 30 should be informed of the increased risk to themselves and their babies during pregnancy and birth and encouraged to lose weight before becoming pregnant (NICE 2008a). It is preferable for weight to be reduced well in advance (at least 3–4 months) of conception to lessen the likelihood of nutritional inadequacy. For pre-pregnancy weight loss NICE recommends providing a structured, tailored programme of ongoing support that combines advice on healthy eating and physical activity and addresses individual barriers to change (NICE 2008a). When weight has been lost it is then important to encourage a diet with adequate energy intake and variety to ensure intake of all essential nutrients to prepare for conception.

Women with Diabetes

Women with diabetes who are planning to become pregnant should establish good glycaemic control before conception and aim to maintain their HbA1c below 6.1 per cent to reduce the risk of congenital malformations. Women with diabetes whose HbA1c is above 10 per cent should be strongly advised to avoid pregnancy (NICE 2008b).

Diabetic women should take a supplement of 5 mg of folic acid daily along with a daily 10 µg vitamin D.

Improving Fertility and the Chance of Conception

Poor nutritional status in males and females can decrease fertility and the chance of conception. Fertility problems affect about 15 per cent of couples and are due to male infertility in about 30–50 per cent of those couples.

Research has shown several key nutritional influences that can decrease fertility and the chance of a woman conceiving:

- body weight
- weight loss and undernutrition
- eating disorders
- poor iron stores
- extreme levels of exercise
- caffeine
- alcohol.

Body weight

Women with a BMI of 20–25 have been shown to have a higher rate of conceiving than those with a BMI higher than 25 or lower than 20 (Zaadstra *et al.* 1993).

Overweight and obesity

Being overweight does not prevent all women from conceiving but overweight and obesity can affect ovulation and also the response to fertility treatment.

Obesity with or without the problem of the polycystic ovarian syndrome (PCOS) is associated with a doubling in the rate of ovulatory infertility (Rich-Edwards *et al.* 1994) In both PCOS and simple obesity weight reduction is associated with a return of ovulation, menstruation and fertility in many cases. A prospective study (Clark *et al.* 1998) showed that when overweight women who were not ovulating followed a weight loss and physical activity programme, the outcome for most women was natural ovulation, conception and successful pregnancy.

Excessive body fat especially central obesity

Central body obesity, indicated by a waist circumference >90 cm (35 inches) is a risk factor for infertility as it takes women with high central obesity longer to become pregnant than women with low central obesity (Zaadstra *et al.* 1993).

Underweight

Conception can occur in women well below average or ideal weight. However, women who have a low BMI (BMI <20) are less likely to conceive (Zaadstra *et al.* 1993).

Low per cent body fat

A study in the 1990s in the United States showed that an improved nutritional status in adolescent girls was associated with an increasingly early date of menarche signalling the onset of fertility. The mean body weight at which menarche occurred in US girls was 48 kg with a mean height of 1.59 m at 12.9 years. Of the mean body weight at the completion of growth (16–18 years) 16 kg was fat, representing an energy reserve for reproduction of 602 MJ (144 000 kcal). Such an energy reserve would provide the theoretical energy requirements of both pregnancy and three months of lactation. Frisch's observation was that body fat proportion of less than 22 per cent of body weight was associated with the absence of ovulation and that healthy fertile women who were ovulating on a monthly basis had an average body fat proportion of 28 per cent.

Weight loss and undernutrition

In normal weight women, weight loss of 10–15 per cent causes hormonal disruption, resulting in amenorrhoea and anovulation. About 30 per cent of impaired fertility cases are related to weight loss. Weight gain is the recommended treatment for amenorrhoea related to low body weight.

Eating disorders

Both anorexia nervosa and bulimia nervosa, which are estimated to affect 1–2 per cent of young women (Hoek 2006), are related to amenorrhoea, anovulation and infertility.

Extreme levels of exercise

High levels of exercise together with a low calorie intake in young women (calorie intake <30 per cent of requirements) can result in a condition known as the 'female athlete triad' with three symptoms: disordered eating, amenorrhoea and osteoporosis (Loucks *et al.* 2006). The latter is as a result of low oestrogen production.

Caffeine

High intakes of caffeine may extend the time it takes to become pregnant. Researchers have found that women who consumed more than four cups of coffee per day – about 500 mg caffeine – were half as likely to conceive as women who had less than two cups of coffee per day (Committee on Toxicity 2008).

Poor iron stores

Iron status prior to pregnancy is related to fertility. Results from a large prospective study of nurses (Chavarro *et al.* 2006) indicated that anovulatory infertility may be related to poor iron status.

Alcohol

A follow-up study of couples planning their first pregnancy found an association between women's alcohol intake and decreased fertility even among women who had five or fewer drinks a week. This would indicate that fertility is reduced in a high proportion of women due to their alcohol intake (Jensen *et al.* 1998). Women experiencing difficulties in conceiving should be advised of the possible advantages of avoiding alcohol completely (Jensen *et al.* 1998). The Department of Health now advises avoiding alcohol altogether but if women choose to drink alcohol it should be limited to one to two units once or twice per week (NHS Choices 2011).

Male Infertility

The causes of male infertility remain largely unknown as it is difficult to identify the role of single factors, and various studies have shown conflicting data. Lifestyle factors such as smoking, alcohol and diet, environment and socio-economic factors may affect sperm motility, fertility or pregnancy outcomes.

Gastrointestinal complaints and low intake of fruit and vegetables have been associated with low sperm counts (Wong *et al.* 2003). Zinc, selenium and vitamin C may be particularly important in sperm production (Tas *et al.* 1996).

Exposure to heavy metals, halogens (pesticides), glycol (antifreeze) and oestrogen-like chemicals (DDT and PCB) in the environment have also been shown to reduce male fertility. The oestrogen-like chemicals reduce the activity of the androgen hormones (e.g. testosterone).

The most prudent advice for men is to:

- consume a balanced and varied diet based on the five food groups, ensuring adequate fruit and vegetable intake

- limit themselves to a moderate alcohol intake of less than 3–4 units per day

- aim for a healthy body weight – very underweight men should gain weight and obese men should lose weight.

Nutritional influences that decrease fertility are summarized in Table 3.1.1.

Table 3.1.1 Nutritional influences that decrease fertility

Nutritional influences that can decrease fertility	In females	In males
Weight loss >15% of normal weight	Y	Y
Negative energy balance	Y	Y
Inadequate body fat	Y	Y
Obesity	Y	Y
Excessive body fat especially central adiposity	Y	Y
Extreme levels of exercise	Y	Y
High alcohol intake	Y	Y
Eating disorders	Y	
High caffeine intake	Y	
High-fibre/low-fat diets	Y	
Poor iron stores	Y	
Coeliac disease	Y	
Diabetes mellitus	Y	
Inadequate zinc status		Y
Inadequate antioxidant status		Y
Heavy metal exposure		Y
Exposure to halogens (pesticides), glycol (antifreeze) and environmental oestrogen-like chemicals (DDT and PCB)		Y

Activity 1

List the nutritional topics you would discuss with the following in a clinic for couples who are failing to conceive:

a) an underweight woman
b) an overweight couple
c) a couple both of normal weight.

Activity 2

What advice would you give to a diabetic woman planning a pregnancy?

References and further reading

Chavarro JE, Rich-Edwards JW, Rosner BA and Willett WC (2006) Iron consumption and the risk of infertility. *Obstetrics and Gynecology* **108**: 1145–1152.

Clark AM, Thornley B, Tomlinson L, Galletley C and Norman RJ (1998) Weight loss in infertile women results in improvement in reproductive outcome for all forms of infertility treatment. *Human Reproduction* **13**: 1502–1505.

Committee on Toxicity (2008) COT statement on the reproductive effects of caffeine. September 2008. **http://cot.food.gov.uk/cotstatements/cotstate mentsyrs/cotstatements2008/cot200804** (accessed April 2012).

Frisch R (1994) The right weight: body fat, menarche and fertility. *Proceedings of the Nutrition Society* **53**: 113–129.

Hoek HW (2006) Incidence, prevalence and mortality of anorexia nervosa and other eating disorders. *Current Opinion in Psychiatry* **19**(4): 389–394.

Jensen TK, Hjollund NH, Henriksen TB, *et al.* (1998) Does moderate alcohol consumption affect fertility? Follow up study among couples planning first pregnancy. *British Medical Journal* **317**: 505–510.

Loucks AB, Stachenfeld NS and DiPietro L (2006) The female athlete triad: do female athletes need to take special care to avoid low energy availability? *Medicine and Science in Sports and Exercise* **38**: 1694–1700.

NHS Choices (2011) Alcohol and drugs during pregnancy. **www.nhs.uk/Planners/pregnan cycareplanner/pages/Alcoholanddrugs.aspx** (accessed April 2012).

NICE (National Institute for Health and Clinical Excellence) (2008a) Public Health Guidance 11. Improving the nutrition of pregnant and breastfeeding mothers and children in low-income households. March 2008. **www.nice.org.uk/ nicemedia/pdf/PH011guidance.pdf** (accessed April 2012).

NICE (2008b) Clinical Guidance 63. Diabetes in pregnancy: management of diabetes and its complications from preconception to the postnatal period. March 2008. **www.nice.org.uk/Guidance/ CG63** (accessed April 2012).

NICE (2010) Public Health Guidance 27. Weight management before, during and after pregnancy. July 2010. **www.nice.org.uk/PH27** (accessed April 2012).

Rich-Edwards JW, Goldman MB, Willet WC, *et al.* (1994) Adolescent body mass index and infertility caused by ovulatory disorder. *American Journal of Obstetrics and Gynecology* **171**: 171–177.

Tas S, Lauwerys R and Lison D (1996) Occupational hazards for the male reproductive system. *Critical Reviews in Toxicology* **26**: 261–307.

Wong WY, Zeilhuis GA, Thomas CM, Merkus HM and Steerrgers-Theuinessen RP (2003) New evidence of the influence of exogenous factors on sperm count in man. *European Journal of Obstetrics Gynecology and Reproductive Biology* **110**: 49–54.

Zaadstra BM, Seidell JC, Van Noord PA, *et al.* (1993) Fat and female fecundity: prospective study of the effect of body fat distribution on conception rates. *British Medical Journal* **306**: 484–487.

Resources

The Centre for Pregnancy Nutrition, University of Sheffield (**www.eatingforpregnancy.co.uk/**)

3.2

Pregnancy

Summary

- During pregnancy, the maternal diet must provide sufficient energy and nutrients to meet the mother's usual requirements as well as those of the growing fetus and stores for use during lactation.

- A healthy balanced diet for pregnancy is based on the five food groups with additional supplements of folic acid and vitamin D.

- Common nutrient deficiencies in UK women prior to conception and during pregnancy include iron, folate and vitamin D.

- Populations at risk of poor pregnancy outcomes due to inadequate nutritional status and/or intake during pregnancy include teenagers, women from low-income groups, vegetarian and vegan women and under- or overweight women.

- More care needs to be taken with food hygiene during pregnancy as fetal development can be adversely affected by food-borne organisms and pollutants.

Introduction

The nutritional status of a woman during pregnancy influences:

- the growth and development of her fetus and forms the foundations for her child's later health (Gluckman *et al.* 2005)

- the mother's own health, both in the short and long term (NICE 2008a).

Poor nutrition during pregnancy has been linked to an increased risk of having a baby with a low birthweight. The link between low birthweight and infant mortality remains strong and, if they survive, low-birthweight babies suffer from higher rates of childhood illness and conditions such as hearing and visual impairment, neurodevelopmental delay and behavioural disorders (Hack *et al.* 1995). Several studies of school age children who had a low birthweight have shown less well-developed language and social skills, more behavioural and attention span problems, and lower IQ, cognitive ability and academic achievement (Dahl *et al.* 2006).

Poor rates of fetal and infant growth have also been linked to higher rates of premature death among adults and higher rates of cardiovascular disease and other conditions such as diabetes and high blood pressure (Barker 2008).

Healthy Eating for Pregnancy

Pregnant women require slightly higher amounts of certain nutrients than non-pregnant women. Most nutrients can be met by eating a balanced nutritious diet based on the five food groups in the 'eatwell plate' shown in figure 1.2.1 (page 16). The nutrients that will not be met even with a balanced nutritious diet are folic acid and vitamin D. A dietary supplement of both these is recommended (Department of Health 1991, Scientific Advisory Committee on Nutrition 2007, NICE 2008a, 2008b).

Table 3.2.1 Recommended daily intake for women during pregnancy

Food groups	Recommended daily intake
Group 1: Bread, rice, potatoes and pasta and other starchy foods	Base each meal and some snacks on these foods. Use wholegrain varieties as often as possible
Group 2: Fruit and vegetables	Include 1 or more of these at each meal and aim for at least 5 portions per day
Group 3: Milk, cheese and yogurt	2–3 portions of milk, cheese, yogurt. Use low-fat varieties if weight gain needs to be limited
Group 4: Meat, fish, eggs, nuts and pulses	2–3 portions. 2 servings of fish per week are recommended, 1 of which should be oily fish
Group 5: Foods and drinks high in fat and/or sugar	Limit these to small quantities and not to be eaten in place of the other 4 food groups. For those trying to lose weight limit them to about 2 small portions per day
Fluids	About 6–8 drinks per day (1½–2 litres) will provide adequate fluid to prevent dehydration. This includes all drinks: water, tea, coffee, milk, soup, fruit juices, squashes and fizzy drinks. More drinks may be needed in hot weather and after physical activity

Recommended daily intakes for women during pregnancy are outlined in Table 3.2.1.

Key Nutrients During Pregnancy

Certain key nutrients are commonly low in women and they need extra consideration during pregnancy to ensure good pregnancy outcomes. They are:

- folate
- vitamin D
- iron
- omega 3 fatty acids
- calcium.

Folate, folic acid and neural tube defects

Research has shown a link between low folic acid/folate intakes and the development of neural tube defects (NTDs) (Medical Research Council Vitamin Study Group 1991). To reduce the risk of NTDs, supplementation with folic acid prior to conception and during the first 12 weeks of pregnancy is recommended. There are two dose levels:

- 5 mg/day (prescription only) for women with spina bifida, with a history of a previous child with an NTD or with diabetes

- 400 µg (0.4 mg)/day for all other women. These supplements are available over the counter and on prescription, but it is cheaper to buy them over the counter.

Mandatory fortification of flour with folic acid has been debated in the UK but has not been recommended despite the example of a fall in NTD rates of up to 40 per cent in the United States and Canada where flour has been fortified with folic acid for over 10 years.

Dietary folates

Folate is the form of folic acid found in food. The folate content of food decreases with long storage times and heat. Cooking may cause a considerable reduction in the folate content of food. As the current average intake from diet is about 200 µg per day, women who may become pregnant should aim to increase their dietary intake of folate, in addition to the folic acid supplement, by:

- eating more folate-rich foods
- avoiding overcooking folate-rich foods
- choosing breads and breakfast cereals fortified with folic acid.

Foods rich in folate include:

- yeast extract
- pulses – peas and beans

- oranges and orange juice
- green leafy vegetables (brussels sprouts, spinach and broccoli)
- potatoes.

Liver is a rich source of folate but is not recommended during pregnancy because it has very high levels of retinol (vitamin A).

Vitamin D

Women have a higher dietary requirement during pregnancy and NICE recommend that:

- all women should be informed at the booking appointment about the importance for their own and their baby's health of maintaining adequate vitamin D stores during pregnancy and while breastfeeding (NICE 2008b)
- all pregnant and breastfeeding women should be advised to take 10 µg vitamin D daily in a dietary supplement (NICE 2008a).

Skin synthesis alone is not always enough to achieve the optimal vitamin D status for all pregnant women; the 'National Diet and Nutrition Survey of British Adults' (Ruston *et al.* 2004) showed that about a quarter of British women aged 19–24 and a sixth of those aged 25–34 are deficient in vitamin D. This rises to 1 in 2 women with dark skins who require more exposure to sunlight to make the same amount of vitamin D in their skin (Datta *et al.* 2002).

During pregnancy, lack of vitamin D may adversely affect fetal bone mineralization and the accumulation of vitamin D stores for the early months of life.

The following groups of women are particularly at risk of low vitamin D status:

- those with black or dark skin (e.g. of Asian, African, Caribbean and Middle Eastern origin)
- those who have limited skin exposure to sunlight (e.g. those who remain covered when outside or are housebound)
- obese women – those with a body mass index (BMI) >30 kg/m^2.

Babies born to women with low vitamin D levels are at higher risk of:

- seizures (hypocalcaemic fits) and breathing problems as young infants
- rickets and growth delay as older infants and toddlers.

The incidence of these preventable diseases appears to be rising in the UK and other northern European countries (Ahmed *et al.* 2011).

In addition, children born to mothers with low vitamin D levels during pregnancy have been found to be more likely to have lower levels of bone minerals at 9 years of age than children born to mothers with normal vitamin D levels (Javaid *et al.* 2006).

Folic acid and vitamin D supplements are listed in Table 3.2.2.

Supplements for pregnant women

The availabilities and relative costs of suitable supplements for women who may become pregnant and who are pregnant are listed in Table 3.2.3.

Iron

Women with good iron status prior to conception and who eat a healthy balanced diet will not need extra iron during pregnancy because the rising demands of iron by the growing fetus are met by:

- diminished losses from the mother as menstrual bleeding is absent during pregnancy
- increased iron absorption during pregnancy – the level of absorption increases progressively as pregnancy advances. Also a greater percentage increase in absorption will occur in anaemic than in non-anaemic women.

The fetus accumulates most of its iron during the last trimester, laying down stores for about the first 6 months of life.

Routine iron supplementation is not recommended for all women (NICE 2008b) and is usually only recommended for those with a history of anaemia who are likely to have low iron stores or

Table 3.2.2 Folic acid and vitamin D supplements

Vitamin	Daily dose	Recommendation
Folic acid	400 µg	For any women and adolescent girls who may become pregnant and up to the 12th week of pregnancy. This supplement can safely be taken throughout the whole of the pregnancy and while breastfeeding
	5 mg	For women at high risk of having an NTD-affected pregnancy. GPs should prescribe for women who are planning a pregnancy, or are in the early stages of pregnancy, if they: • (or their partner) have an NTD • have had a previous baby with an NTD • (or their partner) have a family history of NTD • have diabetes • have coeliac disease • have sickle cell anaemia • are taking anti-epileptic drugs • are overweight
Vitamin D	10 µg	For all women and adolescent girls who may become pregnant, and for those who are pregnant

NTD, neural tube defect.

Table 3.2.3 Suitable supplements for pregnant women and for women who may become pregnant

Supplement	Content	Availability	Relative cost
NHS Healthy Start vitamins for women	400 µg folic acid 10 µg vitamin D3 70 mg vitamin C	From NHS outlets only and some children's centres	Relatively inexpensive
Simple vitamin D supplements	Vitamin D only – dose varies 10–25 µg	From some retail pharmacies and health food stores	Relatively inexpensive
Branded supplements for preconception and pregnancy	Folic acid, vitamin D and a wide range of other nutrients that are normally provided in adequate amounts in a healthy balanced diet	Retail pharmacies and supermarkets	Relatively expensive

who develop clinical signs of anaemia during pregnancy. Women at risk of deficiency during pregnancy are those that start their pregnancy with low iron stores, perhaps due to large menstrual losses and/or low intakes. Iron supplementation may have side-effects such as constipation or nausea.

Iron-rich foods to include are:

- meat, especially red meat, such as beef, lamb or pork
- oily fish – limit to two servings per week (see below)
- pulses (peas, beans and lentils)
- iron-fortified breakfast cereals
- green vegetables
- dried fruit (e.g. apricots, prunes, raisins).

Note: Liver is high in iron but is not recommended during pregnancy because of its high retinol content.

Women following a vegetarian diet and those who eat little meat can increase their iron absorption from cereal and vegetable sources by:

- having food or a drink containing vitamin C with a meal (e.g. orange juice with baked beans on toast)
- avoiding drinking tea at mealtimes as the tannins present in tea bind with the iron, reducing its absorption.

Omega 3 fats/long-chain polyunsaturated fats

Docosahexanoic acid (DHA) and eicosapentanoic acid (EPA) are the long-chain polyunsaturated (LCP) omega-3 fats that are vital for brain growth, visual and neurological development in the fetus and young infant. Women who do not eat fish may not get enough of these fats.

The International Society for the Study of Fatty Acids and Lipids (ISSFAL) recommends that pregnant women should consume:

- 200 mg DHA/day as is recommended for the general adult population (Koletzko *et al.* 2007)
- >500 mg/day of DHA + EPA.

This can be achieved by eating one or two portions of oily fish a week. A portion is about 100 g cooked weight. Oily fish includes salmon, trout, mackerel, sardines, pilchards, herring, kippers, eel, whitebait and fresh tuna. Canned tuna does not count as an 'oily fish' as the fat content is reduced prior to canning.

Pregnant women who do not eat oily fish may choose to take supplements of omega 3 fats to ensure an adequate intake of long-chain omega 3 fats. Supplements containing:

- 200 mg–1 g DHA/day and
- 500 mg–2.7 g in total of omega 3 LCPs (DHA + EPA)

have not caused harm in pregnant women (Koletzko *et al.* 2007).

Note: There is currently no standard preparation for the above dosage. Retail pharmacies stock fish oil supplements and women should look for a suitable preparation which provides quantities within the range above but without vitamin A.

Calcium

Despite high fetal requirements for calcium, additional calcium is not usually needed as the mother's calcium absorption increases during pregnancy. However, some women, particularly teenagers, avoid dairy products and have low calcium intakes. Care should be taken that during pregnancy adequate calcium is consumed by eating 2–3 servings daily of any of the following:

- milk – 1 glass (200 mL)
- cheese – 25 g
- yogurt – 1 pot of 120–150 g
- tofu – 50 g
- calcium-enriched soya milk – 1 glass (200 mL).

Pregnant adolescents have higher needs, however, as they will not have achieved their peak bone mass and should be encouraged to eat at least three servings of these calcium-rich foods each day.

Women who do not eat dairy products or calcium-enriched soya products should be advised to take a calcium supplement of about 700 mg calcium to ensure an adequate calcium intake.

Appropriate Weight Gain During Pregnancy

Additional energy is needed during pregnancy to support the growth of the fetus and to enable fat to be deposited in the mother's body for later use during lactation. However, considerable reductions usually occur in physical activity and metabolic rate to help to compensate for these increased needs. Pregnant women do not need to increase their energy intake and certainly should not 'eat for two'. The Department of Health recommends an extra 200 kcal per day from food for the final three months only (Department of Health 1991) (e.g. two slices of buttered bread provide 200 kcal).

There are currently no UK evidence-based recommendations on appropriate weight gain during pregnancy. However, the American Institute of Medicine (IOM) recommends (Institute of Medicine 1990) the weight gains listed in Table 3.2.4.

Women who gain weight within the IOM ranges are more likely to have better maternal and infant outcomes than those who gain more or less weight (Viswanathan *et al.* 2008). Gaining too little weight during pregnancy can result in infants being born with a low birthweight, which is associated with

Table 3.2.4 Appropriate weight gains during pregnancy

Pre-pregnancy weight	Pre-pregnancy BMI	Appropriate weight gain during pregnancy (kg)
Normal weight	19.8–25.9	11.5–16
Overweight	>30	7
Underweight	<19.8	12.5–18

Adapted from the Institute of Medicine (1990).

health problems for the child. Excess weight gain during pregnancy can increase the risk of gestational diabetes, pre-eclampsia and difficulties during delivery. It is also associated with postpartum weight retention in the short, intermediate and long term (Viswanathan *et al.* 2008).

Overweight and obese women

Around 15–20 per cent of pregnant women in the UK are obese. Maternal obesity is related to health inequalities, particularly socio-economic deprivation, inequalities within ethnic groups and poor access to maternity services (Heslehurst *et al.* 2007a).

NICE (2008a) recommends that obese women are referred to a registered dietitian for assessment and advice and that overweight and obese pregnant women should be advised:

- not to lose weight during pregnancy as this may compromise their nutrient intake and that of the fetus (NICE 2008a)
- to limit the amount of weight gained in pregnancy as those gaining no more than 7 kg during pregnancy have fewer complications (Cedergren 2006)
- to take regular physical activity to help limit their weight gain, as studies have shown that exercise in pregnancy is safe (Artal 2008). Obese pregnant women who are physically active during pregnancy reduce their risk of gestational diabetes by 50 per cent (Dye *et al.* 1997).

Underweight women

Women with a low BMI at the start of pregnancy need to increase their food intake to provide more energy and nutrients for both themselves and their fetus.

Women at Increased Nutritional Risk During Pregnancy

Women with pre-existing medical conditions

Women with pre-existing medical conditions, such as diabetes mellitus, food allergies and malabsorption syndromes, should be referred to a dietitian prior to pregnancy and have their nutritional status monitored closely throughout the pregnancy.

Diabetes

Women with diabetes account for 2–5 per cent of pregnancies in England and Wales. About 90 per cent of these are due to gestational diabetes, while the remainder have become pregnant with pre-existing diabetes. Both forms of diabetes in pregnancy are associated with health risks to both the woman and the developing fetus.

The following conditions are more common during pregnancy in women with pre-existing diabetes (NICE 2008c):

- miscarriage
- pre-eclampsia
- deteriorating diabetic retinopathy
- preterm labour
- stillbirth
- congenital malformations
- macrosomia (abnormally large body size)
- birth injury

- perinatal mortality
- postnatal adaptation problems such as hypoglycaemia.

A recent study suggests that hyperglycaemia during pregnancy is associated with an increased risk of childhood obesity at 7 years of age (Hillier *et al.* 2007).

Gestational diabetes

The risk factors for gestational diabetes are:

- BMI >30
- previous macrosomic baby (4.5 kg or above)
- previous gestational diabetes
- family history of diabetes (first-degree relative with diabetes)
- family origin with a high prevalence of diabetes, such as South Asian (specifically women whose country of family origin is India, Pakistan or Bangladesh), black Caribbean or Middle Eastern (specifically women whose country of family origin is Saudi Arabia, United Arab Emirates, Iraq, Jordan, Syria, Oman, Qatar, Kuwait, Lebanon or Egypt).

Women with any one of these risk factors should be offered testing for gestational diabetes (NICE 2008b).

In most women, gestational diabetes will respond to changes in diet and physical activity. NICE (2008c) recommend that women with gestational diabetes:

- should receive dietary advice including choosing low glycaemic index carbohydrates
- take moderate exercise of at least 30 minutes daily
- are advised to restrict calorie intake (to 25 kcal/kg/day or less) if their pre-pregnancy BMI is above 27 (a registered dietitian can give this advice)
- should aim to keep fasting blood glucose between 3.5 and 5.9 mmol/L and one-hour postprandial blood glucose below 7.8 mmol/L. Oral hypoglycaemic agents or insulin may be

required. Maintaining these levels throughout pregnancy will reduce the risk of miscarriage, congenital malformation, stillbirth and neonatal death. It is important to explain that risks can be reduced but not eliminated (NICE 2008c).

Adolescents

The UK has one of the highest rates of teenage pregnancy in Europe. Studies have shown that teenage pregnancy is associated with:

- lower gestational weight gain
- an increased risk of low birthweight
- pregnancy-induced hypertension (PIH)
- preterm labour
- iron-deficiency anaemia
- maternal mortality.

Nutritional status at conception is more likely to be suboptimal as the diets of teenagers in the UK are poor. National Diet and Nutritional Surveys have shown that a large percentage of teenage girls have inadequate intakes of vitamin A, riboflavin, folate, calcium, iron and zinc. Blood tests showed low blood levels of iron, folate and vitamin D (Gregory *et al.* 2000, Nelson *et al.* 2007).

Factors influencing poor dietary intakes in teenage girls include:

- making own independent food choices
- finalizing their autonomy and rejecting family meals and family food values
- high intake of high-calorie, low-nutrient foods such as sweet drinks and junk foods
- dieting to manage weight – 16 per cent of 15–18 year old girls (Gregory *et al.* 2000)
- following vegetarian diets without substituting alternative sources of iron when meat is eliminated
- low intake of milk and milk products.

Adolescent girls may have increased nutritional requirements because they need to complete their own growth as well as providing for the fetus

(Stevens-Simon and McAnarney 1988). The shorter the length of time between the onset of menarche and pregnancy, the greater the nutritional risk. In particular, teenagers will not have achieved their peak bone mass and should be encouraged to eat at least three servings of calcium-rich foods each day, such as milk, cheese, yogurt and calcium-enriched soya milk.

Around 75 per cent of adolescent pregnancies are unplanned and teenagers are therefore unlikely to be taking folic acid and vitamin D supplements prior to conception or in early pregnancy.

Pregnant teenage girls under the age of 18 years are eligible to join the Healthy Start scheme regardless of their financial circumstances (www. healthystart.nhs.uk). If they join they are entitled to receive free vitamin supplements of folic acid and vitamin D along with vouchers to purchase milk, fruit and vegetables.

Vegetarian and vegan women

Many vegetarian and vegan women have significantly better diets than those of non-vegetarian women, but those particularly at risk are:

- those, often adolescents, who have decided to avoid meat and other animal foods without taking care to ensure alternative sources of nutrients found in meat
- recent immigrants who may not be able to access the foods they would have eaten in their country of origin.

A study of pregnant vegetarian women of Asian background living in the UK in the 1990s found (Reddy *et al.* 1994):

- shorter duration of pregnancy
- more emergency caesarean sections
- lower birthweight
- shorter body length
- smaller head circumference.

Before and during pregnancy, more care needs to be taken to ensure adequate intakes of iron, omega 3 fats, riboflavin, calcium and vitamin B12.

Vegetarian women who avoid red meat need to eat three servings of foods from food group 4 in the 'eatwell plate' (see page 64) to make sure they are eating enough iron. Vegetarian women eating two servings of fish per week and three servings daily of milk, cheese and yogurt will have adequate calcium, vitamin B12 and omega 3 intakes.

Pregnant women who follow a vegan diet normally avoid all sources of animal foods, including milk and milk products, eggs, meat and fish. They should take care to ensure that they consume sufficient:

- iron from good sources such as nuts, pulses and fortified breakfast cereals
- vitamin B12 from good sources such as fortified yeast extracts, fortified soya milk, fortified textured soya protein and fortified cereals (if these are not included in the diet a vitamin B12 supplement may be needed)
- omega 3 – by including walnuts and walnut or rapeseed oil on a daily basis or taking an omega 3 supplement (see page 67)
- calcium from fortified soya milk each day or taking a calcium supplement.

Women who have previously had a low-birthweight baby

It is important to ascertain whether or not the cause of the reduced birthweight in a previous pregnancy had a nutritional component such as poor gestational weight gain and/or a reduced food intake. Short birth intervals predispose to lower birthweights because women may not have had time to replenish their nutrient stores between pregnancies, particularly if they have breastfed their babies (Allen 2005).

Women who are homeless, living in bed and breakfast accommodation or on low incomes

These women may have the combined difficulty of living on state benefits and living with limited cooking facilities. A survey (National Children's Home and Maternity Alliance 1995) demonstrated that there is great difficulty in providing an adequate diet for pregnancy while living entirely on state benefits.

Nutritional risk factors more common in low-income pregnant women are:

- maternal obesity and weight retention after birth (Heslehurst *et al.* 2007b)
- low iron stores
- not taking folic acid or vitamin D supplements prior to pregnancy and during the early stages of pregnancy
- low birthweight <2.5 kg and consequently an increased risk of neonatal morbidity and mortality
- poor diet associated with use of drugs or excess alcohol.

Recent immigrants

Recent immigrants to the UK may not be able to access the foods they would have eaten in their country of origin and may not eat a sufficiently nutritious diet here. They may have poor nutritional status if they have been subjected to famine and/or parasitic infections.

Women with alcohol or drug problems or eating disorders

Women who have alcohol or drug problems are less likely to eat a balanced diet.

Women who give up smoking should take care not to snack on high-calorie foods in place of smoking, as this would put them at risk of gaining excess weight.

Women who are restricting their food intake for reasons such as slimming or self-diagnosed food allergies may cut out whole food groups without advice from a registered dietitian and may be omitting important nutrient sources (NICE 2008a).

Pregnant women with past or current eating disorders such as anorexia nervosa or bulimia nervosa should be viewed as being at high risk and

monitored closely both during and after pregnancy to optimize maternal and fetal outcomes. They are likely to have low body stores of some nutrients and more likely to deliver infants with lower birthweight, smaller head circumference, microcephaly and small for gestational age (Koubaa *et al.* 2005).

Food, Drinks and Supplements to Avoid or Limit

Vitamin A

There are two dietary forms of vitamin A:

- retinol from animal sources
- beta carotene from plant sources – particularly brightly coloured vegetables and fruit.

Both forms are found in a healthy balanced diet and are important during pregnancy. However, high doses of retinol are associated with teratogenesis (malformations in the fetus) (Department of Health 1990).

To avoid high doses of retinol, pregnant women should eat a balanced diet but avoid:

- vitamin supplements containing retinol
- cod liver oil supplements and other fish oil supplements containing vitamin A
- liver and liver products such as liver pâté as liver contains very high amounts of retinol.

Oily fish

Oily fish should be eaten once or twice per week because it is a good source of omega 3 fats for both fetus and mother. It is limited to two servings per week because some of these fish contain dioxins and PCBs (polychlorinated biphenyls) that might affect the nervous systems of the fetus.

Tuna should also be limited to four medium sized cans of tuna a week (with a drained weight of about 140 g per can) or fresh tuna steaks (weighing about 140 g when cooked or 170 g raw).

Swordfish, marlin and shark should be avoided due to the possibility of high mercury levels.

Alcohol

Alcohol intoxication should be avoided at any stage of pregnancy and especially in the early weeks where it is associated with teratogenesis and may cause miscarriage.

The advice around limiting or avoiding alcohol intake during pregnancy varies and although there is no overall consensus opinion there is evidence that:

- the alcohol in the mother's bloodstream crosses the placenta into the bloodstream of the fetus
- drinking heavily throughout pregnancy (more than ten units per day) is linked with an increased risk of fetal alcohol syndrome
- fetal alcohol syndrome is characterized by reduced birthweight and length, a small head size with characteristic facial appearance and a variety of congenital abnormalities
- the safest approach in pregnancy is to choose not to drink at all
- small amounts of alcohol during pregnancy (not more than one or two units, not more than once or twice a week) have not been shown to be harmful
- regular binge drinking (five or more units of alcohol on one occasion) around conception and in early pregnancy is particularly harmful to a woman and her baby
- alcohol has a detrimental effect on the absorption and utilization of folate, thus compounding the problem in women who do not take folic acid supplements.

NICE recommends that pregnant women avoid alcohol but women who do choose to drink should consume no more than one or two units of alcohol, once or twice a week (NICE 2008b).

Alcohol units are defined in Table 3.2.5.

Caffeine

A limit of 200 mg/day of caffeine intake is currently recommended for pregnant women because high levels of caffeine are suspected of causing miscarriage or low birthweights (Food Standards Agency 2010).

Table 3.2.5 Alcohol units

Units of alcohol	Alcoholic drinks
1	Half a pint of ordinary strength beer, lager or cider (3.5% alcohol by volume (ABV)) A 125 mL glass of wine (9% ABV) A 25 mL measure of spirits (40% ABV)
1.5	A 125 mL glass of wine at 11% or 12% ABV 1 bottle of 'alcopop'
2	A 175 mL glass of wine at 11% or 12% ABV

The caffeine content of drinks and chocolate is as follows:

1 shot of espresso coffee	140 mg
1 mug of filter coffee	140 mg
1 mug of instant coffee	100 mg
1 cup of brewed coffee	100 mg
1 mug of tea	75 mg
1 cup of tea	50 mg
1 can of cola	**up to 40 mg**
1 can of 'energy' drink	up to 80 mg
1 bar of plain chocolate	up to 50 mg
1 bar of milk chocolate	up to 25 mg

Certain cold and flu remedies also contain caffeine.

Food Safety

General food hygiene should be followed carefully but extra care should be taken:

- when buying unwrapped foods (e.g. cooked meats and prepared salads) – if scrupulous food handling guidelines have not been followed, these foods can easily become contaminated
- with cook–chill foods – these are ready cooked foods sold chilled and should not be eaten cold, but cooked until piping hot right through. They should be heated once only and the leftovers discarded.

Table 3.2.6 Food-borne illnesses

Food-borne illness	Foods/materials to avoid	Precautions to take
Listeriosis – a flu-like illness caused by the bacteria *Listeria monocytogenes*	Pâté – meat, fish or vegetable unless tinned or pasteurized Mould-ripened soft cheeses (e.g. Brie, Camembert, blue-veined cheeses) Unpasteurized milk and milk products Ready meals especially those containing chicken that are not reheated before consumption	Avoid pâté, soft cheeses and unpasteurized milk products Reheat ready meals to piping hot right through
Salmonella – a bacteria which is the major cause of food poisoning in the UK	Raw or partially cooked eggs and foods containing them such as mayonnaise and mousse Undercooked poultry and other meat	Poultry should be thoroughly defrosted in the fridge and cooked until piping hot right through Eggs should be cooked so both white and egg are solid
Toxoplasmosis – a disease caused by the parasite *Toxoplasma gondii* found in raw meat, soil and cat faeces	Raw or undercooked meat Unpasteurized milk and milk products Soil Cat litter trays	Wash vegetables and salad thoroughly to remove any soil or dirt Wash hands after handling raw meat Thoroughly cook meat
Campylobacter – a bacteria that commonly causes food poisoning in the UK	Undercooked poultry Unpasteurized milk and milk products Untreated water Domestic pets Soil	Wear rubber gloves when emptying cat litter trays Wash hands after handling cats Wear gloves while gardening Do not help with lambing or milking ewes that have recently given birth

Certain food-borne illnesses can cause miscarriage, stillbirth, abnormalities in the developing fetus or severe illness in the newborn (Table 3.2.6).

Raw shellfish (e.g. prawns, cockles and mussels) can cause food poisoning and should only be eaten if they are bought packaged and stamped with a 'use-by' date.

Foods that are safe to eat during pregnancy include:

- cooked shellfish, including prawns that are part of a hot meal and have been cooked thoroughly
- live or bio yogurt
- probiotic drinks
- fromage frais
- crème fraîche
- soured cream
- spicy food
- mayonnaise, ice cream and salad dressing made with pasteurized egg (home-made versions may contain raw eggs and must be avoided)
- honey may be eaten during pregnancy, but is not suitable for infants until over 12 months of age
- many cheeses including hard cheese, such as cheddar and parmesan, feta, ricotta, mascarpone, cream cheese, mozzarella, cottage cheese, processed cheese, such as cheese spreads.

Allergy Prevention Advice

Avoiding foods during pregnancy will not reduce the risk of the fetus developing a food allergy following birth or later in life. As a consequence, the Department of Health changed their advice on peanuts in 2009 to: 'there is insufficient evidence to advise any pregnant women to avoid eating peanuts and peanut products during pregnancy and breastfeeding'.

Common Dietary Problems During Pregnancy

Nausea and vomiting

Nausea in pregnancy is reported in 50–80 per cent of pregnant women; 52 per cent of pregnant women experience symptoms of both nausea and vomiting during early pregnancy, and 28 per cent experience nausea only.

Symptoms commonly start 4–7 weeks after the last menstrual period and cease by 12 weeks in 60 per cent of affected women. About 9 per cent of affected women have symptoms that persist beyond 16 weeks and may persist until 22 weeks of gestation. Symptoms often come and go and can occur at any time during the day. Typical symptoms include nausea, vomiting, fatigue, loss of appetite and weight loss (usually around 5 per cent of pre-pregnancy body weight).

Hyperemesis gravidarum is the most severe form of persistent nausea and vomiting, leading to dehydration, ketonuria, electrolyte imbalance and weight loss greater than 5 per cent of pre-pregnancy weight. It affects between 0.3 per cent and 2 per cent of all pregnant women and they need extra medical care.

The cause of nausea is thought to be the changing pregnancy hormone levels and it can occur at any time of day or night – not just in the mornings. It is often triggered by certain foods, like coffee and fried or spicy foods, or smells, such as perfume, cigarette smoke or petrol. It can also be caused by hunger.

Advice to be given that may help includes:

- eating small, frequent meals based on starchy foods, once every two hours or so throughout the day, including foods such as bread, toast, plain biscuits or ginger biscuits, banana and breakfast cereals
- eating plain or ginger biscuits about 20 minutes before getting out of bed in the morning
- eating cold meals rather than hot meals, which may prevent any smell-related nausea, as cold food does not seem to give off as much smell as hot food
- taking glucose tablets to possibly help prevent blood sugar levels from dropping (low blood sugar levels may cause nausea)
- avoiding any foods or smells that trigger symptoms
- avoiding drinking cold, tart or sweet beverages
- avoiding caffeine and alcohol
- having lots to drink to avoid dehydration but drinking little and often rather than large amounts to prevent vomiting.

Cravings and taste changes

Changes in taste, cravings and appetite may also be related to hormonal changes or due to the removal of energy substrates from maternal blood by the fetus. Unless they alter the balance of a healthy diet they do not present a problem. Pica is a term given to the craving of non-food substances, such as soap, chalk and coal.

Heartburn/oesophageal reflux

This is generally more common in multiple pregnancies and during the last three months of single pregnancies when pressure from the baby in the uterus can cause acid to be pushed back up from the stomach. The following changes may help:

- smaller, more frequent meals
- sitting up straight when eating to relieve the pressure
- not lying down flat after eating
- sleeping propped up by extra pillows if it occurs at night
- avoiding any foods that cause discomfort.

Constipation

This is common at all stages of pregnancy and can be relieved by increasing the amount of high-fibre foods, such as fruit, vegetables, pulses and wholegrain cereals. An increase in fluid intake to 6–8 drinks per day or about 2 litres of all drinks may help. Iron supplements tend to exacerbate constipation.

Promoting Breastfeeding Antenatally

NICE recommends that:

Pregnant women should be offered opportunities to attend participant-led antenatal classes, including breastfeeding workshops. Before or at 36 weeks gestation they should receive breastfeeding information, including technique and good management practices, such as detailed in the UNICEF 'Baby Friendly Initiative' (www. babyfriendly.org.uk). (NICE 2008b)

Activity 1

Develop a plan for a session with pregnant teenage girls. Include five key recommendations.

Activity 2

Write a one-day menu including the appropriate number of servings from each food group to provide a balanced, nutritious diet and appropriate supplements for a women eating entirely from commercially prepared foods.

Activity 3

What are the messages to communicate to avoid food-borne risks?

Acknowledgements

Thanks are due to Fiona Ford, Centre for Pregnancy Nutrition, University of Sheffield.

References

Ahmed SF, Franey C, McDevitt H, *et al.* (2011) Recent trends and clinical features of childhood vitamin D deficiency presenting to a children's hospital in Glasgow. *Archives of Disease in Childhood* **96**: 694–696.

Allen LH (2005) Multiple micronutrients in pregnancy and lactation: an overview. *American Journal of Clinical Nutrition* **81**(5): 1206S–1212S.

Artal R (2008) Weight gain recommendations in pregnancy. *Expert Review of Obstetrics and Gynecology* **3**(2): 143–145.

Barker DJ (2008) Human growth and cardiovascular disease. *Nestlé Nutrition Workshop Services Pediatric Program* **61**: 21–38.

Cedergren M (2006) Effects of gestational weight gain and body mass index on obstetric outcome in Sweden. *International Journal of Gynecology and Obstetrics* **93**(3): 269–274.

Dahl LB, Kaaresen PI, Tunby J, Handegård BH, Kvernmo S and Rønning JA (2006) Emotional, behavioral, social, and academic outcomes in adolescents born with very low birth weight. *Pediatrics* **118**: e449–e459.

Datta S, Alfaham M, Davies DP, *et al.* (2002) Vitamin D deficiency in pregnant women from a non-European ethnic minority population – an interventional study. *British Journal of Obstetrics and Gynaecology* **109**: 905–908.

Department of Health (1990) Women cautioned: watch your vitamin A intake. Department of Health Press Release No 90/507, Department of Health, London.

Department of Health (1991) *Report No 41. Dietary Reference Values for Food Energy and Nutrients for the UK. Report of the Panel on Dietary Reference Values of the Committee on Medical Aspects of Food Policy.* London: HMSO.

Department of Health (1992) *Folic Acid and the Prevention of Neural Tube Defects. Report of an Expert Advisory Group for the Department of Health.* London: HMSO.

Dye TD, Knox KL, Artal R, Aubry RH and Wojtowycz MA (1997) Physical activity, obesity, and diabetes in pregnancy. *American Journal of Epidemiology* **146**(11): 961–965.

Food Standards Agency (2010) High caffeine energy drinks. **www.food.gov.uk/safercating/chemsafe/ energydrinks** (accessed April 2012).

Gluckman PD, Hanson MA and Pinal C (2005) The developmental origins of adult disease. *Maternal and Child Nutrition* **1**: 130–141.

Gregory J, Lowe S, Bates CJ, *et al.* (2000) *National Diet and Nutrition Survey: Young people aged 4–18 years.* London: The Stationery Office.

Hack M, Klein NK and Taylor HG (1995) Long-term developmental outcomes of low birth weight infants. *Future Child* **5**: 176–196.

Henderson L and Hoare J (2004) *National Diet and Nutrition Survey: Adults aged 19–64 years.* London: HMSO.

Heslehurst N, Ellis LJ, Simpson H, Batterham A, Wilkinson JR and Summerbell CD (2007a) Trends in maternal obesity incidence rate, demographic predictors, and health inequalities in 36,821 women over a 15-year period. *British Journal of Obstetrics and Gynaecology* **114**(2): 187–194.

Heslehurst N, Lang R, Rankin J, Wilkinson JR and Summerbell CD (2007b) Obesity in pregnancy: a study of the impact of maternal obesity on NHS maternity services. *British Journal of Obstetrics and Gynaecology* **114**(3): 334–342.

Hillier TA, Pedula KL, Schmidt MM, Mullen JA, Charles MA and Pettitt DT (2007) Childhood obesity and metabolic imprinting: the ongoing effects of maternal hyperglycaemia. *Diabetes Care* **30**(9): 2287–2292.

Institute of Medicine (1990) *Nutrition During Pregnancy: Part I: Weight Gain*. Washington DC: Institute of Medicine.

Javaid MK, Crozier S, Harvey N, *et al.* (2006) Maternal vitamin D status during pregnancy and childhood bone mass at age 9 years: a longitudinal study. *Lancet* **367**: 36–43.

Koletzko B, Cetin I and Brenna JT (2007) Dietary fat intakes for pregnant and lactating women. *British Journal of Nutrition* **98**: 873–877.

Koubaa S, Hällström T, Lindholm C and Hirschberg AL (2005) Pregnancy and neonatal outcomes in women with eating disorders. *Obstetrics and Gynecology* **105**(2): 255–260.

Medical Research Council Vitamin Study Group (1991) Prevention of neural tube defects: results research council vitamin study. *Lancet* **238**: 131–177.

National Children's Homes and Maternity Alliance (1995) *Poor Expectations Poverty and Under Nourishment in Pregnancy*. National Children's Homes Action for Children.

Nelson M, Erens R, Bates B, Church S and Boshier T (2007) *Low Income Diet and Nutrition Survey: Volume 2 Food consumption and nutrient intakes*. London: The Stationery Office.

NICE (National Institute for Health and Clinical Excellence) (2008a) Public Health Guidance 11. Improving the nutrition of pregnant and breastfeeding mothers and children in low-income households. March 2008. **www.nice.org.uk/nicemedia/pdf/PH011guidance.pdf** (accessed April 2012).

NICE (2008b) Clinical Guidance 62. Antenatal care: routine care for the healthy pregnant woman. March 2008. **www.nice.org.uk/Guidance/CG62** (accessed April 2012).

NICE (2008c) Clinical Guidance 63. Diabetes in pregnancy: management of diabetes and its complications from pre-conception to the postnatal period. March 2008. **www.nice.org.uk/Guidance/CG63** (accessed April 2012).

NICE (2010) Public Health Guidance 27. Weight management before, during and after pregnancy. July 2010. **www.nice.org.uk/PH27** (accessed April 2012).

Reddy S, Sanders TAB and Obeid O (1994) The influence of the maternal vegetarian diet on the essential fatty acid status of the newborn. *European Journal of Clinical Nutrition* **48**: 358–368.

Ruston D, Hoare J, Henderson L, *et al.* (2004) *National Diet and Nutrition Survey: Adults aged 19 to 64 years: nutritional status (anthropometry and blood analytes), blood pressure and physical activity*. London: The Stationery Office.

Scientific Advisory Committee on Nutrition (2007) *Position Statement by the Scientific Advisory Committee on Nutrition: Update on vitamin D*. London: Scientific Advisory Committee on Nutrition.

Shaw NJ and Pal BR (2002) Vitamin D deficiency in UK Asian families: activating a new concern. *Archives of Disease in Childhood* **86**: 147–149.

Stevens-Simons C and McAnarney E (1988) Adolescent weight gain and low birth weight: a multifactorial model. *American Journal of Clinical Nutrition* **47**: 948–953.

Tsoi E, Shaikh H, Robinson S, *et al.* (2010) Obesity in pregnancy: a major health issue. *Postgraduate Medical Journal* **86**(1020): 617–623.

Viswanathan M, Siega-Riz AM, Moos MK, *et al.* (2008) *Outcomes of Maternal Weight Gain: Evidence report/technology assessment 168*. Rockville, MD: Agency for Healthcare Research and Quality.

Resources

British Dietetic Association Pregnancy Food Factsheet (**www.bda.uk.com/foodfacts/Pregnancy.pdf**)

Centre for Maternal and Child Enquiries (**www.cmace.org.uk**)

Centre for Pregnancy Nutrition, University of Sheffield (**www.eatingforpregnancy.co.uk**)

Department of Health – *The Pregnancy Book* (**www.dh.gov.uk/en/Publicationsandstatistics/Publications/PublicationsPolicyAndGuidance/DH_107302**)

Folic acid DH leaflet 34627 (**www.dh.gov.uk/en/Publicationsandstatistics/Publications/PublicationsPolicyAndGuidance/DH_4081396**)

Healthy Start (**www.healthystart.nhs.uk**)

International Society for the Study of Fatty Acids and Lipids (**www.issfal.org/statements/pufa-recommendations/statement-4**)

Midwives Information and Resource Service (MIDIRS) information leaflets (**www.infochoice.org**)

Tommy's – Pregnant Teenagers and Diet – A guide for healthcare professionals (mini-guide) (**www.tommys.org**)

Section 4
Infants: 0–12 Months

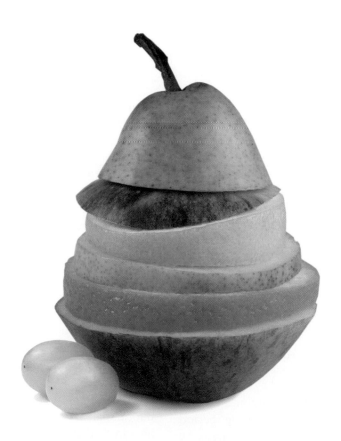

4.1

Milk Feeding

Summary

- Breast milk is the optimal milk feed for infants because it is nutritionally adequate and reduces the risk of illness in infants.

- Breastfeeding mothers may need support to overcome any problems and help them to continue to breastfeed for as long as possible.

- Infant formula is the only alternative to breast milk for the first 6 months. It is nutritionally adequate but does not provide the same protection against illness. It also carries a risk of contamination.

- There are minor differences between brands and types of infant formulas.

- All bottles, teats, pumps and containers must be washed and sterilized before being used for breast milk or infant formula until the infant is 12 months old.

Nutritional Requirements of Infants 0–6 Months

The nutritional requirements of term infants from birth to about 6 months (see Chapter 1.2) can be satisfied by exclusive breastfeeding or infant formula if the mother was well nourished during pregnancy. If a mother did not take a vitamin D supplement during pregnancy then the infant should begin a supplement of vitamin D soon after birth.

Choice of Milk Feeding

Exclusive breastfeeding is the optimal way to feed infants until weaning onto solid food begins at about 6 months of age. It provides:

- the complete nutritional requirements
- protection against illness.

Ideally, the main milk drink should continue to be breast milk throughout the weaning period (Agostoni *et al.* 2008) and beyond for as long as the mother wishes to continue.

Exclusive breastfeeding from birth is possible except for a few medical conditions, and unrestricted exclusive breastfeeding results in ample milk production. (WHO 2003)

Infant formula is the only nutritionally adequate alternative to breast milk during the first 6 months for term infants. Even though it does not provide immunity to protect infants from illness, it has become the more socially acceptable way to feed infants, and by 6 weeks more than half of UK infants are being fed formula milk, resulting in higher hospital admission rates of infants (Bolling *et al.* 2007). It has been estimated that if all UK infants were exclusively breastfed, the number hospitalized each month with diarrhoea would be halved, and the number hospitalized with a respiratory infection would be cut by a quarter (Quigley *et al.* 2007).

When parents have access to reliable advice and information, they can make an informed choice on how to feed their infants. Maternity units that follow the 'Ten Steps to Successful Breastfeeding' developed by UNICEF and the World Health Organization (www.babyfriendly.org.uk/), have higher numbers of mothers breastfeeding on discharge from the unit. The ten steps are:

1. Have a written breastfeeding policy that is routinely communicated to all healthcare staff.

2. Train all healthcare staff in the skills necessary to implement the breastfeeding policy.

3. Inform all pregnant women about the benefits and management of breastfeeding.

4. Help mothers initiate breastfeeding soon after birth.

5. Show mothers how to breastfeed and how to maintain lactation even if they are separated from their babies.

6. Give newborn infants no food or drink other than breast milk, unless medically indicated.

7. Practice rooming-in, allowing mothers and infants to remain together 24 hours a day.

8. Encourage breastfeeding on demand.

9. Give no artificial teats or dummies to breastfeeding infants.

10. Identify sources of national and local support for breastfeeding and ensure that mothers know how to access these prior to discharge from hospital.

Once her decision on how to feed her infant is made, a mother needs to be supported and advised on safe feeding. Breastfeeding mothers often need support to overcome any difficulties and problems that arise, as without appropriate support many give up breastfeeding before they wish to (Bolling *et al.* 2007). Mothers choosing to formula feed need to be shown how to sterilize feeding equipment and make up formula feeds safely.

Milk feeding choices for mothers with HIV

In the UK, women known to be HIV antibody positive, should be advised not to breastfeed but to use infant formula for feeding their baby as the HIV virus can be passed to the infant via breast milk. Mixed feeding – offering both breast milk and infant formula – carries the highest risk of HIV transmission to the infant. Where HIV-positive mothers do not have facilities to make up infant formula safely they are advised to breastfeed exclusively to reduce the risk of death through gastroenteritis from bacterial contamination of infant formula not made up hygienically.

Breastfeeding

Breastfeeding is the natural way of providing nutritional, emotional and social care for the infant. There are also environmental benefits in that no transport or manufacturing costs are involved.

Benefits of breast milk for the infants and their mothers

The health of both mother and child benefit, in the short and long term, and the longer the duration of breastfeeding, the greater the health benefits to both. Exclusive breastfeeding until weaning and then continued breastfeeding while weaning provides maximum health benefits to infants.

Advantages to the infant

The advantages to the infant can be listed as (Quigley *et al.* 2007, 2009; Ip *et al.* 2007; Horta *et al.* 2007):

● optimal growth and development

● reduced incidence of gastrointestinal, urinary tract and respiratory infections

● reduced risk of otitis media until the age of 5–7 years

● reduced incidence of both insulin- and non-insulin-dependent diabetes

● growth factors, which enhance the infant's gut development and maturation

● reduced risk of constipation

● reduced incidence of some childhood cancers (leukaemia and lymphomas, e.g. Hodgkin's disease)

- less likely to succumb to sudden infant death syndrome (SIDS)
- less likely to visit the doctor in the first 2 years of life.

Evidence is controversial around whether breastfeeding reduces:

- risk of obesity (Li *et al.* 2003, Michels *et al.* 2007)
- severity of the allergic conditions asthma and eczema.

Benefits for the mother

Benefits for the mother (Ip *et al.* 2007) include:

- delayed return to menstruation, allowing maternal iron stores to replenish following pregnancy and childbirth
- reduced risk of breast and ovarian cancer (World Cancer Research Fund 2007)
- helps the return to their pre-pregnant weight
- lower risk of postnatal depression.

In addition, women over the age of 65 who have breastfed show a lower incidence of osteoporosis and hip fractures.

Stages of Breast Milk

The composition of breast milk changes at different stages of infant development. The identifiable stages are colostrum, transitional milk and mature milk.

Colostrum

During pregnancy the glandular tissue of the breast proliferates and can produce colostrum from mid-pregnancy. It is ready in the breasts when the baby is born and has the following properties:

- a high-density, low-volume milk, which is ideal for the newborn infant
- less fat, lactose and water-soluble vitamins than mature milk, but more protein, zinc and fat-soluble vitamins A and K

- a laxative effect to aid the passage of an infant's first stool (meconium)
- rich in antibodies and immunoglobulins which provide protection against bacteria and viruses.

Over the first 2 days, infants may be quite sleepy and feed infrequently. Very small volumes of colostrum (10–13 mL/kg per day) are taken and are adequate (Dollberg *et al.* 2001). A net body weight loss occurs, which is mainly fluid as infant's blood volume decreases by about 25 per cent at this time. A weight loss of up to 10 per cent of birthweight is considered normal.

However, blood glucose testing at 2–4 hours after birth should be carried out routinely in infants of women with diabetes. They should also feed as soon as possible after birth (within 30 minutes) and then at frequent intervals (every 2–3 hours) until feeding maintains pre-feed blood glucose levels at a minimum of 2.0 mmol/L (NICE 2008a).

Transitional milk

Transitional milk is colostrum diluted with mature milk and is produced from around the third day after delivery. It has a higher water content, making it a less concentrated feed than colostrum and infants begin to demand increased volumes of this milk. Transitional milk gradually changes into mature milk by about the 14th day as colostrum production gradually diminishes.

Mothers may experience breast discomfort on day 2 or 3 as the blood and lymph flow increases in the breast in preparation for the higher volumes of transitional milk (Jones and Spencer 2007). Breasts may feel full and heavy. At the same time the infant will begin to demand feeds more frequently. Company and support from another adult will be beneficial as a mother may need to feed very frequently throughout that 24 hours. Mothers can be reassured that although they may have an uncomfortable 24 hours, over that time the volume of milk produced will eventually equal the amount that their infant is demanding and their breasts will subsequently become more comfortable again.

Over the subsequent few days infants begin to take larger volumes at each feed and settle into a routine of feeding less frequently. Some feed about every 3–4 hours, however, other babies prefer more frequent feeds until they are older.

More skin-to-skin contact between a mother and her infant is recommended for newborn infants who do not feed well.

Mature milk

Mature milk production is controlled by hormones and feedback mechanisms. Removal of milk from the breast is essential for continued production.

Throughout each feed the composition of the milk changes:

- At the beginning of the feed the milk has a high water content and low fat content satisfying the infant's thirst. It is often called foremilk.

- As the feed progresses the fat content increases, increasing the calorie content of the milk and satisfying the infant's hunger. This high-fat milk produced at the end of the feed is often called hindmilk.

Allowing infants to finish feeding from one breast before being offered the other breast ensures that both foremilk and hindmilk are taken, providing the correct balance of energy and nutrients.

No other food or fluids need to be offered, unless medically indicated, until weaning onto solid foods. Even in hot weather additional water is unnecessary as breastfeeding on demand will satisfy the infant's fluid requirements. Shorter, more frequent feeds may be demanded to satisfy any increased thirst.

Mature milk will provide all the nutrients an infant needs until weaning except for vitamin D in infants whose mothers were vitamin D deficient during pregnancy.

Vitamin D Supplementation Recommendations

The main source of vitamin D is skin synthesis, not food, but the immigration patterns and lifestyles today do not necessarily ensure adequate vitamin D from skin synthesis for all women and infants.

Most term infants are born with adequate vitamin D stores for the first 6 months of life. However, those infants whose mothers were vitamin D deficient during pregnancy are born with inadequate stores and are at risk of tetanic fits or rickets due to vitamin D deficiency.

Groups of women at high risk of vitamin D deficiency are listed on page 65.

The Department of Health (1994) recommends that:

- all breastfeeding mothers should take vitamin D supplements during breastfeeding

- breastfed infants whose mothers did not take vitamin D supplements during pregnancy should be given vitamin D supplements from about 1 month of age

- all other breastfed infants should begin vitamin D supplements from 6 months.

Supporting Mothers to Start and Continue Breastfeeding

When infants are delivered onto the mother's bare skin the period of skin-to-skin contact triggers the onset of lactation, stimulates instinctive feeding behaviour and facilitates bonding. Infants should be offered a breastfeed soon after birth – ideally within the first hour (Jones and Spencer 2007).

Breastfeeding is a skill that mothers and their babies learn together. Reassurance and consistent advice on correct positioning and attachment for breastfeeding will help mothers to breastfeed successfully and overcome problems.

A mother needs to learn the cues her infant gives her to show he or she is hungry. Most newborn infants show the rooting reflex when hungry, turning the head from side to side and making sucking movements. Infants who remain close to their mother can be fed on demand throughout the day and night.

When mothers develop a routine for each feeding session, the baby learns what to expect at each feed.

Example of a feeding session routine

Offer the first breast and allow the infant to feed for as long as he or she wishes, allowing the baby to come off the breast when he or she has had enough. Give the baby a cuddle, holding him or her upright to wind. Next change the nappy and then offer the second breast, allowing the baby to feed for as long as he or she wishes and again to come off this breast when he or she has had enough or falls asleep.

By feeding correctly and on demand a good milk supply should be ensured.

The frequency and length of breastfeeds will vary from infant to infant and changes with age. Some guidance is given in Table 4.1.1.

Positioning and Attachment

Positioning

The infant should be held close to the mother:

- facing her and with the baby's tummy towards her
- with the baby's back, shoulders and neck supported
- such that the baby can easily tilt his or her head back and
- the baby's head is in line with his or her body so that the neck is not twisted.

This can be achieved with the mother sitting or lying. Some mothers like a pillow to support their back and another on their lap to support the infant. Following a caesarean section the underarm method or 'rugby ball hold' may be more comfortable.

Attaching onto the breast

1. The infant should be brought towards the breast with his or her nose level with the mother's nipple, with the chin and lower lip reaching the breast first.

2. As the infant comes close to the breast and touches it, the mouth will gape open. This gape can be encouraged by stroking the top lip.

3. The infant will usually tilt his or her head back bringing the chin to the breast first. At the height of the gape the infant's mouth should be brought onto the nipple and areola with as much of the areola below the nipple being taken into the mouth as possible.

4. There should be no rush to push the infant onto the breast.

5. If the infant is correctly positioned it will not be necessary to press the breast away from the infant's nose and the infant should be able to see the mother's face with his or her top eye.

6. When the infant has fed successfully he or she will come off the breast spontaneously, leaving a totally round, soft nipple.

Note: the photographs in the Department of Health leaflet 'Breastfeeding: Off to the best start' illustrate good attachment (Department of Health 2007).

Indicators of good attachment

Good attachment is indicated if:

- the infant's mouth is wide open while feeding
- the infant's chin is touching the breast

Table 4.1.1 Variability of frequency and length of breastfeeds

Age of baby	Frequency of feeds	Length of feeds
First 48 hours	Infrequent and as few as 3 feeds in first 24 hours	Variable
From day 3 to 7	Increase in frequency on day 3 to up to 12 feeds in 24 hours and then slowly decreasing in frequency	Very variable, both between babies and from feed to feed
After 7 days	Variable between infants but most feed about 6–8 times in 24 hours	Still variable but each baby will begin to develop an individual pattern over a 24-hour period

- the infant's cheeks are full – baby has a great big mouthful of breast
- more of the mother's areola can be seen above the baby's upper lip
- the infant's cheeks stay rounded during sucking
- the infant rhythmically takes long sucks and swallows – although it is normal for the baby to pause sometimes.

Although painless feeding may not be a reliable sign of good attachment, breastfeeding should not hurt after the first few sucks. If discomfort continues, the mother should take the infant off the breast and attach him or her to the breast again, aiming to improve the attachment.

Indicators of poor attachment

Poor attachment is suggested if:

- the infant's lips are pursed
- the infant's mouth is not open wide
- the infant's cheeks are sucked in with each jaw movement
- there is a gap between the infant's chin and the mother's breast
- the infant has not got a big mouthful of breast
- the infant's mouth is central or uppermost on the mother's areola
- nipple pain continues throughout the breastfeed
- the nipple is pointed, flattened, lined or wedge shaped after feeding.

Problems that suggest poor attachment include:

In mothers	In infants
• Breast pain while feeding	• Generally unhappy/ unsettled
• Sore or cracked nipples, engorgement	• Slow weight gain
• Too little milk	• Faltering growth
• Mastitis or breast abscess	• Colic
	• Explosive or green stools

Progression of a Breastfeed

- When correctly attached, sucking will start immediately.
- The sucking action will change from short shallow sucks to long deep sucks.
- Infants will pause from time to time.
- Infants become more relaxed as the feed progresses.
- The feed should be quiet, swallowing may be heard, but any noisy gulping, clicking or kissing sounds may indicate that optimal attachment has not occurred.
- The length of feeds will vary according to the infant's needs in the early days. Feeds may be long but will probably become shorter as baby becomes more efficient at sucking through practice and oral development.
- Infants usually let go of the breast spontaneously on finishing the feed.
- The mother's nipple should be the same shape as it was before the feed – any changes in shape or colour indicate that the nipple should be further back in the baby's mouth.

Breastfeeding Twins and Multiples

In the same way that mothers make enough milk for one infant, it is possible to breastfeed multiples.

Mothers approach this in different ways but most start by feeding each baby separately until they are confident with positioning and attachment. Once that has been achieved, feeding two twins together will shorten overall feeding times. The underarm hold will probably be the easiest to manage both twins at the same time in the early days. The twins should swap breasts at alternate feeds to ensure both breasts are equally stimulated, as one twin may suck more efficiently than the other.

For triplets or more infants, mothers need more individual help. If a mother wishes to give some formula, giving breast milk as well to her infants will benefit them.

Monitoring Breastfed Infants

Frequent weighing of breastfed infants is no longer recommended as small or no discernible weight gain can be distressing for parents and cause them to give up breastfeeding. Small gains in weight can easily be masked by a change in fluid content: an infant with a full bladder can weigh up to 200 g more than after emptying his or her bladder.

A breastfed infant who is feeding adequately will:

- be alert, responsive and healthy in appearance
- take a minimum of six feeds in 24 hours during the day and night
- have at least six wet nappies in 24 hours
- have at least two yellow stools daily.

Overcoming Breastfeeding Problems and Difficulties

Many mothers need support to continue breastfeeding and when discharged from the maternity unit they should be given (NICE 2008b):

- contact details of breastfeeding counsellors they can contact for help and support with breastfeeding in case they encounter problems
- information on local peer support groups since it has been shown that breastfeeding mothers who are in contact with other breastfeeding mothers continue breastfeeding for longer.

The majority of breastfeeding problems are directly or indirectly attributable to incorrect attachment of the infant to the breast. Even if the attachment appears good, it can usually be improved.

To assess breastfeeding problems the healthcare practitioner should:

- take a breastfeeding history – going back to the birth if necessary
- ask about a typical feed
- ask about a typical day, including feed frequency, behaviour in between feeds, including the sleep pattern

- examine the infant, noting general appearance, including the tongue
- check the infant's weight gain and growth chart
- take note of the number of wet nappies and stool frequency and colour
- observe a feed and assess positioning and attachment, noting jaw action, swallow, length of feed and infant's behaviour, and listening for audible swallowing
- examine the mother
- ask about family life and the mother's responsibilities in addition to her infant.

Sore or cracked nipples

Sore nipples are usually due to poor attachment and the pain should decrease when attachment is improved. However, in some instances sore nipples may be due to thrush or Reynaud's syndrome.

Thrush, or *Candida albicans*, is a fungal infection that often follows the use of antibiotics to treat mastitis or other infections. The skin may become sore and itchy. Both mother and baby may be infected and should be referred to the GP for treatment.

Some women's nipples become blanched due to lack of blood supply, known as Reynaud's syndrome. There is no ready cure for this but heat treatment and feeding in a warm room may help.

Cracked nipples may follow from poor attachment. Mothers should be encouraged to continue breastfeeding, as with improved attachment nipple pain should lessen considerably after about the first 20 seconds of feeding. Nipples will then begin to heal.

Occasionally, cracked nipples may bleed and the infant may posit or vomit bloodstained milk. Ingesting blood is harmless for the infant and there is no cause for alarm.

Engorgement

Engorgement occurs when the breast becomes full of milk and the blood and lymph flow slows and enters the breast tissue, causing oedema. Infrequent feeding or abrupt weaning may cause it. One or both breasts may be affected. It may be the areola or the body of the breast or both that are infected. Indications are:

- the breast is warm, painful, throbbing – this may extend up into the mother's armpit
- skin may appear red, shiny, taut and oedematous
- low-grade pyrexia may be present.

Possible actions to deal with engorgement include:

- massaging before feeds; kneading with fingertips using a circular motion, beginning at the chest wall and travelling around the breast in a spiral towards the nipple
- applying warm water before a feed (shower/bowl of water/warm compress)
- combination of massage and heat (e.g. shower and massage together)
- expressing gently, aiming to soften the areola and enabling the baby to attach and feed
- breastfeeding more often, finishing the first breast before moving on to the second
- changing breastfeeding position
- applying cold compresses after feeds to help reduce swelling and relieve pain
- using cabbage leaves – anecdotal evidence says women find these soothing when worn inside the bra next to the skin with a hole cut out for the nipple.

Analgesics such as paracetamol can be used to reduce symptoms. Aspirin should NOT be taken by breastfeeding mothers.

Blocked ducts

Blocked ducts may be caused by engorgement or poor positioning and attachment. The mother should be shown how to massage the affected area and express her breast. Hot flannels and a bath or shower may help. Cold, washed cabbage leaves around the breast are a traditional method still used but without evidence to support it.

Mastitis

Mastitis can be prevented by early diagnosis of and successful treatment of blocked ducts. However, if it does occur the mother should continue to breastfeed, but it is essential that her positioning and attachment be improved. If it fails to respond or gets worse, the mother may need to take antibiotics in addition to correct management. Unless positioning and attachment are improved, mastitis may re-occur. Unresolved mastitis may lead to a breast abscess.

Breast abscess

A breast abscess may require a surgical aspiration or operation and drainage. However, breastfeeding should continue. If the abscess is close to the nipple, the mother may wish to express on the affected side, until it is a little more comfortable.

Inadequate milk supply

Inadequate milk supply is a common reason that mothers cite when they perceive that their milk is not satisfying their infant. This perception may be due to persistent crying or fussing by infants. However, infants do not only cry because they are hungry. They often cry because they are uncomfortable, cold, lonely or bored. A crying infant may just need comforting and someone to talk and interact with them. Some infants experience more discomfort than others (e.g. those who have colic). Comforting an infant who has colic or some other cause for discomfort other than hunger can be very time consuming.

Any of the following measures may help to increase milk supply:

- Different positioning (e.g. underarm or lying down) may help the infant to feed more efficiently.
- The infant needs to feed on both breasts at each feed and for as long as he or she wishes on each breast to ensure adequate intake of the high-calorie hindmilk.
- More frequent feeding may help some infants but it is important they are allowed to feed as long as they wish on both breasts.

- Mothers may need to adapt their lifestyle to allow more time for feeding. Help with their household tasks and looking after other children may encourage some mothers to be more relaxed about the time taken for breastfeeding.

Tongue-tie

On occasions an infant with a marked tongue-tie may experience difficulty with breastfeeding. This can be resolved with minor surgery.

Mixed Breast and Formula Feeding

Introducing any formula milk is likely to decrease an infant's breast milk intake and subsequently the mother's supply of breast milk. If a mother has chosen to supplement with formula milk, one feed per day at a specific time will have less effect on her supply of breast milk than topping up with formula milk after every breastfeed.

Expressing Breast Milk

NICE recommends that all mothers are taught to hand express their breast milk (NICE 2008b). It may be necessary to express breast milk if:

- the mother needs help to attach her infant to a full breast
- the mother's breasts feel full and uncomfortable
- the infant is too small or sick to breastfeed
- the mother needs to be away from her infant for long periods of time such as social engagements or returning to work
- the mother requires surgery
- the mother chooses to bottlefeed her infant with her own expressed milk rather than breastfeeding.

There are three main methods of expressing breast milk:

- hand expression
- using a hand pump
- using an electric pump/battery pump.

Whichever method is chosen it is important that:

- the mother washes her hands thoroughly before she starts
- all containers, bottles and pump pieces are washed in hot soapy water and sterilized before use.

Milk can be expressed from one breast for around five minutes or until the supply slows down or appears to stop. Milk can then be expressed from the other breast. Then the mother can go back to the first breast and start again. Expressing from alternative breasts can continue until the milk stops or drips very slowly.

If there are problems beginning, the following may help the milk to flow:

- the mother should be comfortable and as relaxed as possible – sitting in a quiet room with a warm drink may help
- if possible, skin-to-skin contact with the infant
- having her infant close by or having a photograph of the infant to look at or being able to smell the infant's scent (e.g. on a baby blanket or garment)
- having a warm bath or shower prior to expressing, or applying warm flannels to her breast
- light, gentle massage of the breast by the mother using her fingertips or by rolling her closed fist over her breast towards the nipple. She should work around the whole breast, including underneath. She should not slide her fingers along her breast as this can damage the skin.

After massaging, light stimulation of the nipple between her first finger and thumb encourages the release of hormones which stimulate the breast to produce and release the milk.

As mothers get used to expressing their milk, they will find that they do not need to prepare so carefully. Just like breastfeeding, it gets easier as time goes by.

Hand expressing is free and convenient and is particularly useful if a mother needs to relieve an uncomfortable breast. The best way to learn is to practise (perhaps in the bath) so that the mother can find what works for her. As a guide, the mother should be instructed to try the following steps:

1. Place your first finger under your breast, towards the edge of the areola, with your thumb on top of the breast opposite the first finger. These should then be in about the same position as the baby's mouth. You may be able to feel the knobbly sinuses underneath the areola.

2. Keeping your fingers and thumb in the same places on your skin, press them together for two seconds and release. A hard squeeze will be painful and not effective.

3. This press and release action should be repeated, keeping the thumb and the finger in the same place and taking care not to slide your finger and thumb up or down the breast.

4. Once you have acquired the technique, press and release every few seconds, building up a steady rhythm. The exact rate and rhythm needed to express milk efficiently varies from woman to woman.

5. The milk may take a minute or two to flow. When it does it will drip or spurt from the breast. Collect it in a sterile, wide-mouthed container – a measuring jug is ideal.

6. It is important to rotate your fingers around the breast to ensure that milk is expressed from all the lobes.

7. With practice it is possible to express from both breasts at the same time.

Using a breast pump

It is best to establish a good breastfeeding routine if possible before beginning to use a pump. There are three main types of pump available – hand, battery and electric. There are many varieties for personal preferences and circumstances. For mothers with infants in special care it may be necessary to hire a hospital-grade electric pump.

Simultaneous pumping may be recommended in some circumstances. This is expressing both breasts at the same time. It is thought that this significantly raises the prolactin and fat and volume levels and may be useful for long-term expressing.

Expressing milk for newborn infants

It is important to start expressing as soon as possible after birth for infants who cannot be put to the breast. Mothers who have infants in Neonatal Intensive Care Unit (NICU) should be encouraged to express at least 6–8 times in 24 hours, including at least once during the night. From 2–3 days after birth, milk production is related to milk removal and if milk remains in the breasts too long, there is a build-up of a protein called the 'feedback inhibitor of lactation', which may decrease the milk supply.

Storing expressed breast milk

After expressing into a sterilized container, the container should be covered with a tight-fitting lid and labelled with the date (NICE 2008b). It should then be put into the fridge or freezer as quickly as possible. Breast milk stored in a fridge retains the properties more effectively than freezing.

In a fridge

Breast milk should be stored at the back of the fridge where it remains coldest. It should not be stored on the door of the fridge where it is more likely to be warmer. It can be stored for up to five days if the parents are confident that the fridge remains at 4°C or lower. This cannot necessarily be guaranteed in a domestic fridge that is frequently opened. Hence in a busy household it may be preferable to freeze the beast milk if it is not going to be used within 48 hours.

In a freezer

Breast milk can be stored for up to two weeks in the freezer compartment of a fridge or for six months in a domestic freezer, at minus 18°C or lower.

In hospital

Storage times within hospital guidelines should be followed.

Thawing frozen breast milk

Frozen breast milk should only be defrosted in the fridge and then used within 24 hours. It should not be re-frozen once it has begun to thaw. A microwave oven should not be used to warm or defrost breast milk.

Continuing Breastfeeding when Returning to Work

Mothers returning to work after giving birth can consider continuing breastfeeding by:

- expressing milk so that someone else can feed her infant while she is away
- finding childcare close to her work and arranging to breastfeed during breaks in her work day
- asking her employer for flexible hours around breastfeeding; employers now have a duty to consider such requests
- asking her employer for support and logistics to express and store her milk while she is at work. The Workplace Regulations and Approved Code of Practice require employers to provide suitable facilities for pregnant and breastfeeding mothers to rest.

Information on the rights of mothers returning to work is available on the Maternity Alliance website (www.maternityalliance.co.uk).

Infants reluctant to take a bottle

An infant who steadfastly refuses a bottle from his or her mother may be more likely to take it from someone else when the mother is not around. However, for infants who refuse any bottle the following may work:

- trying a different teat
- running the teat under warm water to raise it to body temperature
- breast milk given in a cup or beaker or on a teaspoon
- wrapping something that smells of the mother around the bottle or cup.

Introducing a cup or beaker

Infants can learn to drink from a cup from the time they are capable of sitting (around 5–6 months). Many infants are never bottlefed as they go directly from breastfeeding to taking milk from a cup.

Nutritional Needs for Breastfeeding Mothers

Although requirements for some nutrients are increased during lactation, eating a healthy balanced diet based on the five food groups as for during pregnancy (see Table 3.2.1 page 64) will usually ensure nutritional requirements are met, except for vitamin D – a daily supplement of 10 μg vitamin D is recommended (Department of Health 1991).

Pregnancy and breastfeeding are times when families are often well motivated to adapt their lifestyles and change to healthier eating habits.

The nutritional quality of breast milk is only affected by the mother's diet if she is undernourished. Strict dieting regimes with restricted food choices in order to lose weight while breastfeeding are not appropriate. Undernourished women and those on very restrictive diets may require some extra nutrient supplementation. Vegan mothers who are breastfeeding need to plan their diets well and may need additional supplements of calcium and vitamin B12 in addition to vitamin D.

Foods to limit

Oily fish and large fish should be limited as for pregnancy (see Chapter 3.2, page 71).

Alcohol is absorbed directly into the bloodstream and passes into breast milk. The highest level of alcohol in milk will occur between 30 and 90 minutes after ingesting alcohol. Breastfeeding mothers who choose to drink alcohol should not ingest alcohol for about two hours before breastfeeding and should keep alcohol intake to a minimum (e.g. one or two units once or twice a week). Regular or binge drinking should be avoided.

Caffeine in tea, coffee, chocolate and energy drinks does not need to be avoided but some mothers find large amounts of caffeine unsettle their baby.

Food hypersensitivity

Very occasionally, a food that the mother eats can cause an allergic response in the infant. Common triggers are dairy products, eggs and nuts. If a mother needs to exclude a whole food group (e.g. milk and dairy products) then she should be referred to a registered dietitian for advice to make sure her diet remains adequate in all nutrients, particularly calcium.

Infant Formula

The standard infant formulas are made from skimmed milk powder with added fats and nutrients to make the composition nutritionally adequate for infants. Formula milks have been modified as knowledge and technology progresses. However, their composition must always comply with strict criteria set by European Union regulations, which are updated from time to time as scientific research advances. Current regulations can be found at http://ec.europa.eu/food/food/labellingnutrition/children/formulae_en.htm and their interpretation for England at www.legislation.gov.uk/uksi/2007/3521/contents/made.

The EU regulations allow the protein in formula milks to be from either cow's milk protein or soya protein. Goat's milk is not allowed as a source of protein as the evidence to support its use that has been presented to the European Food Safety Authority was considered insufficient.

Choosing an infant formula suitable from birth

Infant formulas based on cow's milk protein

There are three main types of milk-based infant formulas:

- *Whey-dominant infant formula*: This is often labelled with a '1' and is promoted for newborn babies. The protein has the same whey-to-casein ratio (60 : 40) as mature breast milk.
- *Casein-dominant infant formula*: This is labelled with a '2' in some brands and is promoted as suitable for hungrier babies. The protein has the same whey-to-casein ratio (20 : 80) as cow's milk. The energy content of casein-dominant formula is the same as that of whey-dominant formula. There is no evidence to support the claim that these formulas are suitable for hungrier babies but there is some evidence that they may take longer to empty from the stomach and infants may therefore feel satisfied for longer (Taitz and Scholey 1989, Billeaud *et al.* 1990).

Overall there is insufficient evidence to suggest changing from whey- to casein-dominant formula or for switching brands.

- *Modified infant formulas* for infants with mild digestive problems such as colic have recently been introduced. They contain partially hydrolysed protein, prebiotics, modified fat and thickeners and are promoted for babies with minor digestive problems. Some have only partially hydrolysed whey protein and no casein while others have a 50 : 50 mixture or partially hydrolysed whey and casein proteins.

Differences between brands

There are four different brands of infant formula in the UK. The formula manufacturers research and develop their milk formulas in different ways and each company promotes the benefits of their formula to healthcare professionals based on different additions such as nucleotides, prebiotics and different milk proteins such as alpha-lactalbumin. However, these differences are minimal and healthcare professionals cannot promote one brand over another.

Some of the nutrients in typical infant formula milks are listed in Table 4.1.2. The list of nutrients is not complete but the table highlights key differences between breast milk and different brands of infant formula milks.

Numbering system

Any infant formula is nutritionally adequate for infants throughout their first year of life. However, the current labelling on formula milks implies that a baby should progress by stages through the different types of formula milks, with the use of

Table 4.1.2 Nutritional components in breast milk and infant formula milks

Nutrients		Breast milk	Infant formulas – suitable from birth
Proteins	Whey and casein	Main proteins in breast milk Whey : casein ratio changes and is 60 : 40 in mature breast milk	Present in whey-dominant formula in the ratio 60 : 40 Present in casein-dominant formula in ratio 20 : 80
	Alpha-lactalbumin	Main component of whey protein	Added to some
	Beta-lactalbumin	Very small proportion of the whey protein	Main component of whey protein in other formula milks
	Lactoferrin	An iron-binding protein. It binds the iron, rendering it unavailable to pathogenic gut bacteria. Their growth is thereby inhibited, reducing the risk of gastrointestinal infections	Not present
	Immunoglobulins (anti-infective proteins)	Remain relatively constant throughout lactation regardless of the amount of breast milk provided by the mother. This happens because concentrations increase as total volume diminishes	Not present
	Taurine	An amino acid essential for the myelination of the central nervous system and brain. In newborns, bile acids are almost exclusively conjugated with taurine, which helps excretion	Present
Fats	Total fat	Provides about 50% of the energy content of breast milk	Present at same level
	Long-chain polyunsaturated fatty acids: docosahexaenoic acid and arachidonic acid	Important in brain and retina development and in myelination of the nervous system	Present
Carbohydrate	Lactose	This is the sugar in breast milk and is about 7% by weight. It is digested to the monosaccharides galactose and glucose	Present at same level

Growth factors	These are especially high in the breast milk of mothers who give birth prematurely. Epidermal growth factor, for example, is a polypeptide that stimulates the proliferation of epidermal and epithelial tissues in the gut lining	Not present
Interferon	Antiviral factor present in breast milk	Not present
Nucleotides	Essential precursors for DNA and RNA and important for the function of cell membranes and the normal development of the brain. They may act as co-factors for the growth of *Lactobacillus bifidus* bacterium which reduces the presence of pathogens, such as *Escherichia coli*, in the faecal flora	Present
Lysozyme	This has a role in the antibacterial activity of breast milk and is also responsible for the development of intestinal flora	Not present
Iron	Low in breast milk but in a form that is highly absorbable – about 70% is absorbed	Added in higher amounts as there is only about 10% absorption from infant formula. The excess iron remaining in the gut promotes bacterial growth
Vitamin D	Naturally low as the main source of vitamin D is from skin synthesis when outside – only during the summer months, April–September in the UK	Added in higher amounts as a supplement
Carnitine	Essential for the catabolism of long-chain fatty acids. It enables fatty acids and ketone bodies to be oxidized to provide alternative fuels to glucose. This helps prevent neonatal hypoglycaemia	Present
Prebiotics	Types of fibre that remain undigested in the gut. They promote the growth of bacteria (e.g. bifidobacteria) in the gut flora that have a positive effect on digestion and absorption	Galacto-oligosaccharides and fructosaccharides are added to some formulas

numbers 1–4 implying the different stages. These numbered stages are not uniform across all brands which may confuse parents. Some examples are listed in Table 4.1.3.

Soya-based infant formulas

Soya-based infant formulas were previously recommended as an alternative to cow's milk-based infant formulas, but they are no longer recommended for infants in the UK under 6 months as they have a high content of phyto-estrogens and may have an oestrogenic effect. The consequences of this are uncertain.

Phytoestrogens are naturally occurring chemicals similar to human oestrogen and are found in some foods of plant origin (e.g. soya beans). One study found that the production of testosterone was suppressed in neonatal marmoset monkeys that were partially fed soya formula. No study has definitely proven that soya formula can cause long-term damage to human infants, and a paediatrician, GP or dietitian may recommend them if there is a clinical need while the infant is still under 6 months of age. In 2004 the Chief Medical Officer advised that: 'Soya-based formulae should only be used in exceptional circumstances to ensure adequate nutrition. For example, they may be given to infants of vegan parents who are not breastfeeding or infants who find alternatives prescribed for allergy treatment unacceptable.'

Follow-on formulas

Follow-on formulas are only suitable for infants over 6 months as they are higher in protein and some nutrients than infant formula. Either infant formula or follow-on formula can be given as the main milk drink between 6 and 12 months.

Specialized infant formulas

There are a range of specialized infant formulas available for infants with certain medical conditions (see Table 4.3.1 pages 119–120). They should only be used on the advice of a doctor or dietitian.

Table 4.1.3 Infant and follow-on formulas based on cow's milk protein

Formulas	Examples	Number on the packaging	Manufacturer
Whey-dominant infant formula – whey-to-casein ratio is 60 : 40	Aptamil First milk	1	Milupa
	Cow & Gate First Infant Milk	1	Cow & Gate
	Hipp Organic First Infant Milk	1	Hipp
	SMA First Infant Milk	1	SMA Nutrition
Casein-dominant infant formula – whey-to-casein ratio is 20 : 80	Aptamil Hungry milk	2	Milupa
	Cow & Gate Infant Milk for Hungrier Babies	2	Cow & Gate
	Hipp Organic Hungry Infant Milk	2	Hipp
	SMA Extra Hungry Infant Milk	–	SMA Nutrition
Modified infant formulas for minor digestive problems Protein is partially hydrolysed, fat is modified, some of the lactose is replaced with starch Have added thickeners	Aptamil Comfort	–	Milupa
	Cow & Gate Comfort	–	Cow & Gate
Follow-on milks Suitable from 6 months	Aptamil Follow On milk	3	Milupa
	Cow & Gate Follow-on Milk	3	Cow & Gate
	Hipp Organic Follow On Milk	3	Hipp
	SMA Follow-on Milk	2	SMA Nutrition
	Hipp Organic Good Night Milk	3	Hipp

Making up and storing infant formula

To reduce the risk of bacterial contamination, up until an infant is 12 months old all bottles and teats must be washed in hot soapy water and then sterilized before formula milk is added to them.

All formula milks are offered in two formats: dry powder and liquid ready-to-feed. They are compared in Table 4.1.4.

Making up powdered formula

Current guidelines for making up powdered infant formula can be accessed on the Food Standards Agency website (www.food.gov.uk/multimedia/pdfs/formulaguidance.pdf). Only safe water should be used for making up formula feeds:

Safe water sources in the UK	Unsafe water sources
• Freshly drawn cold tap water	• Water from the hot tap
• Bottled water that complies with tap water regulations – it may be labelled as 'suitable for making up infant formula'. The sodium content should be less than that allowed in tap water which is 200 mg/L	• Spring or mineral water that does not comply with tap water regulations
	• Carbonated water
	• Water that has been softened with a sodium exchange pump
	• Well water

Water for feeds, whether freshly drawn tap water or bottled water, should be boiled, but only once, and allowed to cool, covered, for up to 30 minutes. This ensures it is still above 70°C. Each bottle should be made up according to the instructions on the packaging. Ideally each bottle should be made up just before feeding to the infant and discarded if not consumed within two hours. To make up a feed outside the home, parents should take the powdered milk and a vacuum flask of water that has been boiled and poured into the vacuum flask within 30 minutes of boiling. The feed can then be made up in a sterilized bottle when needed.

Care should be taken not to over- or under-concentrate the feed:

- the scoop supplied with the milk powder should always be used
- 1 level scoop of powder should be added for each 30 mL boiled water
- care should be taken not to overpack the milk powder in the scoop as this will over-concentrate the feed.

Over-concentration of feeds can result in constipation, vomiting and excess weight gain. Under-concentrating feeds will not provide the infant with sufficient calories or nutrients for growth and development.

Making up formula feeds while travelling or on holiday outside the UK

The customer care line of each formula milk company can advise on a suitable formula milk

Table 4.1.4 Ready-to-feed and powdered formulas compared

	Liquid ready-to-feed formula	Powdered formula
Sterile	Yes – until opened	No – because it cannot be manufactured and packaged without the chance of some bacterial contamination
Making up	Ready-to-feed	Must be made up with boiled water as per instructions on the packaging
Storage	Once opened it can be stored in a refrigerator kept at 5°C or below for up to 24 hours	Keep tin in cool dry cupboard Once made up it can be stored in a refrigerator kept at 5°C or below for up to 24 hours Ideally it should be made up just before feeding to the infant
Cost	More expensive	Less expensive

available in the country to which a family is travelling. Taking at least one unopened can of powder with them will allow some time in which to find a supply abroad.

As in the UK, tap water and bottled water should be boiled for making up a formula feed using powdered formula. The label on the bottled water should be checked to make sure that the sodium level is less than 200 mg/L. Bottled water should be still and unflavoured.

Storing prepared infant formula is no longer recommended but there may be times when feeds need to be prepared in advance. The prepared feeds must be stored in a refrigerator kept at 5°C or below. The maximum storage time is 24 hours and any prepared feed not used after this time should be discarded.

Warming refrigerated feeds

Refrigerated feeds can be warmed to room temperature by standing in a jug of hot water for a few minutes. Microwaving formula feeds is NOT recommended practice and should be discouraged because of:

- ongoing cooking – the milk will continue to heat after removal from the microwave
- 'hot spots' – hot fluid in the centre of the bottle may be undetected and scald the infant.

Bottlefeeding Infants

Total fluid requirements for 24 hours are:

Age	mL/kg body weight/24 hours
0–2/3 days	minimal
3/4 days–6 months	150
7–12 months	120

Newborns may take very small volumes of formula. From day 3 the volume of feeds demanded will gradually increase to around a total of 150 mL per kg every 24 hours. The total volume increases as infants gain weight. As with breastfed babies, younger infants feed more frequently than older infants. At each feed infants should be allowed to regulate their own intake of formula feeds. Parents should:

- learn the cues that their infant uses to show he or she is hungry
- wait for the infant to open his or her mouth and accept the feed and never force the teat into the mouth
- cuddle their infant and use skin-to-skin contact when feeding to ensure the same closeness as when breastfeeding
- tilt the bottle so there is always milk in the teat
- allow the infant to pause from time to time while feeding from a bottle, and to wind him or her at some stage during the feed to allow a break before offering more
- allow their infant to stop feeding when he or she has had enough rather than encouraging him or her to finish each bottle, which may lead to excess weight gain which is a risk factor for childhood obesity
- discard any leftover milk at the end of the feed.

Solid foods should never be added to a bottle of milk and infants should never be left alone with a bottle.

Extra fluid

In exceptionally hot weather formula-fed infants may become thirsty in between their usual feeds as the water content of formula feeds does not vary as during breastfeeding. They can be offered drinks of cooled, boiled water. Flavoured or sweetened waters are not suitable.

Introducing a cup

From about 6 months of age a feeding cup can be introduced and encouraged for milk feeds.

Bottles of milk should be phased out from around the age of 12 months as toddlers may begin to associate bottles of milk with comfort and can become stubborn about giving them up.

Vitamin Supplementation for Formula-fed Infants

All formula milks are fortified with vitamins A and D and most formula-fed infants will receive enough of these two vitamins in their formula milk during the first 6 months of life. All formula-fed infants should begin a supplement of vitamins A and D from 6 months once they are drinking less than 500 mL formula per day (Department of Health 1994). Local policies may vary; in some areas where vitamin D deficiency and rickets are seen more frequently vitamin supplementation for formula-fed infants may be recommended from birth.

Those families who are entitled to receive Healthy Start vouchers are entitled to free Healthy Start children's vitamin drops (www.healthystart.nhs.uk). Some NHS Trusts also sell the vitamin drops but for families who cannot access these a range of infant supplements are available in pharmacies and some large supermarkets.

References and further reading

Agostoni C, Decsi T, Fewtrell M, *et al.* (2008) Complementary feeding: a commentary by the ESPGHAN Committee on Nutrition. *Journal of Pediatric Gastroenterology and Nutrition* 46: 99–110.

Billeaud C, Guillet J and Sandler B (1990) Gastric emptying in infants with or without gastro-oesophageal reflux according to the type of milk. *European Journal of Clinical Nutrition* 44: 577–583.

Bolling K, Grant C, Hamlyn B and Thorton (2007) *Infant Feeding Survey 2005.* London: The Information Centre. www.ic.nhs.uk

Dell S and To T (2001) Breastfeeding and asthma in young children: findings from a population-based study. *Archives of Pediatrics and Adolescent Medicine* 1(55): 1261–1265.

Department of Health (1991) *Report on Health and Social Subjects No. 41. Dietary Reference Values for Food Energy and Nutrients for the United Kingdom.* London: The Stationery Office.

Department of Health (1994) *Weaning and the Weaning Diet. Report on Health and Social Subjects: 45.* London: HMSO.

Department of Health (2004) HIV and Infant Feeding: Guidance from the UK Chief Medical Officers' Expert Advisory Group on AIDS. www.dh.gov.uk/en/publicationsandstatistics/publications/publicationspolicyandguidance/dh_4089892 (accessed April 2012).

Department of Health (2007) Breastfeeding: Off to the best start. www.dh.gov.uk/en/Publicationsandstatistics/Publications/PublicationsPolicyAndGuidance/DH_074095 (accessed April 2012).

Dollberg S, Lahav S and Mimouni FB (2001) A comparison of intakes of breast-fed and bottle-fed infants during the first two days of life. *Journal American College of Nutrition* 20: 209–211.

Greer FR, Sicherer SH, Burks AW, *et al.* (2008) Effects of early nutritional interventions on the development of atopic disease in infants and children. *Pediatrics* 121(1): 183–191.

Heikkilä K, Sacker A, Kelly Y, Renfrew M and Quigley M (2011) Breast feeding and child behaviour in the Millennium Cohort Study. *Archives of Disease in Childhood* 96(7): 635–642.

Horta BL, Bahl R, Martines JC, *et al.* (2007) *Evidence on the Long Term Effects of Breastfeeding: Systematic reviews and meta-analyses.* Geneva: World Health Organization.

Ip S, Chung M, Raman G, *et al.* (2007) *Breastfeeding and Maternal and Infant Health Outcomes in Developed Countries. Evidence report/technology assessment 153.* Rockville, MD: Agency for Healthcare Research and Quality.

Jones E and Spencer SA (2007) The physiology of lactation. *Paediatrics and Child Health* 17: 244–248.

Li L, Parsons TJ and Power C (2003) Breast feeding and obesity in childhood: cross sectional study. *British Medical Journal* 327: 904–905.

Martin RM, Ness AR, Gunnell D, *et al.* (2004) Does breastfeeding in infancy lower blood pressure in childhood? *Circulation* 109: 1259–1266.

Mayer EJ, Hamman RF and Gay EC (1988) Reduced risk of IDDM among breastfed children: the Colorado IDDM registry. *Diabetes* 37: 1625–1632.

Michels KB, Willett WC, Graubard BI, *et al.* (2007) A longitudinal study of infant feeding and obesity throughout life course. *International Journal of Obesity* **31**: 1078–1085.

NICE (National Institute for Health and Clinical Excellence) (2008a) Clinical Guidance 63. Diabetes in pregnancy: management of diabetes and its complications from preconception to the postnatal period. March 2008. **www.nice.org.uk/Guidance/CG63** (accessed April 2012).

NICE (2008b) Public Health Guidance 11. Improving the nutrition of pregnant and breastfeeding mothers and children in low-income households. March 2008. **www.nice.org.uk/nicemedia/pdf/PH011guidance.pdf** (accessed April 2012).

NICE (2008c) Clinical Guidance 62. Antenatal care: routine care for the healthy pregnant woman. March 2008. **www.nice.org.uk/nicemedia/pdf/CG062NICEguideline.pdf** (accessed April 2012).

Oddy W (2009) Breast feeding and childhood asthma. *Thorax* **64**: 558–559.

Quigley MA, Kelly YJ and Sacker A (2007) Breastfeeding and hospitalisation for diarrheal and respiratory infection in the UK Millennium Cohort Study. *Pediatrics* **119**: 837–842.

Quigley MA, Kelly YJ and Sacker A (2009) Infant feeding, solid foods and hospitalisation in the first 8 months after birth. *Archives of Disease in Childhood* **94**: 148–150.

Taitz LS and Scholey E (1989) Are babies more satisfied by casein-based formulae? *Archives of Disease in Childhood* **64**: 619–662.

WHO (World Health Organization) (2003) *Global Strategy for Infant and Young Child Feeding.* Geneva: WHO.

World Cancer Research Fund (2007) *Food, Nutrition, Physical Activity and the Prevention of Cancer: A global perspective.* London: World Cancer Research Fund.

Resources

British Dietetic Association: Breastfeeding (factsheet) (**www.bda.uk.com/foodfacts/Breastfeeding.pdf**)

Department of Health: Breastfeeding: Off to the best start (leaflet 278957) (**www.dh.gov.uk/en/Publicationsandstatistics/Publications/PublicationsPolicyAndGuidance/DH_074095**)

Department of Health: Breastfeeding and work (leaflet 279472) Workplace booklet 04/08 200k (**www.breastfeeding.nhs.uk/en/materialforclients/downloads/leaflet_4.pdf**)

Food Standards Agency. Guidance for health professionals on safe preparation, storage and handling of powdered infant formula (**www.food.gov.uk/multimedia/pdfs/formulaguidance.pdf**)

Healthy Start scheme (**www.healthystart.nhs.uk**)

NHS Choices: Healthy lifestyle and breastfeeding (**www.nhs.uk/Conditions/pregnancy-and-baby/Pages/lifestyle-breastfeeding.aspx**)

DVDs

Breastfeeding: A Guide to Successful Positioning. Produced by Mark-it Television

Breastfeeding: Dealing with the Problems. Produced by Mark-it Television

Prolog: *From Bump to Breastfeeding* (DVD). Order from Prolog: Tel: 0300 123 1002.

Resources for healthcare professionals

Further information on the Safety Guidelines issued by the European Food Safety Authority's (EFSA) Scientific Panel on Biological Hazards in infant and follow-on formulas (**www.efsa.europa.eu/en/efsajournal/pub/113.htm**)

4.2

Weaning onto Solid Foods – Complementary Feeding

Summary

- Infants develop at different rates and parents should be supported to decide when their infant is ready to begin solid foods.

- Most term infants are ready to begin between 4 and 6 months and the UK Department of Health recommends that they begin around 6 months but not before 4 months.

- Breast milk is the ideal main milk drink during weaning but most infants in the UK are already on formula milks by this age.

- Introducing finger foods from the beginning of weaning encourages the development of self-feeding skills.

- A positive feeding environment allowing the infant to decide how much they eat and drink enhances weaning progression. Milk feeds should decrease as more food is eaten.

- Progression through the weaning stages onto more complex textures and a wide variety of tastes of family foods by 12 months decreases the likelihood of feeding problems in toddlers.

Terminology

In the UK the term 'weaning' means the introduction of solid foods alongside an infant's milk feeds, rather than the process of moving an infant from feeding from the breast altogether.

Both the terms 'introduction of complementary foods' and 'complementary feeding' are used internationally for the introduction of solid foods alongside an infant's milk feeds.

Why Wean?

The purpose of introducing solid foods alongside an infant's milk feeds is to:

- provide extra energy (calories) and nutrients when breast milk or infant formula no longer supplies them in sufficient amounts to sustain normal growth and optimal health and development

- provide infants the opportunity to learn to like new tastes and textures, based on family foods, at a time when they are receptive to learning to like them.

Ideally, breast milk should continue as the main milk drink throughout weaning (Agostoni et al. 2008).

When to Begin Introducing Solid Foods

Over the last few decades recommendations on the suitable age to begin weaning have changed and conflicting advice is sometimes given to parents in the UK. The key recommendations from various agencies are summarized in Table 4.2.1.

Infants all develop at different rates and healthcare professionals need to support parents to decide when their individual infant is ready to wean. Oromotor skills to support weaning onto solid food are noticeable in infants between 3 and 6 months of age (Carruth and Skinner 2002).

Table 4.2.1 Summary of advice on weaning

Year	Organization	Recommendation
1994	UK Department of Health	'The majority of infants should not be given solid foods before the age of 4 months and a mixed diet should be offered by the age of 6 months' (Department of Health 1994)
2001	World Health Organization	1. Exclusive breastfeeding until 6 months of age to reduce the incidence of gastroenteritis, which causes death in developing countries 2. But each baby should be considered individually because exclusive breastfeeding to 6 months could lead to iron deficiency in susceptible infants, and growth faltering and other micronutrient deficiencies in others
2001	UK Scientific Advisory Committee on Nutrition (SACN)	'There is sufficient scientific evidence that exclusive breast feeding for 6 months is nutritionally adequate', however, 'early introduction of complementary foods is normal practice in the UK' and there should be flexibility in the advice but that any complementary feeding should not be introduced before the end of 4 months (17 weeks)
2004	UK Department of Health	'Although there is no evidence to suggest that giving a baby solid food before 6 months has any health advantage, it is important to manage infants individually so that any deficit in growth and development is identified and managed appropriately'
2008	European Society for Paediatric Gastroenterology, Hepatology and Nutrition (ESPGHAN)	'Exclusive breast feeding for around 6 months is a desirable goal. Weaning on to solids should begin by 6 months but not before 4 months' (Agostoni et al. 2008)
2009	European Food Safety Authority (EFSA)	'The introduction of complementary foods into the diet of healthy infants between 4 and 6 months is safe and does not pose a risk for adverse health effects' 'Exclusive breast-feeding is nutritionally adequate up to 6 months for the majority of infants, while some infants may need complementary foods before 6 months (but not before the age of 4 months) in addition to breast-feeding to support optimal growth and development.' 'Breast milk may not provide sufficient iron and zinc in some infants after the age of 4–6 months, and these infants require complementary foods' If complementary food is introduced after 4 months of life it does not constitute a problem for the digestive system or the renal function of the infant Iron deficiency in fully breastfed 6-month-old infants is more likely to occur in male infants and in infants with a birthweight of 2500–2999 g

Within Europe, national recommendations vary from country to country, with most recommending beginning weaning between 4 and 6 months of age (EFSA 2009). The UK Department of Health recommends term infants should be considered individually and should begin around 6 months or 26 weeks, beginning by this age but not before 4 months or 17 weeks. Mothers tend to choose to wean male babies and larger infants earlier than smaller and female babies (Wright *et al.* 2004).

This is probably because they perceive that babies growing more quickly are ready for more than just milk at an earlier age.

In practice, the developmental signs that suggest that an infant is ready to accept solid foods are:

- able to sit with support and with good head and neck control
- putting toys and other objects in the mouth

- watching others with interest when they are eating
- seeming hungry between milk feeds or demanding feeds more often even though larger feeds have been offered.

Between 4 and 6 months seems to be the best time to start solids because from this age infants learn to accept new tastes and foods relatively quickly.

Night-time waking and crying are not necessarily signs of hunger at this age. Around this time sleeping patterns change and some infants are more easily aroused and may begin to wake during the night. Many parents hope that weaning onto solid food will help their infant sleep through the night, but no evidence supports this hopeful theory.

Progressing Through the Weaning Stages

Weaning is a learning process and infants only learn to develop their feeding skills and accept and enjoy new tastes and textures if they are given the opportunity to try them. A study found that when infants are kept on puréed foods for too long and not offered lumps and finger foods by 10 months they are more likely to be fussy eaters at the age of 3 years compared to those weaned appropriately (Northstone *et al.* 2001).

The types and textures of foods to be introduced at each weaning stage are summarized in Table 4.2.2.

Weaning Stage 1: Beginning solids

Solids may be introduced at any time during the day that is convenient for the carer and infant. For the first few tastes it is best to give some of the milk feed first, then offer first tastes of solids before offering the rest of the milk feed. Before a milk feed infants might be too hungry and thirsty and not prepared to try anything new, while at the end of their feed they may be too satisfied to bother with anything else in their mouth. As the infant becomes accustomed to solids, he or she can be offered solids before the milk feed.

The amount of solid food given should always be as much as the infant is happy to eat. As the infant's feeding skills become more adept he or she will gradually take more and other foods can be offered for one and then two other meals.

Texture of foods

A smooth purée or well-mashed food is best for the first few tastes, offering it from a shallow teaspoon or plastic weaning spoon. Parents can then make thicker purées or mashed food as the baby becomes used to taking food from a spoon. Some infants may begin with soft finger foods but they should not be restricted to finger foods only as the infant is unlikely to be able to eat enough to

Table 4.2.2 Types of food to be introduced at different weaning stages

Stage	Age guide	Skills to learn	New food textures to introduce
1	Around 6 months but not before 4 months (17 weeks)	Taking food from a spoon Moving food from the front of the mouth to the back for swallowing Managing thicker purées and mashed food	Smooth purées Mashed foods
2	6–9 months	Moving lumps around the mouth Chewing lumps Self-feeding using hands and fingers Sipping from a cup	Mashed food with soft lumps Soft finger foods Liquids in a lidded beaker or cup
3	9–12 months	Chewing minced and chopped food Self-feeding attempts with a spoon	Hard finger foods Minced and chopped family foods

Adapted from Shaw and Lawson (2007).

successfully increase the energy (calories) and nutrients he or she derives from food.

Foods to offer

Any appropriate nutritious family foods from the list below can be introduced as the first weaning food, but most parents begin with cereal, potato, root vegetables or fruit, often mixed with a little of their infant's usual milk:

- all vegetables
- all fruits
- all cereal foods
- well-cooked lean meat, poultry, fish and eggs
- dhal, lentils, hummus, chick peas and other pulses
- plain yogurt or fromage frais.

Herbs and mild spices can be used to flavour food but salt should not be added.

Freshly prepared foods may be frozen in small quantities, in ice cube trays or bags as a convenience measure.

Previous guidance was to avoid some foods before 6 months of age but this advice has changed since the European Society for Pediatric Gastroenterology, Hepatology and Nutrition (ESPGHAN) Committee on Nutrition made the following recommendations in 2008 (Agostoni et al. 2008):

- Introducing gluten* between 4 and 7 months while breastfeeding may reduce the risk of coeliac disease, type 1 diabetes and wheat allergy. (*Foods containing gluten are wheat, rye, barley and oats.)
- High-allergen foods such as milk, eggs, fish and nut pastes can be offered from the beginning of the weaning process – there is no evidence that delaying their introduction until after 6 months of age will reduce the likelihood of allergies.

The Scientific Advisory Committee on Nutrition (SACN) and the Committee on Toxicity (COT) also considered the timing of the introduction of gluten and concluded that there was not enough evidence to support a recommendation for any timing of introduction of gluten into the diet except that it should be later than 3 months of age (www.sacn.gov.uk/pdfs/sacn_cot_statement_timing_of_introduction_of_gluten_into_.pdf).

Menu Planner

First meals

	Day 1	Day 2	Day 3
Before a morning feed	Baby cereal with milk	Porridge with milk	Baby cereal with milk
Before a middle-of-the-day feed	Puréed or well-mashed potato and carrot	Puréed or well-mashed sweet potato and cauliflower	Puréed or well-mashed parsnip and broccoli
Before an evening feed	Puréed or well-mashed cooked apple	Puréed or well-mashed peach	Puréed or well-mashed avocado

More nutritious first meals as the infant begins to eat more than 1–2 teaspoons

	Day 1	Day 2 – vegetarian	Day 3
Breakfast	Baby cereal with puréed pear and milk	Baby porridge with puréed or well-mashed banana and milk	Wholegrain wheat breakfast cereal with puréed cooked apple and milk
Midday meal	Puréed lamb with spinach and sweet potato	Puréed or well-mashed lentils with carrot and coriander	Puréed beef with potato, broccoli and red pepper
Evening meal	Puréed or well-mashed mango and yogurt	Puréed or well-mashed apple and pear	Puréed or well-mashed peach and apricot

Weaning stage 2: 6–9 months

Texture

At this stage foods should be a thicker mash with soft lumps and soft finger foods can be introduced. Meat may still need to be puréed at first but can be mashed if it is very soft.

Infants who begin weaning at or just before 6 months of age should be moved onto mashed food as quickly as possible to ensure nutritional adequacy and for them to learn to cope with new textures. Finger foods offered with all meals will keep infants engaged in the meal and give them the opportunity to develop self-feeding skills.

Some infants are more sensitive to texture changes and benefit with slow gradual changes. Those who spit out lumps need more practice managing them rather than being moved back to smooth purées.

Examples of soft finger foods

Soft fruit pieces (e.g. mango, melon, banana, soft ripe pear, peach, papaya and kiwi)

Cooked vegetable sticks (e.g. carrot sticks, green beans, courgette sticks, potato and sweet potato)

Cooked vegetable pieces (e.g. cauliflower and broccoli florets)

Cooked pasta pieces

Crusts of bread or toast

Cheese cubes

Soft roasted vegetable sticks (e.g. potato, sweet potato, parsnip, pepper, carrot, courgette)

By this age infants can move their tongue from side to side and can therefore manage to move soft lumps to between their hard gums to be chewed. Teeth are not necessary for chewing lumps.

Foods to offer

Different foods should be offered at the three different meal times. For example:

- breakfast: cereal and fruit with milk
- midday meal: meat/fish/dhal with potatoes/rice and vegetables
- evening meal: egg/grated cheese with bread or pasta, a vegetable and some fruit.

Over the three meals in a day, a variety of foods from all the four food groups should be included (Table 4.2.3).

By the age of 6 months, an infant's iron stores that were laid down during pregnancy are no longer adequate to meet the infant's iron requirements. Breast milk is low in iron and so the iron-rich foods from food group 4 as well as iron-fortified breakfast cereals and green leafy vegetables should be encouraged. Foods rich in vitamin C will increase the absorption of iron from plant-based foods.

Drinks with meals

Once infants are eating thickly mashed food they will need to be offered some water with all meals to satisfy their thirst. Sips of water from a cup without a valve allow the infant to learn to sip.

Table 4.2.3 Appropriate items from each food group

Food groups	Appropriate foods to introduce
Group 1: Bread, rice, potatoes, pasta and other starchy foods	Potato, toast crusts, rice, couscous, pasta, porridge and other breakfast cereals
Group 2: Fruit and vegetables	Soft ripe fruits, cooked harder fruits, cooked vegetables
Group 3: Milk, cheese and yogurt	Yogurt, cheese, custard and milk puddings
Group 4: Meat, fish, eggs, nuts and pulses	Meat, fish, well-cooked eggs, pulses (peas, beans and lentils) and nut butters or pastes of finely ground nuts

Fruit juices are not necessary for infants and if used they should always be well-diluted and offered in a cup not a bottle. High-vitamin C juices do aid iron absorption from plant-based foods at vegetarian meals but high-vitamin C fruits and vegetables in the meal will be just as effective.

Meals can finish with the usual milk feed or a milk pudding.

Menu planner for 6–7 months

	Day 1	Day 2	Day 3 – vegetarian
Breakfast	Wheat biscuit with mashed pear and milk Finger food: ripe pear slices	Porridge with mashed banana and milk Finger food: banana sticks	Breakfast wheat biscuit (e.g Weetabix) with mashed strawberries and milk Finger food: strawberries
Midday meal	Puréed lamb with mashed potato and broccoli Finger food: cooked broccoli florets	Poached white fish with vegetables Finger food: cooked broccoli florets	Courgette, cauliflower and chick pea curry Finger food: cooked parsnip sticks
Evening meal	Mashed mango and yogurt Finger food: mango slices	Mashed cooked apple and pear Finger food: ripe pear slices	Mashed peach and apricot Finger food: peach slices

Menu planner for 7–9 months

	Day 1	Day 2	Day 3 – vegetarian
Breakfast	Baby rice with mashed peach and milk Finger food: ripe peach slices	Baby porridge with sultanas and milk Finger food: banana slices	Scrambled egg with toast Finger food: toast fingers

Midday meal	Baked mackerel with roasted sweet potato and vegetables Finger food: roasted potato pieces Rice pudding with cooked plums and slices of ripe plum as finger food	Chicken casserole with potato and leeks Finger food: cooked carrot sticks Egg custard and slices of ripe pear	Vegetable curry with dhal and rice Finger food: cooked carrot sticks Strawberries with yogurt
Evening meal	Scrambled egg with toast Finger food: toast fingers Mashed kiwi fruit with fruit slices	Poached fish with mashed potato Finger food: potato chips Mashed peaches and slices of ripe peach	Pasta with red pepper and lentil sauce Finger food: cooked pasta pieces Mashed banana and banana slices

Weaning stage 3: 9–12 months

Foods to offer

A variety of foods from all the four food groups over the three meals should be offered at this stage. Two courses at the two main meals will provide a wider range of nutrients and tastes. These should comprise:

- a savoury first course with starchy food, vegetables and one of meat, fish, eggs or pulses
- a fruit or milk-based second course.

The average numbers of servings to be included from each food group per day are listed in Table 4.2.4.

Table 4.2.4 Average number of servings from each food group at 9–12 months

Food groups	Daily servings
Group 1: Bread, rice, potatoes, pasta and other starchy foods	3–4 servings (i.e. at each meal)
Group 2: Fruit and vegetables	3–4 servings (i.e. fruit at breakfast and a vegetable and fruit at the 2 main meals)
Group 3: Milk, cheese and yogurt	1–2 servings
Group 4: Meat, fish, eggs, well-ground nuts and pulses	1–2 servings or 2–3 for vegetarians

When infants join in family meals they learn to like the taste of family foods. They also develop their own feeding skills by watching and copying other family members' eating habits.

Family foods offered to them should have been prepared without the addition of salt and should not be based on convenience foods that are high in salt.

Texture

Minced and chopped foods can be introduced along with harder finger foods such as raw ripe fruit and vegetable sticks. Family foods such as sandwiches are also suitable.

Examples of harder finger foods

Pieces of raw fruit (e.g. apples, pears)

Fruits with the pips or stones removed (e.g. cherries, halved grapes,[a] and segments of oranges, satsumas and clementines)

Raw vegetables (e.g. sticks of cucumber, carrot, peppers, courgette)

Breadsticks and crackers

Pitta bread strips with hummus

Rice cakes

Sandwiches with soft fillings

Slices of hard boiled egg

Mini sausages

[a] Soft round foods are a choking hazard and should be cut in half.

Menu planner for 9–12 months

		Day 1	Day 2	Day 3 – vegetarian
Breakfast		Porridge with mashed fruit	Baby muesli with milk	Boiled egg with toast
	Finger foods	Banana slices	Blueberries	Kiwi fruit slices
		Milk feed	Milk feed	Milk feed
Midday meal	1st course	Beef casserole with green beans	Fried fish fillet with mashed sweet potato and peas	Vegetable curry with dahl
	Finger foods	Green beans	Steamed sweet potato sticks	Cooked vegetable sticks
	2nd course	Banana with custard	Rice pudding with apple and cinnamon	Yogurt and mashed peach
	Finger foods	Banana slices	Apple slices	Ripe peach slices
	Drink	Water	Water	Water
Evening meal	1st course	Scrambled egg with toast	Macaroni cheese	Peanut butter sandwiches
	Finger foods	Toast fingers and button mushroom pieces	Cooked macaroni pieces and cherry tomatoes	Carrot and cucumber sticks
	2nd course	Fruit compote	Yogurt and mashed raspberries	Strawberries and fromage frais
	Finger foods	Clementine segments	Raspberries and grapes	Fresh strawberries
	Drinks	Water and milk feed to finish	Water and milk feed to finish	Water and milk feed to finish

Vegetarian Diets in Infancy

Infants can successfully be weaned onto a vegetarian diet as long as a food high in iron is offered at each meal. For example:

- iron-fortified breakfast cereal, oats or egg at breakfast
- eggs/pulses/finely ground nuts at the other two main meals.

Foods from food group 4 should be offered 2–3 times per day and a food high in vitamin C should be included at all meals.

Activity 1

Make a menu plan for a week for an infant being weaned onto vegetarian food.

Weaning Infants at High Risk of Allergy

Infants are at higher risk of allergy if they have a parent or sibling with eczema, asthma, hay fever and/or food allergies. Ideally, breastfeeding should be continued throughout weaning and the highly allergenic foods should be introduced one at a time so that any reaction to these foods can be noted.

Highly allergenic foods are:

- cow's milk
- egg
- nuts
- fish and seafood
- wheat
- soya
- sesame seeds
- lupin
- celery
- mustard.

There is no evidence to delay introducing these foods beyond specified ages (Zutavern *et al.* 2006, Anderson *et al.* 2009), but some parents may prefer to introduce them slightly later than less allergenic foods. More research is needed in this area before more specific recommendations can be made.

Milk Feeds for Infants 6–12 Months

Breast milk or formula milk continue to be an important part of an infant's nutritional intake, however, these milk feeds should decrease as the quantity of solid food increases:

- The amount of breast milk taken should naturally decrease as the infant is able to regulate his or her own milk intake if allowed to continue feeding on demand.
- Early morning milk feeds should be discontinued from around 9 months to encourage more food to be eaten at breakfast. A milk feed can be offered after breakfast.
- When two courses are offered at the other two main meals, the milk feed can be dropped at one meal – particularly if a milk pudding is given as the second course.

Formula-fed infants need to decrease their milk intake in the same way. Parents feeding formula milk should be advised to offer less milk after meals and not to encourage finishing the whole bottle but to let the infant stop when he or she indicates they have had enough. By 9 months formula milk intake should be about 500–600 mL milk per day (Department of Health 1994).

Expected intakes at each weaning stage are listed in Table 4.2.5.

Table 4.2.5 Expected milk and food intake at each weaning stage

Stage	Age guide	Milk feeds	Meals	Variety of foods
1	Around 6 months. Begin by 6 months but not before 4 months	5–4	1–2	From one or two food groups
2	6–9 months	4–3	3	Three different meals with foods from all four nutritious food groups One or two courses per meal Offer water in a cup with each meal Vitamin A and D supplement for breastfed babies
3	9–12 months	3–2	3	Three different meals from four nutritious food groups Two courses per meal Offer water in a cup with each meal Vitamin A and D supplement for breastfed babies

Follow-on formula can be given in place of infant formula after 6 months but this is not a necessary change for infants being weaned appropriately. However, using it may provide a useful source of extra nutrients for infants who do not readily accept solid foods or have feeding problems.

Suitable drinking cups

Drinks can be offered from a cup from about 6 months. Non-valved lidded cups are the ideal as they allow infants to learn to sip. Cups with valved lids that infants must suck from should be discouraged. It is ideal to phase out all drinks from bottles around an infant's first birthday. This is to help prevent tooth decay known as 'bottle caries' in the toddler years which can occur in toddlers who use bottle feeding for comfort.

Commercial Baby Foods

Commercial baby foods, such as pouches, cans, jars and dried food, may be convenient in some circumstances but their exclusive use should be discouraged as they provide much less variety of taste and texture. Learning to like family foods is a key aim of weaning but the family foods when used for infants need to be nutritious and balanced as described above. Some families may need a lot of support to improve their cooking skills and knowledge of healthy eating.

Organic baby foods have become much more popular in recent years but they are low in iron content. Most manufacturers only add the minimum amounts of meat required by the regulations governing the nutritional content of baby foods, which is 8–10 per cent. Non-organic baby foods are usually fortified with iron and have a higher content, but few parents now choose to buy non-organic for their infants.

Positive Feeding Environment

Feeding infants in a positive and responsive environment allows infants to eat to their appetite and enjoy mealtimes. Many parents find it disappointing and frustrating when their infant eats less than they expect. Some parents need a lot of reassurance to allow their infant to decide when he or she has had enough food or enough milk to drink.

Infants who are coerced or forced to eat more than they need may gain weight rapidly and cross centiles upwards on their growth chart. Excess weight gain in infancy is a risk factor for future obesity (Reilly *et al.* 2005) (see Chapter 7.2, page 199).

Infants who are able to see and to play with their food at mealtimes learn more about it and develop a positive relationship with food. Finger foods give this opportunity, but touching and playing with soft or liquid foods in their bowl or plate is also important. Some parents find the mess involved hard to accept and may need to be encouraged to allow this important part of an infant's learning experience.

Offering finger foods and allowing infants to have their own spoon with which to try feeding encourages the development of self-feeding skills. Infants who are allowed to become involved in learning to self-feed will feel more engaged in the feeding process and will be less likely to want to end the meal because they have become bored.

Although offering only finger foods to infants has been promoted in recent years, there is no evidence to support the energy and nutritional adequacy of this method (Wright *et al.* 2011). Younger infants need more help with feeding as they may not be able to feed themselves adequate quantities of food fast enough to satisfy their hunger.

Components of a responsive feeding environment include:

- infant sitting with support for both back and feet
- infant and carer facing each other
- pleasant and positive interaction between infant and carer
- allowing infant to set the pace and following his or her cues
- having food where the infant can see it and allowing the infant to touch and play with food

- offering finger foods from early weaning
- no distractions such as TV or toys so that the infant can concentrate on eating
- use bibs/cloths/plastic sheets/newspaper to 'contain' mess so that it can be cleaned up at the end of the meal.

Following infant cues

Infants can regulate their calorie needs if allowed to. When happy to eat more food, infants will:

- open their mouth to accept a spoon of food
- pick up food and put it in their mouth themselves.

When they have had enough, infants will:

- keep their mouths shut when food is offered
- turn their head away from food offered
- put their hand in front of their mouth
- push away a spoon, bowl or plate
- hold foods in their mouth and refuse to swallow
- spit out food repeatedly
- cry, shout or scream
- try to climb out of their high chair
- gag or retch.

When offered a new taste, infants may show surprise and be reluctant to take more at that meal. However, if new tastes are offered repeatedly infants will usually learn to like that taste as they become more familiar with it. Parents often give up offering new foods if they perceive that their infant does not like that food. However, this narrows down the range of foods the infant has the opportunity to learn to like. By persevering in offering small tastes of a new food every few days the infant will have the opportunity to learn to like that food (Birch 1998, Maier *et al.* 2007).

Gagging and coughing

When infants are learning to manage new textures they may gag or cough back food that needs more chewing. This is part of the learning process and

parents should be advised not to panic; the infant might just need more experience to cope easily with that texture. If an infant gags or coughs frequently, families may need further assessment from a speech and language therapist.

Food Safety

Preventing choking

Infants must never be left unattended with foods or drinks as they can easily choke. Tragic cases of choking do occur and having infants seated and in a calm atmosphere at all times when eating is a safeguard against this. Cutting finger foods into short lengths rather than round pieces will also reduce the risk. Soft round foods such as cherry tomatoes and grapes should be cut in half.

Hygiene

- Bottles and teats for formula milks should always be sterilized.
- Plates, bowls, drinking cups and cutlery do not need to be sterilized but should be scrupulously clean.
- Freshly cooked food can be stored for up to 24 hours in the fridge.
- Food for infants should be reheated until piping hot right through and then cooled before feeding. Food should not be reheated more than once.
- Frozen food should be thawed in the fridge. Thawed frozen food should not be refrozen.
- Eggs, meat, fish and shellfish should all be well cooked right through.

Foods to limit and avoid

Foods that should be limited and/or avoided are listed in Table 4.2.6.

Vitamin Supplements

The Department of Health (1994) recommends that all infants begin a vitamin A and D supplement:

Table 4.2.6 Foods to limit and avoid

Foods	Reason
Foods to limit	
Foods with added sugar	They provide excess calories with fewer nutrients Infants are born with a preference for sweet foods and weaning is a time for learning to like other tastes In homemade puddings and cooked fruit a small amount may be added if necessary to reduce the tart flavour of sharp fruits
Foods with added salt such as adult ready meals and commercial sauces, soups and packet snacks	An excess of salt could cause dehydration if an infant becomes ill. However, nutritious foods that are preserved with salt, such as bread and cheese, do not need to be limited as infants need a certain amount of sodium to grow. See Chapter 1.2, page 19
Liver	Should be limited to one small serving per week because of the high levels of vitamin A
Foods to avoid	
Honey	Carries a very small risk of botulism
Under-cooked eggs, meat, fish and shellfish Unpasteurized soft cheeses	Likely to cause gastroenteritis
Large fish such as marlin, swordfish and shark	May contain mercury
Whole nuts	A choking hazard and can cause severe reactions if inhaled

- Breastfed infants should begin from 6 months if their mother was well nourished during pregnancy. If there is any doubt about a mother's vitamin status during pregnancy then breastfed infants should begin this supplement at 1 month of age.

- Formula-fed infants should begin taking a supplement once they are over 6 months and drinking less than 500 mL formula per day. This is because infant formula is supplemented with vitamins A and D. This is usually about 11–12 months.

This policy may vary locally: in areas where the incidence of rickets is high due to low vitamin D status of mothers and infants, some NHS Trusts/Boards recommend this supplement from birth for all infants.

Unfortunately, in some areas a vitamin A and D supplement is not widely recommended to parents and the recent rise in rickets is linked to the poor uptake of this supplement. Infants in the UK most at risk of low vitamin D are those of Asian, Black or Middle Eastern origin whose mothers did not take a vitamin D supplement during pregnancy.

Suitable supplements available

Healthy Start children's vitamin drops are available free for Healthy Start beneficiaries through some, but not all, NHS Trusts/Boards. A variety are available in retail pharmacies and outlets, but most are expensive because they contain additional vitamins and minerals. Some are prescribable.

Activity 2

Make up some weaning meals for each of the three weaning stages, taking care to mix them to the correct texture. Buy some commercial baby foods and compare the flavour and texture to those you have prepared from fresh ingredients.

References and further reading

Agostoni C, Decsi T, Fewtrell M, *et al.* (2008) Complementary feeding: a commentary by the ESPGHAN Committee on Nutrition. *Journal of Pediatric Gastroenterology and Nutrition* **46**: 99–110.

Anderson J, Malley K and Snell R (2009) Is 6 months still the best for exclusive breastfeeding and introduction of solids? A literature review with consideration to the risk of the development of allergies. *Breastfeeding Review* **17**(2): 23–31.

Birch LL (1998) Development of food acceptance patterns in the first years of life. *Proceedings of the Nutrition Society* **57**(4): 617–624.

Booth IW and Aubett MA (1997) Iron deficiency in infancy and early childhood. *Archives of Disease in Childhood* **76**: 549–554.

Butte NF, Lopez-Alarcon MG and Garza C (2002) *Nutritional Adequacy of Exclusive Breastfeeding for the Term Infant During the First Six Months of Life.* Geneva: WHO.

Butte N, Cobb K, Dwyer J, *et al.* (2004) The Start Healthy feeding guidelines for infants and toddlers. *Journal of the American Dietetic Association* **104**(3): 442–454.

Carruth BR and Skinner JD (2002) Feeding behaviours and other motor development in healthy children (2–24 months). *Journal of the American College of Nutrition* **21**(2): 88–96.

Daly A, McDonald A and Booth IW (1998) Diet and disadvantage: observations on infant feeding from an inner city. *Human Nutrition and Dietetics* **11**: 381–389.

Department of Health (1994) *Weaning and the Weaning Diet. Report on Health and Social Subjects No. 45.* London: HMSO.

EFSA (European Food Safety Authority) Panel on Dietetic Products, Nutrition and Allergies (NDA) (2009) Scientific opinion on the appropriate age for introduction of complementary feeding of infants. *EFSA Journal* **7**(12): 1423.

Lanigan JA, Bishop JA, Kimber AC and Morgan J (2001) Systematic review concerning the age of introduction of complementary foods to the healthy full term infant. *European Journal of Clinical Nutrition* **55**: 309–320.

Maier A, Chabanet C, Schaal B *et al.* (2007) Food-related sensory experience from birth through weaning: Contrasted patterns in two nearby European regions. *Appetite* **49**(2): 429–440.

Mughal MZ, Salama H, Greenway T, *et al.* (1999) Florid rickets associated with prolonged breastfeeding without vitamin D supplementation. *British Medical Journal* **318**: 39–40.

Northstone K, Emmett P, Nethersole F and the ALSPAC study team (2001) The effect of age of introduction to lumpy solids on foods eaten and reported feeding difficulties at 6 and 15 months. *Journal of Human Nutrition and Diet* **14**: 43–54.

Quigley MA, Kelly YJ and Sacker A (2009) Infant feeding, solid foods and hospitalisation in the first 8 months after birth. *Archives of Disease in Childhood* **94**: 148–150.

Reilly JJ, Armstrong J, Dorosty AR, *et al.* (2005) Early life risk factors for obesity in childhood: cohort study. *British Medical Journal* **330**: 1357–1359.

Shaw V and Lawson M (2007) *Clinical Paediatric Dietetics*, 3rd edn. London: Blackwell.

Ward Platt MP (2009) Demand weaning: infants' answers to professional dilemmas. *Archives of Disease in Childhood* **94**: 79–80.

WHO (2001) *World Health Organization 54th World Health Assembly 2001. Global strategy for infant and young child feeding. The optimal duration of exclusive breastfeeding.* A54/INF.DOC./4. Geneva: WHO.

WHO/UNICEF (1998) *Complementary Feeding of Young Children in Developing Countries: A review of current scientific knowledge.* Geneva: WHO.

Wright CM, Parkinson KN and Drewett RF (2004) Why are babies weaned early? Data from a prospective population based cohort study. *Archives of Disease in Childhood* **89**: 813–816.

Wright CM, Cameron K, Tsiaka M and Parkinson KN (2011) Is baby-led weaning feasible? When do babies first reach out for and eat finger foods? *Maternal and Child Nutrition* **7**: 27–33.

Zutavern A, Brockow I, Schaaf B, Bolte G, Von Beg A and Diez U (2006) The timing of solid food introduction in relation to atopic dermatitis and sensitisation considering reverse causality: results from a prospective birth cohort study. *Pediatrics* **117**: 401–411.

Resources

British Dietetic Association Factsheet Weaning (**www.bda.uk.com/foodfacts/index.html**)

Department of Health (2009) *Birth to Five Book*. London: The Stationery Office.

Healthy Start scheme (**www.healthystart.nhs.uk**)

More J (2010) *Teach Yourself Stress-Free Weaning*. London: Hodder Education.

NICE (National Institute for Health and Clinical Excellence) (2008) Public Health Guidance 11. Improving the nutrition of pregnant and breastfeeding mothers and children in low-income households. March 2008. **www.nice.org.uk/ nicemedia/pdf/PH011guidance.pdf** (accessed April 2012)

Common Feeding Problems in Infancy

Summary

- Early feeding difficulties may be related to slow development of feeding skills or neurodevelopmental delay.

- The most common feeding problems in infants are colic, posetting and vomiting, gastro-oesophageal reflux disease, diarrhoea and gastroenteritis, food hypersensitivity, constipation and faltering growth.

- Better attachment and positioning may help with breastfeeding problems.

- There are several specialist infant formulas that can be prescribed for formula-fed infants with specific conditions.

Many parents have concerns and anxieties about feeding infants. In breastfed infants, poor feeding may be a consequence of poor attachment, as discussed in Chapter 4.1. When seen in bottlefed babies it may simply be a consequence of slow feeding skills development. Most feeding problems resolve with time but those that may need support from healthcare professionals and possibly intervention include:

- oromotor delay
- colic
- gastro-oesophageal reflux
- persistent diarrhoea and gastroenteritis
- food hypersensitivity
- faltering growth.

Slow Development of Feeding Skills and Oromotor Delay

Difficulty in feeding and food refusal is commonly seen during infancy. From birth, some infants are slow to develop feeding skills and coordinate their suck, swallow and breathing. Without adequate fluid intake they can dehydrate quickly and may need medical intervention. They may lose more than 10 per cent of their birthweight and may take longer to regain their birthweight. Breastfeeding mothers find this distressing and are often persuaded to change to bottlefeeding, which is a more passive mode of feeding for the infant.

For some infants, poor feeding may be the first indication of oromotor delay or neuro-developmental delay. In research, about a fifth of mothers reported poor appetite and oromotor delay in their 6-week-old infants (Wright *et al.* 2006).

Slow development of feeding skills is evident in weaning infants that take longer to manage solid food and may be much slower moving from smooth to lumpy textures.

Unsettled Infants/Colic

Many young infants have a period during the day when they are unsettled and cry with discomfort but appear not to be hungry. This is often referred to as 'colic'. It occurs commonly in the late afternoon and evening. It usually resolves by the time the infant is about 5 months of age.

Causes of colic are unknown but it is thought to be due to swallowing large amounts of air during feeding which then becomes trapped in the digestive tract and causes bloating and severe abdominal pain.

Comforting and soothing the baby with a massage or a warm bath sometimes helps.

Healthcare professionals should:

● ask about the infant's feeding routine and bowel movements

● observe a feed and correct positioning and attachment in breastfed infants

● check that formula feeds are being made up correctly and not over- or under-concentrated

● check the teat hole size of bottlefed infants

● check that infants are being winded correctly during and after the feed.

Colic preparations are available in retail pharmacies but there is no scientific evidence to support their use.

Posseting and Gastro-oesophageal Reflux

Posseting is seen in most young infants. It occurs when the immature valve mechanism where oesophagus and stomach meet (gastro-oesophageal sphincter) allows the stomach contents to regurgitate back up into the mouth without any harmful effects. Infants with mild posseting will gain weight and thrive normally (Puntis 2000).

More severe reflux/regurgitation, resulting in distress to the infant is called gastro-oesophageal reflux disease (GORD). In this case the stomach contents come up into the oesophagus but not always into the mouth. This causes discomfort or pain to the infant but the carer will not necessarily be aware that it is happening. Screaming episodes may be caused by GORD.

Both conditions usually resolve with time as the infant grows and the length of the oesophagus increases and the gastro-oesophageal sphincter becomes more efficient. GORD may continue throughout infancy and beyond in some children. Symptoms often improve when weaning onto solid food begins, or when the infant starts to walk and is in a more upright position.

Management by the primary healthcare team is usually sufficient and should include explanation and reassurance to the parent. In addition:

● better positioning and attachment of breastfed babies may help improve GORD

● changing breastfed infants to infant formula will not help

● volume and concentration of formula feeds should be checked to make sure infants are not being overfed with large volumes or over-concentrated feeds.

A thickened feed can be considered for formula-fed infants. This can be done by either:

● adding a thickener, such as Thixo-D or Instant Carobel (Cow & Gate) to the normal formula just before feeding; or

● changing to a formula that thickens in the stomach (e.g. Enfamil AR (Mead Johnson) or SMA Staydown (SMA Nutrition)).

A medical practitioner may sometimes prescribe anti-reflux medications such as Gaviscon. It acts in a similar fashion to the formulas Enfamil AR (Mead Johnson) or SMA Staydown (SMA Nutrition).

If the problems persist, despite having taken the above measures, or if the infant has faltering growth, referral to a paediatrician is recommended.

GORD is sometimes caused by intolerance to cow's milk protein (Farahmand et al. 2011) and a trial of a diet free from cow's milk protein can be tried for 1–2 weeks to see if symptoms resolve:

● The mother of a breastfed infant would need to exclude milk and foods containing milk from her diet.

- Formula-fed infants can be changed to a specialized milk formula, such as an extensively hydrolysed milk formula.
- Infants who have begun weaning need to be referred to a dietitian for advice on milk-free weaning foods.

Diarrhoea and Gastroenteritis

Diarrhoea or loose stools occur frequently in infants. It is often seen in those experiencing pain during teething and resolves as the pain subsides.

Acute gastroenteritis is an infectious disease of the alimentary tract, producing damage to the mucosa, either structural or functional and of variable extent and severity. The main aim in managing gastroenteritis in infants is the correction of dehydration and maintenance of hydration and electrolyte balance. Infants under 6 months are particularly vulnerable to gastroenteritis and dehydration and may require hospital admission.

Gastroenteritis is uncommon in infants who are exclusively breastfed. In the rare event that it occurs, it is important that breastfeeding is continued, as discontinuation of breastfeeding is a major risk factor for the development of dehydration (Faruque *et al.* 1992). Severe cases may require the addition of oral rehydration fluids.

Infant formula feeds may be stopped for a short time (6–24 hours) and an oral rehydration solution (e.g. Dioralyte or Rehydrat) given to replace lost fluids (i.e. after vomiting or diarrhoea) and provide the infant's fluid requirement. Formula feeds should then be re-commenced at full strength and not diluted (Guarino *et al.* 2008).

If infants have started on solids, it may also be necessary to discontinue these for a similarly short period of time.

Continued diarrhoea after acute gastroenteritis may be associated with a temporary intolerance to lactose in a very small minority of infants (McDonald 2007). Breastfeeding should continue, but formula-fed infants could be changed to a lactose-free formula. Advice on excluding foods containing milk and lactose will be needed for infants who are already being weaned.

Constipation

Constipation can be simply defined as 'difficult passage of hard stools'; it may also present as:

- abdominal pain
- rectal bleeding which may indicate anal fissure
- soiling from 'overflow' diarrhoea
- passage of very large stools that are difficult to flush away
- stool withholding behaviour.

In the first 3–4 months infants should pass frequent, loose, bright yellow stools, at least 2–3 times in 24 hours. From 3 to 4 months, stools will become less frequent. It is not unusual for an infant to go several days without a bowel movement, and providing the infant is well and happy this is of no significant concern. After the introduction of solid food, stools may change in frequency and colour.

Most constipation in infants and young children is idiopathic in origin – that is to say there is no underlying cause that can be identified. Dietary factors can cause or exacerbate it.

Constipation is rare in breastfed infants but if it occurs it may indicate:

- inadequate milk intake due to poor attachment or positioning. If this can be improved it may resolve the problem but additional fluids other than breast milk are not recommended
- cow's milk protein intolerance – this is more likely in infants that have asthma or eczema. If so it should resolve if the breastfeeding mother removes milk and dairy products from her own diet. She will need to begin a calcium supplement to ensure her own nutritional adequacy.

Constipation is a more frequent problem in formula-fed infants and causes can be:

- the calcium salts in the formula harden the stools in susceptible infants – this often develops when infants change from breastfeeding to formula feeding or from a whey-dominant formula to a casein-dominant formula

- over-concentrating of the infant formula
- inadequate fluid intake, including underfeeding
- cow's milk protein intolerance.

Constipation may also begin with weaning onto solid food.

Management of constipation in formula-fed infants

- Fluid intake: Ask parents to keep a feed diary for 2–3 days. Check the volume of feed given/kg actual body weight/24 hours against recommended intake (see page 96).
- Check that the infant formula is being made up according to the manufacturer's instructions and not being over-concentrated or under-concentrated.
- Casein-dominant milks can be more constipating than whey-dominant milks so a change from casein-dominant to whey-dominant formula may help.
- Changing to a modified formula for minor digestive problems may help as the fats in these formula are different to standard formulas (Moro *et al.* 2002, Schmelzle *et al.* 2003).
- A two-week trial of a hydrolysed protein or amino acid-based formula will indicate if the cause is cow's milk protein intolerance.
- Additional drinks of cooled boiled water can be offered in between milk feeds and particularly in hot weather.

If the infant is being weaned then check that a balanced weaning diet including fruit, vegetables and cereals are being offered. More wholegrain cereals can be offered such as porridge or wheat-based breakfast cereals (e.g. Weetabix or Shreddies). However, bran should not be given to infants. Also check that drinks or water are being offered with meals.

If conservative management with diet fails to resolve constipation, then the infant should be referred for further medical opinion.

Food Hypersensitivity (Food Allergy and Food Intolerance)

About 2–5 per cent of infants are sensitive to certain foods, but many more parents suspect that a food is causing problems for their infant (Venter *et al.* 2006).

The foods that most commonly cause problems are milk, eggs, soya, fish, wheat and peanuts. Many infants grow out of it by 12 months so it is important that the condition is monitored carefully to ensure special diets are not continued for longer than necessary.

Symptoms

Symptoms of immediate-onset allergy may occur up to one hour after food ingestion and include skin manifestations (urticaria, itching, rash), vomiting, angioedema and anaphylaxis. Delayed-onset reactions are harder to diagnose and may not manifest until hours or days after the ingestion of the offending food. Possible symptoms include eczema, chronic diarrhoea, colic/abdominal pain and faltering growth.

Diagnosis

The gold standard test is the placebo-controlled double-blind food challenge. In clinical practice, however, open challenges are usually performed where parents and practitioners know what is in the food. Food challenges are an integral part of diagnosis in order to:

- detect a specific food which causes symptoms – a positive result confirms the need to exclude that food from the diet; or
- prove that a specific food is not responsible – an absence of symptoms confirms that a restricted diet is not needed.

Once diagnosed, a food causing symptoms should be excluded.

In breastfed infants the mother may need to exclude foods from her diet and take a calcium supplement to ensure nutritional adequacy. Formula-fed infants can usually be changed to an appropriate specialized feed if necessary.

Advice from a registered dietitian is needed to ensure the infant's milk and weaning food intake continues to provide all the necessary nutrients for optimizing growth and development.

Excluding cow's milk protein

The infant formula of choice is an extensively hydrolysed infant formula. In some cases, if an improvement in symptoms is not seen, an amino acid infant formula can be trialled.

Some mothers choose to try a soya formula, but these are not recommended for infants under 6 months of age (see Chapter 4.1, page 94).

Faltering Growth

Infants who are not drinking enough milk for their needs will not grow as expected. The Avon Longitudinal Study of Parents and Children (Emond *et al.* 2007) showed the following feeding problems to be associated with poor growth:

- sucking problems and slow feeding in the first few weeks
- difficulties in weaning onto solids at around 6 months.

Oromotor dysfunction may be the cause of both these feeding problems.

Faltering growth is defined as weight falling through 2 centile spaces. However, interpreting growth charts of infants requires training as various factors impact on growth rates:

- Infants lose weight in the first few days of life but should have regained it by 2 weeks of age.
- Over the first 6 weeks of life infants with a weight above the 50th centile may cross centile lines downwards and small infants with a birthweight below the 50th centile may cross centile lines upwards, moving closer to the 50th centile line.

- Breastfed and formula-fed infants have slightly different growth patterns during the first year of life. Breastfed infants grow more quickly in the first 3–4 months and then grow more slowly from about 5 months when compared to formula-fed infants. Infants should all be plotted on the UK WHO growth charts based on breastfed infants.
- Infants should not be weighed more frequently than every two weeks as shorter intervals are not necessarily indicative of accurate weight gain or loss.

Other indications of inadequate milk intake are:

- apathetic or weakly crying infant
- poor muscle tone and skin turgor
- concentrated urine, a few times/day
- infrequent, scanty stools
- fewer than 8 short breastfeeds/day.

The management of faltering growth is different for breast- and formula-fed infants.

Management of faltering growth in breastfed infants

A person skilled in breastfeeding management should assess mother and infant feeding.

- The infant should feed at least eight times in 24 hours (including at night).
- Infants should be fed until they come off the breast spontaneously. If sleepy, a nappy change may help to rouse them and the infant can then be fed on the second breast.
- The mother and infant should be in skin-to-skin contact as often as possible.
- The mother should be encouraged to express milk from her breasts after the infant has finished feeding as after completely emptying the breast more milk will be produced for the next feed.
- Different positioning for feeding (e.g. under-arm, or especially with mother lying down) may help the infant to feed more efficiently.

- If the mother's milk supply has diminished, she may benefit from taking domperidone 10 mg three times a day in consultation with a lactation specialist.

- If the infant is sleepy or reluctant to feed it may be necessary for the mother to express her milk for some time and feed her infant with her expressed breast milk by syringe, cup or bottle until the infant is passing frequent yellow stools and is more alert. The infant can then be re-introduced to the breast.

- A healthcare professional should check that the mother is eating a balanced diet and drinking adequate fluid.

- The interaction between the mother and infant should be considered.

- The mother should be asked about any emotional stress or anxieties as this can reduce her milk production.

- The social circumstances of the family should be assessed and support arranged where necessary.

Management of faltering growth in formula-fed infants

The healthcare professional should first take a diet history and/or ask parents to keep a feed and food diary.

- Check frequency and volume of feeds taken.

- Check that the appropriate formula is being used and that it is being made up correctly with good hygienic practices.

- Check the size of the teat on the bottle is appropriate.

- Check the infant is not constipated.

- If the infant was born preterm, check that the parents are continuing to use a preterm formula as directed by the paediatrician or dietitian.

- If weaning foods are being offered check their suitability.

If there are no obvious dietary causes of faltering growth or the above measures do not result in improvement in weight gain, the infant should be referred to a paediatrician.

Some infants with certain diseases or syndromes have particularly high energy requirements and those unable to take sufficient volumes of standard infant formula should be referred to a paediatric dietitian. A 'high-energy' infant formula may be recommended (e.g. Infatrini or SMA High Energy). These should only be used with dietetic and/or medical recommendation and ongoing assessment.

Vitamin D Deficiency

Infants born to mothers with low vitamin D levels before and during pregnancy may be born with low vitamin D levels themselves. This can lead to low plasma calcium and they may present with:

- stridor or seizures

- tetany

- cardiomyopathy

- reduced muscle tone – floppy infant.

They may also present with delayed closure of anterior fontanelle – prominent forehead.

Even infants who are not breastfed and receiving small amounts of vitamin D in formula milk have presented with these symptoms.

Rickets may be seen in late infancy but is usually seen in toddlers.

Specialist Infant Formulas

Specialist infant formulas are prescribable for certain medical conditions as specified in the British National Formulary (www.bnf.org, Appendix 7, Borderline Substances) (Table 4.3.1). Only a qualified doctor can prescribe them, although doctors often do so on the advice of a paediatric dietitian. The formulas are available over the counter if a parent asks a pharmacist to order them. However, they are much more expensive than standard formulas and therefore most parents would ask for them to be prescribed.

Table 4.3.1 Some specialized infant formulas – suitable from birth or, where stated, from 6 months of age

Type of formula	Examples	Manufacturer	Relevant compositional details	Used for infants with:
High-energy for faltering growth	Infatrini	Nutricia	100 kcal/100 mL	Faltering growth when a more modified formula is not required
	Similac High Energy	Abbott Nutrition	100 kcal/100mL	
	SMA High Energy	SMA Nutrition	91 kcal/100 mL	
Thickening feeds for GORD	Enfamil AR	Mead Johnson Nutrition	Rice starch thickens on contact with gastric acid	Gastro-oesophageal reflux disease
	SMA Staydown Infant Milk	SMA Nutrition	Corn starch thickens on contact with gastric acid	
Lactose-free	Enfamil O-Lac	Mead Johnson Nutrition	Lactose is replaced with glucose	Lactose intolerance
	SMA LF	SMA Nutrition		
Soya formulas	Cow & Gate Infasoy	Cow & Gate	Protein is from soy bean and carbohydrate is glucose	Infants over 6 months of age with cow's milk protein allergy or lactose or sucrose intolerance
	SMA Wysoy	SMA Nutrition		
Extensively hydrolysed formulas	Nutramigen Lipil 1 Nutramigen Lipil 2 – suitable from 6 months	Mead Johnson Nutrition	Protein is extensively hydrolysed casein	Whole protein or disaccharide intolerance
	Pepdite	Nutricia/SHS	Protein is hydrolysed pork collagen and soya; 3% of fat is MCT	Whole protein and/or disaccharide intolerance, multiple malabsorption, short bowel syndrome
	MCT Pepdite	Nutricia/SHS	Protein is hydrolysed pork collagen and soya; 75% of fat is MCT	Pancreatic insufficiency, multiple malabsorption, short bowel syndrome, whole protein intolerance requiring MCT
	Aptamil Pepti 1 Aptamil Pepti 2 – suitable from 6 months	Aptamil	Protein is 100% hydrolysed whey. Carbohydrate is 41% lactose in Aptamil Pepti 1 and 36% in Aptamil Pepti 2	Cow's milk protein allergy without suspected lactose intolerance
	Pepti-Junior	Cow & Gate	Semi-elemental; 50% of fat is MCT; trace lactose	Whole protein and/or disaccharide intolerance, multiple malabsorption, short bowel syndrome
	Pregestimil Lipil	Mead Johnson Nutrition	Extensively hydrolysed casein; 55% of fat is MCT	Whole protein and/or disaccharide intolerance, multiple malabsorption, short bowel syndrome

(Continued)

Table 4.3.1 Some specialized infant formulas – suitable from birth or, where stated, from 6 months of age (*Continued*)

Type of formula	Examples	Manufacturer	Relevant compositional details	Used for infants with:
Amino acid formulas	Neocate LCP	Nutricia/SHS	Protein is a mixture of free amino acids with no peptide chains; 4% of fat is MCT	Whole protein/hydrolysate intolerance, multiple malabsorption, short bowel syndrome
	Nutramigen Lipil AA	Mead Johnson Nutrition	Protein is a mixture of free amino acids with no peptide chains	
Galactomin range for carbohydrate disorders	Galactomin 17	Nutricia/SHS	Carbohydrate is glucose	For lactose intolerance, galactosaemia and glucokinase deficiency
	Galactomin 19	Nutricia/SHS	Carbohydrate is fructose	For glucose–galactose intolerance
Modified fat	Caprilon	Nutricia/SHS	12% carbohydrate is lactose; 75% fat is MCT	Liver disease, fat malabsorption, pancreatic insufficiency
	Monogen	Nutricia/SHS	90% fat is MCT	Fat malabsorption
High-fat, low-carbohydrate	Ketocal Infant	Nutricia/SHS	73% fat	Infants on a ketogenic diet for treatment of epilepsy
Formula for renal disease	Kindergen	Nutricia/SHS	Higher in energy (101 kcals/100 mL), fat, carbohydrate and sodium but lower in potassium than standard infant formulas	For chronic renal failure and where peritoneal rapid overnight dialysis (PROD) or continuous cycling peritoneal dialysis (CCPD) is required
Very low-calcium formula	Locasol	Nutricia/SHS	Very low in calcium and vitamin D	For infants with hypercalcinaemia

GORD, gastro-oesophageal reflux disease; MCT, medium-chain triglycerides; LCP, long-chain polyunsaturated fatty acids.

References and further reading

Crotteau CA, Wright ST and Eglash A (2006) Clinical inquiries. What is the best treatment for infants with colic? *Journal of Family Practice* **55**: 634–636.

Emond A, Drewett R, Blair P and Emmett P (2007) Postnatal factors associated with failure to thrive in term infants in the Avon Longitudinal Study of Parents and Children. *Archives of Disease in Childhood* **92**: 115–119.

Farahmand F, Najafi M, Ataee P, Modarresi V, Shahraki T, Rezaei N (2011) Cow's milk allergy among children with gastroesophageal reflux disease. *Gnt and Liver* **5**(3): 298–301. Epub 2011 Aug 18.

Faruque AS, Mahalanabis D, Islam A, *et al.* (1992) Breastfeeding and oral rehydration at home during diarrhoea to prevent dehydration. *Archives of Disease in Childhood* **67**: 1027–1029.

Guarino A, Albano F, Ashkenazi S, *et al.* (2008) ESPGHAN/ESPID Evidence-based guidelines for the management of acute gastroenteritis in children in Europe. Expert Working Group. European Society for Paediatric Gastroenterology, Hepatology, and Nutrition/European Society for Paediatric Infectious Diseases. *Journal of Pediatric Gastroenterology and Nutrition* **46**(suppl 2): S81–122.

Joneja JM (2012) Infant food allergy: Where are we now? *Journal of Parenteral and Enteral Nutrition* **36**(suppl): 49S–55S.

Lucassen PL, Assendelft WJ, Gubbels JW, van Eijk JT, van Geldrop WJ and Neven AK (1998) Effectiveness of treatments for infantile colic: systematic review. *British Medical Journal* **316**: 1563–1569.

McDonald S (2007) Gastroenterology. In: Shaw V and Lawson M (eds) *Clinical Paediatric Dietetics*, 3rd edn. London: Blackwell.

Moro G, Minoli L, Mosca M, *et al.* (2002) Dosage-related bifidogenic effects of galacto- and fructooligosaccharides in formula-fed term infants. *Journal of Paediatric Gastroenterology and Nutrition* **34**: 291–295.

Puntis JWL (2000) Posseting. *Professional Care of Mother and Child* **10**(5): 128–133.

Rudolf M (2011) Predicting babies' risk of obesity. *Archives of Disease in Childhood* **96**: 995–997.

Schmelzle H, Wirth S, Skopnik H, *et al.* (2003) Randomised double-blind study of the nutritional efficacy and bifidogenicity of a new infant formula containing partially hydrolysed protein, a high β-palmitic acid level and non-digestible oligosaccharides. *Journal of Paediatric Gastroenterology and Nutrition* **36**: 343–351.

Shaw V and Lawson M (2007) *Clinical Paediatric Dietetics*, 3rd edn. London: Blackwell.

Vandenplas Y, Rudolph CD, Di Lorenzo C, *et al.* (2009) Pediatric gastroesophageal reflux clinical practice guidelines: joint recommendations of the North American Society for Pediatric Gastroenterology, Hepatology, and Nutrition (NASPGHAN) and the European Society for Pediatric Gastroenterology, Hepatology, and Nutrition (ESPGHAN). *Journal of Paediatric Gastroenterology and Nutrition* **49**: 498–547.

Venter C, Pereira B, Grundy J, *et al.* (2006) Incidence of parentally reported and clinically diagnosed food hypersensitivity in the first year of life. *Journal of Allergy and Clinical Immunology* **117**: 1118–1124.

Wright CM, Parkinson KN and Drewett RF (2006) How does maternal and child feeding behavior relate to weight gain and failure to thrive? Data from a prospective birth cohort. *Pediatrics* **117**(4): 1262–1269.

4.4

Preterm Infants

Summary

- Preterm infants are those born before 37 weeks gestation.

- The nutritional needs of preterm infants are higher per kg body weight than those of term infants and vary depending on the infant's gestation and size.

- Babies who are born very preterm and/or very small are likely to require neonatal parenteral nutrition while establishing enteral feeds.

- Maternal breast milk, either enterally via a feeding tube or orally, provides health benefits.

- Mothers may need skilled support to express breast milk for their preterm infant.

- Most infants weighing less than 1500 g (1.5 kg) at birth require breast milk fortifiers added to

maternal breast milk to aid growth and ensure adequate nutritional status.

- If breast milk is unavailable there are preterm formulas and nutrient-enriched postdischarge formula milks which have been designed to meet the specific nutritional needs of preterm infants.

- Development of oral feeding is individual and dependent on many factors, including gestation and size at birth and the medical condition and history of the baby.

- Weaning can begin at an earlier post-conception age than in term infants as preterm infants need a more nutrient-dense diet earlier.

Classification of Preterm and Small-for-Gestational-Age Infants

Infants born preterm (less than 37 weeks gestation) or with a low birthweight (LBW), below 2500 g (2.5 kg), have special nutritional needs which vary according to the infant's maturity and any medical complications that are present at birth or develop subsequently. The terms used to classify preterm and low-birthweight infants are defined in Table 4.4.1.

Nutritional Requirements

The energy and nutrient requirements for any infant are calculated based on their body weight in kilograms and the need to support energy expenditure and growth. As preterm infants have not accumulated the body stores of nutrients that term infants accumulate during the third trimester of pregnancy, they have higher nutrient needs per kilogram of body weight than term infants. Adequate protein and energy are required for growth. An optimal protein:energy ratio is at least 3 g protein/kg for every 100 kcal/kg.

The nutritional requirements of preterm infants are compared with those of term infants in Table 4.4.2.

Recent enteral nutrition guidelines for the neonate have been published by the European Society of Paediatric Gastroenterology, Hepatology and Nutrition (ESPGHAN) in 2010 (ESPGHAN

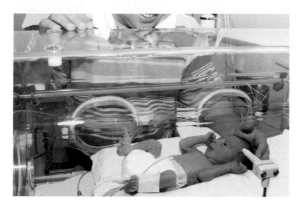

Figure 4.4.1 Preterm infant in an incubator

Committee on Nutrition 2010), which provides recommendations for 1000–1800 g preterm infants. These guidelines differ from those described in Table 4.4.2 in that they recommend higher protein and vitamin D intakes.

Feeding Routes for Preterm Infants in the Neonatal Unit

The feeding route or routes used for preterm infants will depend on gestation, size and condition at birth (Table 4.4.3). Where possible, all infants will receive enteral nutrition as soon as clinically indicated.

Table 4.4.1 Classification of preterm and low-birthweight infants

Preterm	Born before 37 weeks gestation
Low birthweight (LBW)	Birthweight: 1500–2500 g
Very low birthweight (VLBW)	Birthweight: 1000–1500 g
Extremely low birthweight (ELBW)	Birthweight: <1000 g
Small for gestational age (SGA)	Birthweight below the 9th centile for gestational age. Can result from a number of causes such as infection and genetic reasons
Intrauterine growth restriction (IUGR)	Born with a low weight but may show normal head and length growth depending on how long there has been a placental deficiency. Often at high risk of feeding problems as there may have been redirection of blood flow from the gut to brain and other organs

Table 4.4.2 Comparison of daily nutritional requirements of term infants with preterm infants feeding orally or enterally

	Term	Low birthweight and very low birthweight	Extremely low birthweight
Fluid (mL/kg)	150	150–220	150–220
Energy (kcal/kg)	96	110–130	130–150
Protein (g/kg)	2.1	3.4–4.2	3.8–4.4
Sodium (mg/kg)	35	69–115	69–115
Potassium (mg/kg)	133	78–177	78–177

From Tsang et al. (2005).

Table 4.4.3 Feeding routes for preterm infants

	Route	Feeds used	
Parenteral nutrition	Administered directly into the bloodstream usually via peripherally sited central venous access	A sterile complete feed delivered as an aqueous solution with a standardized composition of dextrose, amino acids, electrolytes, vitamins and minerals. Alongside this, a lipid solution containing fat-soluble vitamins is also infused	Infants who are born at <1000 g, and some <1500 g Some intrauterine growth restriction infants
Enteral nutrition	Milk feed via a nasogastric (NG) tube (from nose to stomach) or an orogastric tube (mouth to stomach)	In order of preference: Expressed breast milk (EBM) Banked expressed breast milk (BEBM) Breast milk fortifiers may be added to either EBM or BEBM Preterm formula	Begin as soon as clinically indicated as trophic feeding (minimal enteral feeding) and increase as tolerated
Breastfeeding	Oral feeding direct from the mother's breast	Breast milk	Can begin when infant starts to coordinate suck, swallow and breathing for short periods
Bottlefeeding	Oral feeding using sterilized bottles and teats	Expressed breast milk Preterm formula Nutrient-enriched post-discharge formula	

Parenteral nutrition (Figure 4.4.2)

Parenteral nutrition has been used in neonatal units for many decades to feed infants born too early to tolerate an adequate amount of enteral feeds. It is now common practice on neonatal units. There is no consensus on which babies should receive parenteral nutrition but it is mainly used for the following groups of infants:

- those with a birthweight less than 1250 g, as studies have shown that they can take up to four weeks to establish full enteral feeds
- infants <30 weeks gestation
- where there is a non-functioning gastrointestinal system either pre or post operation
- those with short bowel syndrome.

Some parenteral nutritional requirements are lower than those for enteral and oral nutrition because absorption across the gut wall is not complete. Most stable preterm infants on a neonatal unit will have nutrient requirements for growth as described in Table 4.4.4 (Tsang *et al.* 2005, ESPGHAN Committee on Nutrition 2010).

Enteral nutrition

Enteral nutrition is used for infants with:

- immature suck/swallow
- mechanical ventilation with an endotracheal tube in place preventing oral feeding
- limited oral intake that is less than adequate and requires top-up of feeds via a nasogastric or orogastric tube (see Figure 4.4.2).

The route of the tube will depend on how the baby is receiving ventilation or oxygen support.

Trophic feeds or minimal enteral feeding

Trophic feeds or minimal enteral feeding is often used in neonatal units, especially for the smallest

Table 4.4.4 Daily nutritional requirements via parenteral or enteral nutrition

	Parenteral nutrition	Enteral nutrition for infants 1–1.8 kg
Fluids (mL/kg)	150–220	135–200
Energy (kcal/kg)	90–100	110–135
Protein (g protein/kg)	3.2–3.8	3.5–4.0
Sodium (mg/kg)	69–115	69–115
Potassium (mg/kg)	78–177	66–132
Calcium (mg/kg)	60–80	120–140
Phosphorus (mg/kg)	45–60	60–90
Magnesium (mg/kg)	4.3–7.2	8–15
Iron (µg/kg)	100–120	2000–3000
Vitamin A (µgRE/kg)	210–450	40–100
Vitamin D (IU)	800–1000	150–400
Vitamin E (mg/kg)	2.8–3.5	2.2–11
Vitamin K (µg/kg)	10	4.4–28
Thiamine (µg/kg)	200–350	140–300
Riboflavin (µg/kg)	150–200	200–400

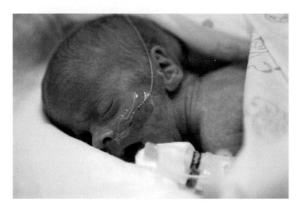

Figure 4.4.2 A young baby with a nasogastric tube

sickest infants on parenteral nutrition. Very small amounts of feed of ≤24 mL feed/kg per day are given. Meanwhile parenteral nutrition provides all the nutrition for the infants.

The benefits of trophic feeding include:

- gut priming
- a reduced dependence on parenteral nutrition as there is a more rapid tolerance to enteral feeds
- lower peak bilirubin and alkaline phosphatase levels
- enhanced gut motility
- increased lactase activity
- less hyperglycaemia
- reduced rate of sepsis.

Maternal breast milk is the first choice for trophic feeding but where this is unavailable and the infant is thought to be at risk of developing necrotizing enterocolitis, donor breast milk may be used if available. If neither source of breast milk is available, a preterm formula milk (discussed below) can be used.

Increasing enteral feeds will commence once clinicians are confident that the infant is tolerating trophic feeds. There is no consensus on the best way to advance feeds but there is evidence that the use of standardized feeding regimens on the neonatal unit can help prevent necrotizing enterocolitis.

Breast Milk

The health benefits of breast milk for term infants also apply to preterm infants and are described in Chapter 4.1. Additional specific benefits for preterm infants include:

- reduced incidence of necrotizing enterocolitis
- reduced incidence of sepsis
- improved neurodevelopmental outcomes
- associated with later improved bone mineralization.

Breast milk is also better tolerated than formula milk so can reduce the duration of parenteral nutrition.

These benefits are dose-dependent so the more breast milk an infant receives the greater the benefit to them.

Expressing breast milk for preterm infants

Until their infant is old enough or well enough to feed directly from the breast, in order to supply breast milk mothers must express their milk. This has benefits for both mother and child. Mothers often say that it is the one thing they can do for their preterm infant in an intensive medical environment where skilled staff do most of the care for their infant. It also helps bonding and attachment between mother and infant.

Mothers of even the most preterm infants are able to provide all or some of the milk needed by their baby to grow and develop (Bonet *et al.* 2011). When infants are born extremely prematurely, breast development will be at an earlier stage than those of the mothers of term infants. Compensatory breast growth can be achieved by efficient early and frequent milk removal by expressing. When mothers have given birth before 28 weeks gestation, expressing their milk about 10–12 times in 24 hours for the first 2 weeks supports catch-up growth of the breast and effective initiation of lactation.

Ideally, mothers should initiate expressing within 6 hours after delivery. Initially, hand expression will provide the first few drops of colostrum. After 2–3 days, as maternal milk increases in volume, mothers can move to electric pumping to express their breast milk. A trained member of staff should ensure that mothers have the correctly fitting equipment and should show them how to use the pump.

Maintaining lactation through expression for an infant born prematurely can be a long and tough process, so mothers need good, consistent advice and support from the outset. The following tips may help them through the process:

- Prepare the breast through gentle massage before beginning to express.
- Hand expression can be useful before pump expressing or breastfeeding to initiate milk flow.
- Express regularly: a minimum 8–10 times per day.
- Don't leave the gap between expression longer than six hours.
- Express once at night – preferably between 2 and 4 am.
- Ensure the breast is fully emptied before stopping expressing.
- Make sure you are fully confident about using the breast pump.
- Check the funnel size as they come in different sizes and can cause trauma if not fitting correctly.
- Where possible double pump from both breasts at the same time.
- Engage in regular skin-to-skin contact (e.g. kangaroo care).
- Sensory stimulation encourages oxytocin hormone levels and the let-down reflex. This may be by expressing beside the infant's cot or expressing with a picture of the infant and/or toys/muslin cloths with the infant's smell.

Evidence suggests that mothers should be encouraged to express 750–1000 mL of breast milk in 24 hours by 2 weeks post delivery in order to enable them to maintain long-term lactation. Once lactation has been established, some mothers may be able to express less frequently to achieve this volume. The volume produced at each expression depends on the glandular tissue content of the breasts, which varies from mother to mother. Some mothers can therefore produce larger volumes than others at each expression.

Nutrient content of preterm breast milk

Preterm breast milk, like term breast milk, starts out as colostrum rich in protein and immunoglobins specifically designed to help protect the preterm infant from infection. After 2–3 days the milk goes through a transitional phase for about 15 days and then becomes mature milk.

The composition varies during the course of an expression/feed and also depends on:

- time since birth
- the time of the day
- expressing technique
- how much the milk is handled after expressing.

Energy

As the transitional and mature milks increase in fat and energy throughout the feed, mothers are encouraged to 'empty' both breasts each time they express to include the high-fat, high-energy content at the end of the feed.

Protein

The maternal protein is of a higher bioavailability compared to formula milk and so is better absorbed by the preterm infant. The protein content is higher at 1.8 g/100 mL in the transitional milk from the mothers whose infants were born 31 weeks gestation. It then falls to about 1.3 g/100 mL in mature milk – similar to that of mature milk in mothers of term infants. The higher content in transitional milk promotes better growth.

Calcium and phosphorus

These are also better absorbed from breast milk than from formula milk. However, phosphorus can become a limiting nutrient for bone development and is therefore always given to the infant as a supplement.

Vitamin and iron

The vitamin and iron content of breast milk is lower than preterm requirements so preterm infants feeding only on breast milk need a vitamin supplement once on full enteral feeds and then an iron supplement from around 4 weeks of life. Local policies for supplementation can vary.

Most infants less than 1500 g grow satisfactorily on maternal breast milk and vitamin supplements for the first weeks of life, however, some may need additional phosphorus and sodium. Beyond this, many will require additional protein as the breast milk levels decrease over time.

Breast milk fortifiers

Breast milk fortifiers may be added to expressed breast milk in the neonatal unit if the infant is not gaining sufficient weight on breast milk alone. These are powdered supplements which are added to the maternal breast milk to increase the nutrient and energy content to aid growth. They contain protein, sodium, potassium, calcium and phosphate, trace minerals and vitamins, but in the UK provide no iron.

Infants on breast milk fortifier require iron as a separate supplement and some neonatal units also give an extra vitamin supplement.

There is no consensus on the stage at which to add breast milk fortifiers, however, they are probably not required in early breast milk while the protein level is high.

There are also no current recommendations on when breast milk fortifiers should be added to expressed breast milk. Manufacturers recommend that they can be added to each batch of milk feeds for the next 24 hours. Local policies vary but ideally they should be added to the breast milk just prior to feeding if possible.

Most units use multicomponent breast milk fortifiers but single components are available. Disadvantages to adding protein, phosphorus, sodium, calcium and trace elements all separately include a higher risk of contamination, unacceptably high osmolarity and poor use of nursing time.

Breast milk fortifiers are usually discontinued before discharge from the neonatal unit.

Oral Feeding

Feeding development in the preterm infant is individual and dependent on many factors, including gestation and size at birth, the medical condition and history of the baby.

Breastfeeding

With appropriate support preterm infants may be able to start breastfeeding attempts from as early as

28 weeks gestation as an extension of 'kangaroo care', but they are unlikely to achieve full nutritive breastfeeding until around 36 weeks gestation.

Kangaroo care (Figure 4.4.3) involves the infant being secured against the mother's skin – usually on her chest between her breasts. This maintains the infant's body heat and the benefits for the infant include reduced morbidity and mortality.

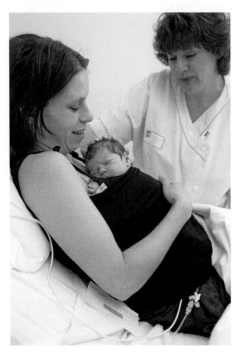

Figure 4.4.3 A baby being held in kangaroo care

As breastfeeding development is reliant on the mother and infant dyad, every effort should be made to enable mothers to be with their infant as much as possible. A general overview of breastfeeding progression is summarized in Table 4.4.5.

Patience, practice and persistence are needed in the transition from tube feeding to breastfeeding. Ongoing practical and emotional support from staff trained in breastfeeding care is needed. They can observe and support breastfeeding attempts and help mothers to:

- understand normal feeding behaviours of preterm infants
- understand the development to effective attachment and positioning on the breast and sucking behaviours
- assess success and progress of their infant's breastfeeding.

Physiological benefits for preterm infants of breastfeeding rather than bottlefeeding include:

- improved temperature control
- improved oxygen saturations
- improved suck swallow breathe coordination.

There is some evidence that breastfeeding facilitates earlier discharge from neonatal units than bottlefeeding (Altman *et al.* 2009). Bottlefeeding may interfere with the development of breastfeeding if introduced before breastfeeding is fully established.

Bottlefeeding

If a mother chooses not to breastfeed, preterm infants can start attempting bottlefeeding once the infant is old enough and well enough to coordinate suck, swallow and breathing; this is usually around 34 weeks gestation.

Table 4.4.5 Overview of breastfeeding progression in preterm infants

Gestational age	Breastfeeding skills of preterm infants
Less than 30 weeks	Smell, open mouth, protrude tongue, dribble saliva, lick milk from the nipple, take some breast tissue into the mouth, and make a few weak sucks
30–32 weeks	Attach to the breast and may make some weak to strong sucks with long pauses in between
32 weeks and over	Root, organize sucking bursts with long pauses, take part of a feed from the breast and as he or she becomes older may take one to all complete feeds from the breast
36 weeks and over	Breastfeed in a well-coordinated way

From Lang (2002).

Preterm infants often need slow milk flow teats, supportive positioning and careful monitoring to achieve safe and efficient feeding, especially if their breathing and bottlefeeding are less well coordinated. Parents will therefore need support to feed safely and effectively. As they progress, bottlefed infants can be fed according to their hunger cues as for term infants.

Formula Milks for Preterm Infants

There are two types of formula used on neonatal units for preterm infants. They are summarized in Table 4.4.6.

1. Preterm formulas

Preterm formulas are for supervised hospital use only and only available in a sterile, ready-to-feed format. They have been designed to meet the nutritional requirements of preterm infants providing:

- adequate energy and protein levels with a protein-to-energy ratio to optimize growth
- phosphate and calcium levels at the optimum ratio for bone mineralization
- required vitamin, mineral and iron content.

Preterm formulas are usually given to infants who are <2 kg at birth.

There are three brands available but most neonatal units usually just stock one brand.

2. Nutrient-enriched post-discharge formula

Nutrient-enriched post-discharge formula may be given to preterm infants still in hospital who have been on a preterm formula and have reached 2–2.5 kg. They contain less energy and protein than preterm formulas but are higher in energy, protein, vitamins and minerals, especially calcium and phosphorus and iron, than standard formulas for term infants. They are used to support the higher nutritional requirements for catch-up growth in preterm infants once they have been discharged home.

They are available both as:

- sterile ready-to-feed and
- non-sterile powder that must be reconstituted with boiled water.

There are two brands available.

After Discharge Home from the Neonatal Unit

Once discharged home there is no consensus on the optimal nutritional requirements for a preterm infant. Some preterm infants may go home with some nutritional deficits but most will demand feed orally and should be allowed to 'catch up' any growth deficit in their own time. Their nutritional intake and growth should be regularly assessed and monitored.

Breastfed infants require additional vitamin and iron supplements, as directed by the consultant paediatrician or dietitian.

Table 4.4.6 Types of formula milk available for preterm infants

Type of formula milk	Examples	Manufacturer	Relevant compositional details	Used for infants with:
Preterm formula	Aptamil Preterm	Milupa	Higher in energy and nutrients than term formulas and nutrient-enriched post-discharge formulas	Preterm or low-birthweight infants in hospital
	Nutriprem 1	Cow & Gate		
	SMA Gold Prem 1	SMA Nutrition		
Nutrient-enriched post-discharge formulas	Nutriprem 2	Cow & Gate	Higher in nutrients than term – particularly vitamin D and iron	Discharged preterm and low-birthweight infants
	SMA Gold Prem 2	SMA Nutrition		

Formula-fed infants do not usually require extra supplements as the nutrient-enriched post-discharge formula is fortified with all nutrients. It is usually prescribed until 6 months after the infant's expected date of delivery or until adequate catch-up growth has been achieved. However, the evidence for benefit beyond three months after their expected date of delivery is limited (Young *et al.* 2012).

Some neonatal units recommend that the sterile ready-to-feed formula should be used until 4 weeks corrected age to reduce the risk of food-borne infections. After this infants can be switched onto the cheaper powdered formula. Preparation and storage recommendations for these formula milks are the same as for standard formulas for term infants.

Weaning Preterm Infants

The time to begin weaning a preterm infant may be a clinical decision made by the paediatrician. Preterm infants have high nutritional needs that are unlikely to be satisfied from milk alone for the 4–6 months after their estimated date of delivery. Current recommendations are that weaning should begin at an earlier post-conception age than for term infants. It is usually between 5 and 8 months old – the age from the preterm infant's actual birth date and not based on their corrected age (King 2009, King and Aloysius 2009).

As the infant's gut is being used for milk feeds from an earlier gestational age, it matures earlier and will have adapted to cope with solid foods.

Some preterm infants will not have good head control when it is time to begin weaning and parents need to be advised to make sure the head and neck are well supported during feeding, as seen in Figure 4.4.4.

Weaning should then progress as for term babies, introducing new textures to give infants the opportunity to learn to manage them in their mouth. Preterm babies are more likely to have feeding problems than term babies.

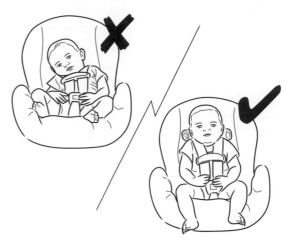

Figure 4.4.4 Safe positioning for weaning pre-term infants

Activity 1

Calculate the fluid, energy and nutrient requirements of a preterm baby weighing 1.8 kg and being fed by a nasogastric tube. Compare this to the nutrients provided in a suitable volume of expressed breast milk and a nutrient-enriched post-discharge formula. The compositional details of the formula milk can be found on the company website.

Activity 2

If a baby is born at 27 weeks gestation, between which post-EDD (expected date of delivery) ages would you consider beginning weaning?

Acknowledgements

With thanks to Caroline King, Specialist Neonatal Dietitian, Hammersmith Hospital, London, and Karen Hayes, Neonatal Dietitian, Addenbrooke's Hospital, Cambridge.

References and further reading

Altman M, Vanpée M, Cnattingius S and Norman M (2009) Moderately preterm infants and determinants of length of hospital stay. *Archives of Disease in Childhood; Fetal Neonatal Edition* **94**(6): F414–F418.

Bonet M, Blondel B, Agostino R, *et al.*; MOSAIC research group (2011) Variations in breastfeeding rates for very preterm infants between regions and neonatal units in Europe: results from the MOSAIC cohort. *Archives of Disease in Childhood; Fetal Neonatal Edition* **96**(6): F450–F452.

Dorling J (2005) Feeding growth restricted preterm infants with abnormal antenatal Doppler results. *Archives of Disease in Childhood; Fetal Neonatal Edition* **90**: F359–F363.

ESPGHAN Committee on Nutrition (2010) Enteral nutrition supply for preterm infants: Commentary from the European Society for Paediatric Gastroenterology, Hepatology, and Nutrition Committee on Nutrition. *Journal of Paediatric Gastroenterology and Nutrition* **50**: 1–9.

King C (2005) Human milk for preterm infants – when and how to fortify. *Nutrition* **1**(2): 14–17.

King CL (2009) An evidence based guide to weaning preterm infants. *Paediatrics and Child Health* **19**(9): 405–414.

King CL and Aloysius A (2009) Joint consensus statement on weaning preterm infants. **http://bapm.org/nutrition/guidelines.php**

King C and Jones E (2005) *Feeding and Nutrition in the Preterm Infant*. Edinburgh: Elsevier Churchill Livingstone.

Klingenberg C, Embleton ND, Jacobs SE, O'Connell LAF and Kuschel CA (2011) Enteral feeding practices in very preterm infants: an international survey. *Archives of Disease in Childhood; Fetal Neonatal Edition* **97**: F56–F61.

Lang S (2002) The position and attachment of the baby at the breast. In: *Breastfeeding Special Care Babies*. Oxford: Elsevier, p. 31.

Tsang RC, Uauy R, Koletzko B, *et al.* (2005) *Nutrition of the Preterm Infant: Scientific basis and practical guidelines*, 2nd edn. Cincinnati, OH: Digital Educational Publishing, 2005.

Turck D and Weaver LT (2006) Feeding preterm infants after hospital discharge: A commentary by the ESPGHAN Committee on Nutrition. *Journal of Pediatric Gastroenterology and Nutrition* **42**: 596–603.

Young L, Morgan J, McCormick FM and McGuire W (2012) Nutrient-enriched formula versus standard term formula for preterm infants following hospital discharge. *Cochrane Database Systematic Reviews* **3**: CD004696.

Resources

BLISS – Breastfeeding your premature baby (**www.bliss.org.uk**)

British Association of Perinatal Medicine (**www.bapm.org**)

Neonatal Dietitians Interest Group (**www.bapm.org/nutrition/**)

Section 5
Preschool Children: 1–4 Years

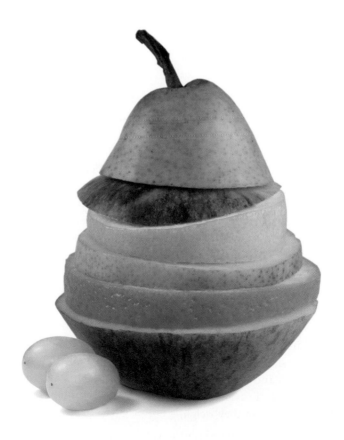

5.1

Preschool Children 1–4 Years

Summary

- 1–4 year olds need a balanced diet based on a combination of foods from the five food groups along with a supplement of vitamins A and D.

- A daily meal and snack routine of 3 meals and 2–3 planned nutritious snacks will provide adequate calories and nutrients and prevent toddlers becoming over hungry or too tired to eat.

- Toddlers' appetites vary from day to day and they should be allowed to eat to their appetite and finish eating when they have had enough.

- Snacks given should always be nutritious snacks as toddlers are unlikely to eat an adequate amount of nutrients in just three meals.

- High-calorie low-nutrient foods should be limited to small quantities and offered as part of a meal.

- Teeth of under-fives are vulnerable to dental decay and sugary and acidic foods should be limited to four occasions per day (e.g. three meals and one snack).

This age group should be offered nutritious family foods and included in as many family meals as possible. Younger toddlers usually need their food cut up for them for some time and some continue to need help with feeding as they may not be able to feed themselves fast enough to satisfy their hunger. However, self-feeding should continue to be encouraged until they can manage by themselves. Finger foods make self-feeding easier for this age group.

Achieving Nutrient and Calorie Requirements

Toddlers and preschool children have high nutrient requirements relative to their size as they are still undergoing quite rapid growth and development and are usually very physically active. They need about 70 kcalories for every kilogram they weigh,

whereas adults only need about a half of this – that is about 30–35 kcalories for every kilogram they weigh.

Toddlers also need larger amounts of most nutrients per kilogram of their body weight than adults. As toddlers' stomachs are quite small they need very nutritious foods at all meals and snacks to ensure a good intake of nutrients. A routine of two or three planned nutritious snacks in addition to three meals each day will help to give them all the calories and nutrients they need in food portions that they can manage comfortably.

Toddlers fed only on the low-fat, high-fibre foods which are recommended for a healthy balanced diet for older children and adults may include too many high-fibre foods that can make this age group feel full and could reduce the amount of food – and therefore energy and nutrients – that is eaten.

Combining the food groups

A balanced nutritious diet for 1–4 year olds is based on the five food groups as discussed in Chapter 1.2. However, this can be more challenging than in older children. Even children 1–4 years old eating well may not consume enough vitamin A and a supplement of vitamin A and D is recommended for under-fives (see page 136).

Food group 1: Bread, rice, potatoes, pasta and other starchy foods

This group provides a good source of energy. It is also a good source of fibre, but under-fives should be offered a mixture of both wholegrain and refined bread and cereals (e.g. white and wholemeal bread and white and brown rice). Too much fibre in younger children can be very filling and fibre binds with certain minerals, thereby reducing their absorption. Wholegrains can be slowly increased for those with constipation, or decreased if they cause a tendency towards diarrhoea.

Food group 2: Fruit and vegetables

This is the food group some young children have most trouble eating, particularly vegetables with a bitter taste. Offering them at every meal is important, even though they may be refused, to teach under-fives that fruit and vegetables are a normal part of each meal. Seeing others, particularly their parents, eating and enjoying them is a powerful encouragement for under-fives to taste and then, with time, learn to like them. Small portions should be offered and more can be given when children request it.

Food group 3: Milk, cheese and yogurt

This food group involves the biggest change from feeding during infancy. Children from 1 year of age will obtain adequate calcium from just three servings of these foods each day. A serving for children 1–4 years old is:

- 1 cup of milk (120 mL)
- cheese in a sandwich or sauce, or on pasta or pizza
- a small pot of yogurt (about 120 g).

These foods are very low in iron and need to be limited to an average of three servings a day to ensure they do not replace iron-containing foods of the food groups 1, 2 and 4.

Bottles of milk should have been discontinued around a child's first birthday. Children who drink excess milk for comfort will be filling up on this at the expense of eating more iron-rich foods and will be at risk of iron-deficiency anaemia. If no yogurt or cheese is eaten then three cups of milk a day, about 350 mL in total, is adequate.

Full-fat cow's milk is higher in vitamin A than low-fat milks and is given until a child is at least 2 years old. Semi-skimmed milk can be introduced from this age providing the toddler eats a wide variety of foods. However, full-fat milk can continue to be given and will provide more vitamin A than semi-skimmed milk. Skimmed milk is not suitable as the main drink for children under 5 years of age as it contains very little vitamin A.

Follow-on or toddler milks may be used for milk drinks in place of cow's milk to provide extra nutrients for toddlers who eat poorly. They provide the same range of nutrients as cow's milk but in addition they are fortified with iron and higher levels of zinc and some vitamins. The disadvantage is that they are more expensive than cow's milk.

Food group 4: Meat, fish, eggs, nuts and pulses

This food group is the richest source of iron and under-fives have high iron requirements. A significant number become anaemic from not having enough food from this group (see Chapter 5.2).

Chicken is a popular texture in this group and darker meat from the thigh and leg provide more iron.

Toddlers often reject hard, chewy red meats and prefer softer cuts and minced meat in burgers, meatballs, meat loaf and sausages. When good-quality products with a high lean meat content are used, adequate iron will be provided. Liver, if offered, should be limited to one small serving per week because of the high levels of vitamin A.

Fish in fishcake and fish pies are popular alternatives to fried fish products such as fish fingers. The Food Standards Agency advises that:

- Oily fish should be limited for girls to two servings per week as these fish can contain dioxins and polychlorinated biphenyls. Girls can retain an excess of these chemicals into their childbearing years. Boys may have up to four servings per week.
- Swordfish, marlin and shark should not be given to under-fives because of their mercury content.

Pulses include baked beans, kidney beans, other starchy beans, chickpeas, hummus, lentils and dhal.

Ground and chopped nuts and nut butters can be offered but whole nuts should not be given as they can cause choking or severe lung inflammation if inhaled.

Food group 5: Foods and drinks high in fat and/or sugar

These energy-dense foods should be limited to small amounts and not given in place of foods from the other four more nutritious food groups. However, a sweet nutritious pudding can be given as the second course at both main meals. A nutritious pudding is one that contains one or more of the following: milk, fruit, eggs, flour and ground or chopped nuts. Food and drinks sweetened with sugar should be limited to four times per day to reduce the risk of dental decay – that could be the three meals and one snack per day.

Recommended Vitamin Supplementation for 1–4 Year Olds

The Department of Health recommends that all young children are given a vitamin supplement containing vitamins A and D as they have high requirements for these two vitamins. Food is not the main source of vitamin D and many under-fives do not eat enough food containing vitamin A (see below).

Suitable supplements are available over the counter in most pharmacies. The Healthy Start children's vitamin drops are the least expensive but they are not widely available. Healthy Start beneficiaries are entitled to them free but must access them via their NHS Trust which may not be convenient. They are not sold in retail pharmacies or supermarkets.

Under-fives who may need a supplement with a wider range of vitamins and minerals include:

- persistent poor eaters
- children who eat a very limited number of foods
- those on restricted diets by choice
- vegans
- children on restricted diets because of food allergy or intolerance.

A dietitian can advise on a supplement for these children after assessing which nutrients are inadequate in their diet.

NHS Healthy Start children's vitamin drops contain the following amounts of vitamins in a daily dose of 5 drops:

- 233 µg vitamin A
- 20 mg vitamin C
- 7.5 µg vitamin D3.

Portion Sizes for Children 1–4 Years

There are no specific portion sizes of food for under-fives as there is a wide variation in the quantities eaten by this age group. It varies from one meal to another, one day to another and depends on how active the child is and whether they like the food or not. The portion size ranges listed in Table 5.1.1 give parents and carers an idea of the quantities to offer. If preschool children are eating amounts within these ranges then parents can be reassured that they are eating an adequately nutritious diet.

The foods in group 5 should always be limited to small portion sizes and should not be offered in place of foods from the other more nutritious food groups.

Table 5.1.1 Portion size ranges recommended for children aged 1–4 years

Food groups	Portion size
Group 1: Bread, rice potatoes, pasta and other starchy foods	½–1 slice wholegrain or white bread, muffin, roll or chapatti
	3–6 heaped tbsp breakfast cereals
	5–8 tbsp of hot cereals like porridge made up with milk
	2–5 tbsp of rice or pasta
	½–1½ egg-sized potatoes or 1–4 tbsp of mashed potato
	½–2 crispbreads or 1–3 crackers
Group 2: Fruit and vegetables	¼–½ apple, orange, pear, banana
	3–10 small berries or grapes
	2–4 tbsp freshly cooked, stewed or mashed fruit
	1–2 tbsp raw or cooked vegetables
Group 3: Milk, cheese and yogurt	100–120 mL whole cow's milk as a drink
	1 small pot (125 mL) yogurt or fromage frais
	2–4 tbsp grated cheese
	Cheese in a sandwich or on a piece of pizza
	4–6 tbsp custard or a milk pudding
Group 4: Meat, fish, eggs, nuts and pulses	2–4 tbsp ground, chopped or cubed lean meat, fish or poultry
	½–1 whole egg
	2–4 tbsp whole or mashed pulses (peas, beans, lentils, hummus, dhal)
	½–1 tbsp peanut butter or 1–2 tbsp ground nuts
Group 5: Foods high in fat and sugar	½–1 digestive biscuit or 1–2 small biscuits
	1 small slice cake
	1 tsp butter, mayonnaise or oil
	1 tsp jam, honey or sugar
	3–4 crisps or 2–4 sweets
	1 small fun-sized chocolate bar

The measures used are 1 tbsp – one 15 mL tablespoon and 1 tsp – one 5 mL teaspoon. These are the spoons found within a set of spoons for standard recipe measures.

Drinks

Children should be offered 6–8 drinks of 100–120 mL per day to provide adequate fluid. They may need more drinks in very hot weather or after extra physical activity as young children can dehydrate quite quickly.

Water and milk are the safest drinks to offer between meals as they do not cause tooth erosion or increase the risk of dental decay. Up to three drinks per day can be milk (see above).

Pure fruit juices do provide nutrients from fruit but they contain large amounts of the fruit sugar, fructose, and they are acidic. Both this sugar and acid can cause dental decay. To lower the acid and sugar content fruit juices should be given diluted to under-fives – by only giving them at mealtimes the risk of dental decay is lowered.

Fizzy drinks and squashes containing added sugar are not necessary in a young child's diet as they add calories without providing nutrients and can contribute to dental caries and obesity.

'No added sugar' drinks may contain natural sugars and/or acids and can therefore still contribute to tooth decay. These include 'baby' juices, natural fruit juices, fruit juice drinks and sugar-free squashes and fizzy drinks.

Tea and coffee are not recommended for young children because the tannins and polyphenols in them bind with iron, reducing the availability of iron to the body. They also contain caffeine.

Children sucking drinks from bottles or cups with teats or valved spouts have the sugar and acid in contact with the teeth for longer. Hence sweet and/or acidic drinks, if offered, should be given in open cups or glasses or those with free-flowing spouts that require the toddler to sip, not suck.

Meal and Snack Routines

With their small stomachs but high energy and nutrient needs, it is preferable to offer toddlers nutritious food about 5 or 6 times a day – that is 3 meals and 2–3 nutritious planned snacks. They would not satisfy their calorie and nutrient requirements with just three meals if they eat small meals. Ideally, a daily routine is planned with meals and snacks at regular times evenly spaced throughout the day around any daytime sleeps.

A daily meal and snack routine:

- prevents toddlers becoming over hungry or thirsty by going too long between eating occasions

- avoids attempts to feed toddlers when they are ready to sleep and too tired to eat

- prevents grazing on less nutritious food throughout the day

- prevents toddlers not being hungry at mealtimes because they have just eaten snacks or had large sweet drinks just before the meal.

If a child has not eaten well at a meal a parent can be reassured that it will only be about two or three hours before another nutritious meal or snack will be offered. If a toddler does not eat well at a meal parents often give snacks or an extra milk drink just to make sure the toddler has at least eaten something. However, toddlers often prefer the snack foods given at these times and may refuse to eat meals in order to have the snack or drink that they prefer.

At meal and snack times:

- children should be sitting comfortably with their feet on the floor or supported on a foot rest

- offer finger foods often to make self-feeding easier

- if used, give cutlery and utensils that are appropriate to the child's age and feeding skills

- toddlers up to about 3 years may still need help to eat

- offer small portions as more can be offered if the first portion is finished quickly

- accept mess as a normal part of the feeding process

- avoid distractions like the TV and games so that toddlers can concentrate on eating and drinking.

Ideally, two courses should be offered at each main meal – a savoury course followed by fruit or a small nutritious pudding. This provides a wider range of nutrients to be eaten and makes the mealtime more of an occasion. The second course should not be used as a bribe or reward for eating the first course.

A positive eating environment helps toddlers to enjoy mealtimes, stay engaged and eat well. Elements of a positive eating environment include:

- making mealtimes happy, social occasions with parents or carers eating with the children

- making eye contact and interacting with the children in a positive way

- making positive comments about the food being offered

- allowing plenty of time for the meal to ensure children are not rushed, but ensuring it is not prolonged beyond about 30 minutes

- allowing children to decide when they have eaten enough. When parents accept that decision and do not try to coerce them to eat more, mealtime battles are not set up and children become more confident in their perception of satiety.

Young children indicate they have had enough to eat by:

- saying 'no' when offered or encouraged to eat more food

- keeping their mouth shut

- turning their head away from food being offered

- putting their hand in front of their mouth

- holding food in the mouth without swallowing it

- crying, shouting or screaming when food is offered

- trying to get out of the chair or away from the table

- vomiting or spitting food out.

When a meal is a positive experience it becomes an opportunity for toddlers to learn good social skills and behaviours associated with eating and drinking (e.g. chatting to other children and adults, developing good table manners, offering and sharing food, learning to respect others).

Meal Plans

The following menus use seasonal food and incorporate a mixture of finger foods and foods requiring a spoon and fork.

Meal plan for spring

		Day 1	Day 2	Day 3
Breakfast		Porridge with dried fruit and milk	Poached egg with toast fingers Kiwi fruit slices	Toasted hot cross bun and slices of pear
	Drink	Milk	Water	Hot chocolate to drink
Midday meal	1st course	Chicken nuggets with new potatoes and purple sprouting broccoli	Salmon fish fingers with pasta pieces Spinach and radish salad	Roast lamb Potato wedges Broccoli florets
	2nd course	Chocolate almond cake with orange segments	Rhubarb crumble with custard	Yogurt and stoned cherries
	Drink	Water	Water	Water
Evening meal	1st course	Hummus and baby spinach sandwich	Baked beans on toast with carrot sticks	Cheese omelette with asparagus spears
	2nd course	Fruit salad and yogurt	Mini muffin and apple slices	Lemon tart with banana slices and ice cream
	Drink	Water	Water	Water

Meal plan for summer

		Day 1	Day 2	Day 3
Breakfast		Muesli with milk and blueberries	Pancake with strawberries	Breakfast wheat biscuit with milk and peach slices
	Drink	Water	Glass of milk	Glass of diluted fruit juice
Midday meal	1st course	Cold chicken pieces with rice salad and fresh peas	Mini lamb burger New potatoes and cherry tomatoes	Tuna pasta Green beans Carrot sticks
	2nd course	Gooseberry fool	Summer pudding with fresh berries and fromage frais	Strawberries and ice cream
	Drink	Water	Water	Water
Evening meal	1st course	Tomato omelette with toast fingers and sliced peppers	Breadsticks with hummus dip and cucumber slices	Ham sandwich with cucumber and courgette sticks
	2nd course	Melon pieces and yogurt	Chocolate biscuit and nectarine slices	Drop scones with raspberries
	Drink	Water	Glass of diluted fruit juice	Water

Meal plan for autumn

		Day 1	Day 2	Day 3
Breakfast		Muesli with milk and blackberries	Boiled egg with toast fingers Grapes	Breakfast wheat biscuit with milk and sliced pears
	Drink	Milk	Glass of diluted fruit juice	Glass of diluted fruit juice
Midday meal	1st course	Chicken nuggets with stir-fried vegetables	Fish and potato cakes, roast butternut squash and parsnips	Mini meatballs Potato wedges Cauliflower florets
	2nd course	Apple crumble with custard	Cooked plums and fromage frais	Apple and blackberry compute with yogurt
	Drink	Water	Water	Water

Evening meal	1st course	Mushroom omelette Toast fingers and cherry tomatoes	Mini pizza topped with ham, tomato and diced peppers Carrot and cucumber sticks	Pasta and red pepper sauce with grated cheese
	2nd course	Chocolate cake and grapes	Mini muffin and plums	Fruit salad and shortbread
	Drink	Water	Water	Water

Meal plan for winter

		Day 1	Day 2	Day 3
Breakfast		Boiled egg with toast fingers Kiwi fruit slices	Porridge with dried apricots and yogurt	Breakfast wheat biscuit with milk Apple slices
	Drink	Water	Glass of diluted fruit juice	Water
Midday meal	1st course	Chicken and vegetable curry and rice	Fish and potato pie Stir-fried leeks	Slow cooked beef stew Potato and swede mash Cauliflower florets and brussels sprouts
	2nd course	Fromage frais and pear slices	Apple crumble and custard	Warm fruit salad with yogurt
	Drink	Water	Water	Water
Evening meal	1st course	Pasta and red pepper sauce with grated cheese	Toast fingers with chicken liver pâté Celery sticks	Butternut squash and lentil soup with a bread roll
	2nd course	Tangerine segments with chocolate biscuits	Slice date and walnut loaf	Drop scones with clementine segments
	Drink	Water	Glass of diluted fruit juice	Water

Nutrients at Risk

Key nutrients that are often low in the diets of under-fives are:

- iron
- vitamin D
- fibre.

The consequences of this are discussed in more detail in Chapter 5.2.

Vitamin A plays a key role in several systems: the immune system, vision, maintenance of skin, hair and membranes. Major sources of vitamin A in the diets of under-fives are meat, milk and carotene in fruits and vegetables and past dietary surveys showed that about 50 per cent of 1–4 year olds do not have an adequate intake of vitamin A (Gregory *et al.* 1995). Consequently the Department of Health recommends that some vitamin A is also provided in a supplement for under-fives (Department of Health 1994).

Vitamin C is usually adequate in the diets of UK toddlers but low-income families have the lowest intakes and for this reason vitamin C is included in the Healthy Start vitamin supplements that should be made available to low-income families qualifying for this scheme (see www.healthystart. nhs.uk).

Vegetarian and Vegan Diets

A vegetarian diet for preschool children needs careful planning to make sure that three servings of foods from food group 4 are offered each day to ensure adequate iron intake. Within each meal a high-vitamin C food will help the absorption of non-haem iron from vegetarian foods.

Meal plans for a vegetarian diet with high-iron and high-vitamin C foods

	Day 1	Day 2	Day 3
Breakfast	Boiled egg with toast fingers Banana slices Small glass of diluted orange juice	Baked beans on toast Small glass of diluted orange juice	Toddler muesli with added ground almonds and strawberries
Midday meal	Chick pea curry with courgette and cauliflower Rice Yogurt and strawberries	Dhal and rice Broccoli and carrot Rice pudding Mango slices	Pasta with lentils in bolognaise sauce Green beans Custard and fresh peaches
Evening meal	Tofu stir fry with noodles, cherry tomatoes and spinach Pancake with raspberries and ice cream	Cheese omelette with toast fingers Pepper slices and courgette sticks Pear slices and a muffin	Pitta bread with hummus Carrot and cucumber sticks Slices of kiwi fruit with a biscuit

Activity

Identify the high-iron and high-vitamin C foods within each of the meals above.

Vegan diets

Vegan diets are not recommended for young children as they are unlikely to provide all the energy and nutrients required in adequate amounts, particularly if the child is a faddy eater or has a small appetite. These children may not be able to eat enough vegan food, which is bulky and high in fibre, to obtain all the energy (calories) and nutrients they need for growth and development.

A child on a vegan diet should always be referred to a dietitian for assessment to ensure that the foods consumed by the child contain all the essential nutrients. Vegan mothers who are breastfeeding should also have their diets assessed as they may need a supplement of calcium, vitamins D and B12.

Dental Health

Under-fives are particularly vulnerable to dental decay (caries) which is the breakdown and wearing away of enamel. Dental care principles and tooth brushing discussed in Chapter 5.2 are particularly important for this age group. When any of the first teeth have to be extracted it increases the likelihood of overcrowding when the adult teeth come through.

Food Safety

Under-fives are still susceptible to food poisoning and can become very ill quickly so great care should be taken with food hygiene. Eggs, meat, fish and shellfish should all be well cooked.

Choking

Children under 3 years are more at risk from choking than older children, however, children above this age can also be at risk. As children get older, they put fewer non-edible items into their mouths but food risks are present at any age.

To minimize the risk:

● children should not run around or play while eating, and all mealtimes and snacks should be supervised
● young children should be seated and in a calm atmosphere when eating
● foods should be cut into small lengths rather than round pieces
● stones and pips should be removed
● soft round foods such as grapes and cherries should be cut into halves or quarters.

The foods frequently implicated in choking incidents are:

● sweets
● popcorn
● grapes and cherries
● hard fruit
● hard vegetables – especially peas, celery, carrots
● hot dogs/sausages
● burgers
● chunks of cheese
● meatballs
● whole nuts and seeds.

Faddy Eating, Selective Eating and Food Refusal

Young children do not eat well when they are:

● tired
● over hungry – they will just feel unhappy without realizing that if they eat they would feel better
● distracted by TV, games, new environment
● not feeling well – teething, sore throat, getting a cold
● anxious, worried, scared, rushed, sad.

In addition to these factors all toddlers go through a phase of becoming quite choosy about what they will and will not eat. It may be most noticeable around 18 months of age but it can begin any time in the second year. Toddlers may:

- eat less than expected
- refuse to taste new foods that are offered
- refuse to eat certain foods including some they have previously eaten well
- refuse to eat a food that looks slightly different to the food they are familiar with e.g. if a piece of apple has a mark on the skin, a yogurt is a different colour or in a different carton, or a biscuit is broken, not whole.

Food Neophobia

Becoming wary of trying new foods is a normal stage in their development and is called food neophobia because 'neophobia' means fear of new. It is more evident in some toddlers while hardly noticeable in others. Parents begin to notice it soon after toddlers have become independently mobile and are becoming more adept at investigating their environment. The fear of new foods is probably a survival mechanism to prevent mobile young toddlers from harming themselves through eating anything and everything: if they were to taste any interesting looking berry on a bush they could well poison themselves.

Once the neophobic stage begins toddlers may refuse to even try a taste of a new food they are not familiar with. They will take much longer to learn to like and eat new foods than during infancy.

Most toddlers will move through this stage in their own time if parents and carers follow some or all of the suggestions below:

- Offer a variety of foods and repeatedly introduce new foods from an early age to allow young children time to learn to accept different tastes and textures. It is the number of times they taste a food not the amount eaten that will determine how long it takes for them to learn to like a new food.

- Eat together as a family and make mealtimes happy, relaxed, social occasions. Parents should offer their toddler nutritious foods but allow the toddler to decide which foods and how much he or she will eat. Without any pressure exerted to eat certain foods or quantities, toddlers will come to enjoy mealtimes and different foods.

- Eat the foods you would like your toddlers to eat. Parents are good role models for their toddlers who learn by copying what others do. If parents eat and make positive comments about foods their toddlers will be more likely to try eating those foods. Siblings, other children and carers are also good role models for toddlers. Some toddlers may need to watch others eating a food that is new to them several times before they become confident to try it themselves.

- Make foods easy to eat by offering finger foods so that toddlers can feed themselves and have more control over how much they eat.

- Praise toddlers when they eat well or try new foods as toddlers respond to praise and tend to repeat behaviours they are praised for.

- Allow enough time to finish eating and drinking but do not extend the mealtime to try to coerce a toddler to eat more than they want to. Average ideal times are around 15 minutes for a snack and 20–30 minutes for a meal.

- Reward toddlers with attention but not food or drinks. Foods used as rewards or treats become more desirable than other foods and this encourages taste preferences for sweet, high-calorie foods that are generally used as rewards.

Some young children are much more likely to take longer to move out of this phase and strategies to help them are discussed in the next chapter.

References and further reading

Birch LL (1998) Development of food acceptance patterns in the first years of life. *Proceedings of the Nutrition Society* **57**(4): 617–624.

Birch LL and Marlin DW (1982) I don't like it; I never tried it: effects of exposure on two-year-old children's food preferences. *Appetite* **3**(4): 353–360.

Cooke L (2004) The development and modification of children's eating habits. *Nutrition Bulletin* **29**: 31–35.

Cooke LJ, Chambers LC, Añez EV and Wardle J (2011) Facilitating or undermining? The effect of reward on food acceptance. A narrative review. *Appetite* **57**(2): 493–497.

Department of Health (1994) *Weaning and the Weaning Diet. Report on Health and Social Subjects No. 45*. London: HMSO.

Gregory JR, Collins DL, Davies PSW, Hughes JM and Clarke PC (1995) *National Diet and Nutrition Survey: Children aged 1½ and 4½ years*, Volume 1. Report of the Diet and Nutrition Survey. London: HMSO.

Harris G (2008) Development of taste and food preferences in children. *Current Opinion in Clinical Nutrition and Metabolic Care* **11**: 315–319.

More J (2010) *Teach Yourself Happy Toddler Mealtimes*. London: Hodder Education.

Moy RJD (2006) Prevalence, consequences and prevention of childhood nutritional iron deficiency: a child public health perspective. *Clinical and Laboratory Haematology* **28**: 291–298.

Remington A, Añez E, Croker H, Wardle J and Cooke L (2012) Increasing food acceptance in the home setting: a randomized controlled trial of parent-administered taste exposure with incentives. *American Journal of Clinical Nutrition* **95**(1): 72–77.

Russell CG and Worsley A (2008) A population-based study of preschoolers' food neophobia and its associations with food preferences. *Journal of Nutrition Education and Behavior* **40**(1): 11–19.

Resources

Bedfordshire Under 5s Healthy Eating Award Project (**www.under5healthyeatingaward.nhs.uk**)

Comic Company (**www.comiccompany.co.uk**): 'Cool Kids Use Cups' leaflet and activity pack.

Department of Health (**www.dh.gov/publications**): Delivering Better Oral Health: An evidence-based toolkit for prevention, September 2007.

Healthy Child (**www.e-lfh.org.uk/healthychild**): Healthy Child self learning programme: Module 8 Growth and nutrition.

Infant and Toddler Forum (**www.infantandtoddlerforum.org**): Factsheets and Resources: 'Ten Steps for Healthy Toddlers'; Factsheet 1.1 Healthy Eating for Toddlers; Factsheet 1.2 Combining Food for a Balanced Diet; Factsheet 1.3 Portion Sizes for Children 1–4 years; Factsheet 2.1 Why Toddlers Refuse Food.

National Daycare and Nurseries Association (**www.ndna.org.uk**): Publications: *Your Essential Guide to Nutrition, Serving Food and Oral Health*; *Your Essential Guide to Cooking Healthy, Tasty Food*.

Common Nutritional Problems in Preschool Children

Summary

- The common nutritional problems seen in 1–4 year olds are dental caries, iron-deficiency anaemia, obesity, constipation, diarrhoea, gastro-oesophageal reflux disease, selective eating, faltering growth and rickets.

- Following the healthy eating guidelines for children aged 1–4 will prevent most of these conditions except selective eating and constipation.

- Many parents need support to improve healthy eating, management of mealtimes and challenging eating behaviours in their young children.

- If their feeding problems affect health and growth, some children may need a referral to a specialist feeding clinic.

Dental Caries

Dental caries is common in under-fives and is mainly due to poor dental healthcare in the home.

Thirty per cent of children 3–5 years old have some experience of dental decay (Hinds and Gregory 1995, Department of Health 2009) and in the National Diet and Nutrition Survey in 1995 the risk was higher in children:

- from lower socio-economic groups
- whose teeth brushing began at a later age
- whose teeth were brushed less frequently than twice a day
- who always brushed their own teeth compared to those who had an adult helping them
- who used a bottle, dinky feeder or dummy
- who more frequently ate sugar and confectionery and carbonated drinks
- who had a drink containing non-milk extrinsic sugars in bed at night.

The most important preventative measure in preschool children is brushing teeth twice a day with fluoridated toothpaste. This procedure should be supervised as young children lack the dexterity to brush properly and care should be taken to avoid swallowing toothpaste and excessive rinsing (Gibson and Williams 1999).

More recently, dentists report that increasing rates of dental erosion are caused by frequent consumption of fruit juice in under-fives. Many dentists advise against giving under-fives any drinks of fruit juice as well as sweetened squashes and fizzy drinks.

Sweet, acidic foods should be limited to just 4 feeding episodes each day and children should not be allowed to graze on food throughout the day but should follow a routine of 3 meals and 2–3 planned nutritious snacks. Water is the best drink to offer outside these times.

Saliva has a protective effect on teeth but saliva production reduces during sleep. Hence sweet or acidic drinks given at bedtime are very harmful.

Most harmful are sweet and acidic drinks given in a bottle which is left with the child to suck as they fall asleep and during the night. This is also a choking risk.

Iron-Deficiency Anaemia

Between 10 and 11 per cent of all preschool children in the UK and up to one-third of Asian toddlers are thought to be iron deficient (Moy 2006). It is not unique to any population although its incidence tends to be higher in inner city areas and among Asian populations (Lawson *et al.* 1998).

Diagnosis of iron-deficiency anaemia is based on blood tests. The World Health Organization definition of iron-deficiency anaemia is a haemoglobin of <11.0 g/dL. Low plasma ferritin levels indicate very low stores of iron.

An iron supplementation is usually prescribed to correct anaemia.

A poor diet is by far the most common cause of iron-deficiency anaemia in children 1–4 years old. The dietary risk factors are:

- late weaning or inappropriate weaning foods during infancy
- changing to cow's milk as their main drink before 12 months of age
- consuming excessive amounts of cow's milk – frequently from a bottle (an excess is more than 600 mL per day)
- eating an unbalanced diet with excess milk, confectionery, or low-nutrient snack foods and eating too few high-iron foods.

Iron deficiency may cause:

- pallor, spoon-shaped nails (koilonychia), sores at the corner of the mouth (angular stomatitis), a sore tongue (glossitis)
- tiredness, irritability
- poor appetite
- reduced exercise tolerance
- increased risk of infection
- developmental delay
- poor educational achievement
- breath holding
- swallowing difficulty with food sticking (pharyngeal web)
- pica (e.g. licking newspapers, eating soil, carpet underlay, wood, etc.).

To correct iron deficiency an iron supplement may be prescribed, but for the long term a diet as discussed above with the appropriate number of servings of foods from food groups 1–4 will prevent iron deficiency.

Maintaining iron stores and preventing deficiency in children 1–4 years old can be promoted by:

- advising against the change to cow's milk as the main milk drink before 12 months of age and then restricting it to 360 mL/day or less if the toddler is eating yogurt and cheese
- encouraging consumption of iron-rich foods (e.g. red meat, oily fish, eggs, iron-fortified breakfast cereals, beans and pulses, nuts, dark green vegetables and dried fruit). (NB: Liver is a good source but should be limited to once per week as it has a high vitamin A content.)
- giving vitamin C-rich fruit and vegetables with meals as this promotes iron absorption, for example, citrus fruit, tomatoes, peppers, kiwi fruit, strawberries and potatoes
- advising against giving tea as a drink with meals and snacks as it contains tannin, which decreases the absorption of iron from food (Booth and Aubett 1997).

Parents who have trouble reducing an excess cow's milk intake in their young child could consider changing from cow's milk to an iron-fortified formula such as a follow-on formula or a growing-up milk. However, the ultimate aim should be to cut down milk consumption so that more iron-rich foods will be eaten.

Obesity

Obesity in children 1–4 years old is becoming increasingly prevalent. The prevention, consequences and treatment are discussed in detail in Chapter 7.2.

Constipation

A simple definition of constipation is 'the difficult passage of hard stools' and it is often a complex problem. Usually there is no one underlying cause that can be identified. Infrequent passing of stools is not always indicative as normal stool habit in children 1–4 years old is considered to be within the range of passing a stool three times per day to one stool every three days. The average is passing one stool a day.

Factors exacerbating constipation include:

- insufficient intake of dietary fibre and/or fluid
- cow's milk protein allergy – probably more common in children with atopic disorders (e.g. eczema and asthma)
- emotional disturbances
- childhood infection
- a change in routine
- an intentional or subconscious withholding of a stool after a traumatic event.

It may have begun in infancy but may begin in some children at around 2 years of age when potty training begins.

Symptoms include:

- abdominal pain
- bleeding from the bottom (anal fissure)
- passage of very large stools that are difficult to flush away
- stool-withholding behaviour which can be misinterpreted as 'straining' to open bowels
- soiling (from 'overflow' diarrhoea) – usually a result of chronic faecal retention in children over 3 years old.

Chronic faecal retention desensitizes the rectum wall, which exacerbates the problem as large stool volumes are then required to signal the need for a bowel movement.

Constipation may cause poor eating if a child feels discomfort when constipated. Fibre and fluid intake will then decrease, possibly exacerbating the constipation.

Treatment

NICE (2010) recommends that treatment should begin with emptying the large bowel and then maintaining regular passage of soft stools with laxatives so that the fear of painful defecation subsides. Parents need to be reassured that laxatives are both necessary and safe. Stress in the family over a child's constipation, and poor compliance with treatment can both delay recovery. Families need frequent support and encouragement; in difficult cases involvement of the clinical psychology or child and adolescent mental health team may be essential. Coercive potty training is to be avoided.

Once the constipation is being treated young children may begin to eat better and dietary changes can be considered. In time and on an individual basis, slow weaning from laxative treatment can begin as most children will eventually grow out of constipation.

Dietary changes to suggest

Encourage the child to eat more foods with higher fibre content, such as:

- wholegrain breakfast cereals and wholemeal bread
- fruit and vegetables
- beans, pulses and lentils (e.g. baked beans)
- ground and chopped nuts.

Offer 6–8 drinks per day of about 100–120 mL each. More may be required in hot weather and after physical activity.

Unprocessed bran should not be given to young children as it can cause bloating and interferes with the absorption of micronutrients, such as iron, calcium and zinc.

Diarrhoea

Toddler diarrhoea may occur in children who are otherwise healthy and growing well. The condition is thought to be due to a degree of immaturity of gut function and often improves spontaneously at around 3 or 4 years of age. Frequent loose stools containing recognizable food matter (peas, carrots, sweetcorn) may be passed up to eight times a day.

Dietary causes include:

- the consumption of large quantities of some squashes and fruit juices (e.g. clear apple juice) because they contain large quantities of non-absorbable monosaccharides and oligosaccharides (Hoekstra 1998)
- cow's milk protein allergy – a trial elimination diet will prove whether this is the cause or not (see Chapter 7.1, page 192).

Dietary advice should be a healthy balanced diet with a limit on squash and fruit juice intake.

Continued diarrhoea (>7 days) after acute gastroenteritis may be associated with a temporary intolerance to lactose (Davidson *et al.* 1984). This might require the exclusion of dairy products and other lactose containing foods for a few weeks. Lactose-free milks, such as Lactofree or calcium-fortified soya milk, can be used as a direct substitute for cow's milk.

Gastro-Oesophageal Reflux Disease

Most children grow out of gastro-oesophageal reflux disease (GORD) around their first birthday, however, for a small minority it may continue and may be diagnosed after the age of 1 year rather than during infancy. It may be:

- a symptom of cow's milk protein allergy
- a cause of faltering growth.

Investigations to aid diagnosis include:

- X-ray of a barium swallow to rule out something wrong with the way the gut has formed (e.g. hiatus hernia; narrowing in the bowel;

malrotation/twisting of the small intestine – usually giving rise to green bile in the vomit)

- 24-hour pH (acid) monitoring with a probe inserted through the nose with acid-sensitive tip in the lower oesophagus, giving a continuous 24-hour record of when acid stomach contents spill back into lower oesophagus
- endoscopy (flexible 'telescope') examination under anaesthetic of the oesophagus and stomach, with tissue samples to look at under the microscope for inflammation, including allergy.

Drug treatment is usually instigated in children aged 1–4 and includes:

- suppressing acid secretion in the stomach (e.g. ranitidine; omeprazole)
- stimulating stomach emptying (e.g. domperidone).

Dietary treatments include giving 5–6 small meals each day rather than 3 larger meals and small snacks. Continuous nasogastric tube feeding may be tried in children with this disease who have faltering growth as a result of eating insufficient calories and nutrients.

Anti-reflux fundoplication surgery is reserved for severe complications resistant to medical management. It is major surgery that carries inherent risks and is performed much less frequently now than in previous decades.

Selective Eating and Food Refusal

As discussed in the previous chapter, most toddlers pass through this normal developmental stage of food neophobia and eventually widen the range of foods they eat if their parents manage mealtimes well.

Older toddlers from 2 years may refuse foods for other reasons:

- They may begin to associate things that look similar and may associate a food with something that is disgusting to them. Noodles may resemble 'worms' or sausages may look like 'dog poo'. They will be unable to bring themselves to eat a food that reminds them of something disgusting.

● A liked food may be contaminated with a disliked food or a food they are wary of. If a disliked food is touching or even just on the same plate as food usually eaten all the food, including the liked foods, may be rejected.

Toddlers who are much slower to grow out of this phase of food neophobia and eat very selectively and consequently cause more parental anxiety include:

● those who during infancy had little experience of different food textures and family foods

● toddlers who, as infants, were mainly fed on commercial baby foods and who did not eat many family foods during weaning

● those fed on a narrow range of foods during infancy because they were only offered a narrow range

● those who were not offered food with lumps by 9 months of age

● those who were tube-fed for medical reasons.

Some toddlers lack experience of food because they were not allowed to touch and play with food or to develop their self-feeding skills. Some parents prefer to do all the spoon feeding themselves and do not offer finger foods. Sometimes this is to minimize mess but it may be because they prefer to retain full control.

Negative experiences at mealtimes may result from pain with reflux, coercion and force feeding or poor interaction with parent or carer. Sometimes toddlers have had negative experiences around their mouth during infancy, for example preterm infants who had tubes inserted in their mouth and medication via syringe.

Stubborn, strong-willed children are less likely to copy what parents, siblings and others are doing.

Occasionally, children have high oral sensitivity, which may have been noticed when lumpy foods were first introduced and infants took much longer to accept them and move onto more complex food textures. These children may be also be sensitive to sound, touch or smells. They may dislike getting their hands and face dirty. It is especially important that these children are not forced to eat foods that they dislike as it may lead to vomiting.

Poor oromotor development may or may not be associated with other developmental delay or cerebral palsy. These children may prefer puréed food and may choke or gag on other textures which make the feeding process uncomfortable or frightening.

Underlying medical problems, such as constipation, anaemia, gastro-oesophageal reflux and delayed gastric emptying, can all cause toddlers to limit the quantity or type of food they will eat. Medical treatments to resolve these conditions need to be implemented before helping parents with other interventions to change mealtime behaviours.

When young children do not eat as well as expected, parents can become very anxious. Their concerns that their child may become malnourished and not grow and develop normally may lead to management strategies that exacerbate the situation. This includes:

● expecting their child to eat more than is needed

● having unrealistic expectations of growth rates which are lower in 1–4 year olds than in infants

● becoming very anxious at mealtimes

● mismanaging mealtimes.

Mismanagement of mealtimes can include the following:

● Giving frequent drinks of milk or juice: many young children prefer drinking to eating and readily fill themselves up with drinks (Smith and Lifshitz 1994, Houlihane and Rolls 1995). Useful advice is that drinks should be limited to water in between meals. Cups should replace any bottles still being given as this will help to reduce fluid intake.

● Frequent snacking: Some children end up eating most of their food between meals and the snack food often tends to be high in fat and sugar. There is often little or no incentive for the child to eat an appropriate meal if they are allowed to fill up on confectionery, biscuits and crisps. Less frequent snacking and more appropriate snacks such as fruit or small sandwiches can be offered.

- Snacks being given when a meal is refused. Children may prefer snack foods and refuse meals in order to be given snacks instead.
- Coercing children to eat more and/or extending mealtimes when the child has indicated they have had enough to eat.

Management of selective eating behaviour

A consistent approach is essential and all those involved in the care of the child, including relatives and child minders, need to cooperate with any management plan that is agreed.

If a food offered at mealtimes is rejected, it should be removed without comment but nothing substituted in its place or offered before the next planned snack or mealtime. There is never a place for threats or other measures to force a child to eat specific foods.

Some toddlers may need to be offered a new food ten or more times before they are brave enough to taste it. The food may then need to be tasted several times before the toddler learns to like it.

Dos and don'ts for managing challenging eating behaviour	
Do	**Reason**
Develop a daily routine of 3 meals and 2–3 planned nutritious snacks around a toddler's sleeping pattern	Toddlers don't eat well if they become over hungry or very tired. A routine gives children the security of knowing what to expect
Always offer something you know your toddler will eat at each meal. In addition offer the foods other family members are eating	Toddlers will be able to eat and enjoy some food while having the opportunity to watch others eating the foods that they are wary of trying
Offer two courses at meals: one savoury course followed by a sweet course	This gives two opportunities for the toddler to take in calories and nutrients and offers a wider variety of foods. It also makes the meal more interesting
Always give the second course whether the first course is eaten or not	The second course will provide nutrients and calories
Allow toddlers to finish the course or meal when they signal they have eaten enough and remove uneaten food without comment	Toddlers should be allowed to decide what and how much they eat. If very little is eaten it will only be 2–3 hours before the next planned snack or meal is offered
Eat with your child as often as possible	Toddlers learn by copying their parents and other children. Parents are their strongest role models
Praise toddlers when they eat well	Toddlers respond positively to praise
Make positive comments about the food	Parents and carers are strong role models. Toddlers are more likely to try foods about which they hear positive comments
Give small portions. If these are finished, praise the toddler and offer more	Toddlers can be overwhelmed by large portions and lose their appetite
Offer finger foods as often as possible	Toddlers enjoy having the control of feeding themselves with finger foods
Eat in a calm relaxed environment without distractions such as TV, games and toys	Toddlers concentrate on one thing at a time. Distractions make it more difficult to concentrate on eating

(Continued)

Dos and don'ts for managing challenging eating behaviour

Do	Reason
Finish the meal after about 20–30 minutes and accept that is all the toddler is going to eat	Dragging the meal on for a long time is unlikely to result in a toddler eating much more. It is better to wait for the next snack or meal and offer more nutritious foods then
Arrange for toddlers to eat with other toddlers as often as possible	Some toddlers eat better when they are with their own age group. Their eating habits often improve dramatically once they begin eating with other children on starting nursery or school
Involve toddlers in food shopping and preparing for the meal, such as putting things on the table	This will encourage a positive attitude to food
Involve toddlers in simple cooking and food preparation	Handling and touching new foods without pressure to eat them will help a toddler become familiar with new foods and become more likely to try them
Change the venue of meals and have an impromptu picnic with everyone in the garden or on the playroom floor	This will make eating and food a fun experience for the toddler

Don't	Reason
Rush a meal	Some toddlers eat quite slowly and rushing a toddler to eat can reduce their appetite
Insist a toddler finishes everything on his or her plate	Toddlers should be allowed to eat to their appetite and parents and carers should respect this
Coerce toddlers to eat more when they have indicated that they have had enough	
Take away a refused meal and offer a completely different one in its place	Toddlers will soon take advantage if you do this. In the long run it is better to offer family meals and accept that your child will prefer some foods to others. Always offer one food at each meal that he or she will eat
Offer the sweet course as a reward	That will make the sweet course seem more desirable
Offer large drinks of milk, squash or fruit juice within an hour of the meal	Large calorific drinks will reduce appetite for food. Give water instead
Offer snacks just before a meal	Snacks will reduce appetite
Give a snack very soon after a meal if a toddler hasn't eaten well at the meal	Many parents may do this just to ensure their toddler has eaten something. However, it is best to have a set meal pattern and wait until the next snack or meal before offering food again
Assume that because a toddler has refused a food he or she will never eat it again	Tastes change with time. Some toddlers need to be offered a new food up to 12–15 times before they feel confident to try it

Growth and dietary intake can be assessed in children with selective eating by:

● measuring weight and height accurately on calibrated scales and plotting on growth charts

● asking parents to record a 3–7-day food diary that can then be assessed in terms of food group content (see Chapter 2.2, page 48–54).

In most cases parents can be reassured that the child is eating adequately and growing normally. If the child is not eating adequately then a vitamin and mineral supplement can be given to cover any low intakes of specific nutrients until the child widens their intake of food.

If growth is faltering then a child needs to be referred to a paediatrician for assessment. Referral to a specialist feeding team may be possible where a multidisciplinary team can support parents to manage the feeding problem.

A very small number of children do not grow out of this phase and continue to restrict the foods they eat throughout their childhood years. If they eat enough of their preferred foods to meet their energy requirements and take a vitamin and mineral supplement to address any deficiencies, they will grow and develop normally despite a very restricted diet.

Faltering Growth

When children do not eat enough their growth may falter. This is defined as weight or height crossing down through 2 centile spaces on a growth chart.

Causes of faltering growth are:

- malnutrition through not eating enough food
- diseases involving malabsorption or decreased appetite
- hormonal syndromes (e.g. hypothyroidism, Turner syndrome, growth hormone insufficiency)
- physical or emotional neglect.

Most faltering growth in children 1–4 years old is due to poor eating. Only 5 per cent is due to disease or hormonal disorders. It is estimated that a further 5 per cent is due to neglect and will need the support of those involved in child protection.

If faltering growth is due to fussy faddy eating as described above then the first aim should be to agree a strategy for managing meal and snacktimes so that the child does not become anxious around mealtimes and is allowed to decide what and how much they eat.

The second aim is to increase calorie intake and this is best achieved by increasing the calorie content of foods and meals that the child is happy to eat. Often the appetite is suppressed and so strict healthy eating guidelines should be put aside until the child is gaining weight and has an improved appetite.

Increasing fat intake using oil, butter, cream and mayonnaise are the most effective ways of increasing calories:

- Foods can be roasted or fried in butter or oil rather than grilled, steamed or boiled.
- Butter or oil can be added or mixed into hot foods such as pasta, rice, vegetables and mashed potatoes.
- Mayonnaise can be added to dishes in larger quantities.
- Butter and margarine can be spread more thickly on bread or crackers.
- Cream can be added to puddings, fruit and breakfast cereals.

Increasing carbohydrate is usually most effective by adding extra sugar to cold foods, drinks, puddings and breakfast cereals.

If children enjoy high-calorie foods such as cheese, peanut butter, fatty meats, cakes and biscuits, these can be offered more frequently and in larger portions.

Powdered supplements for adding to food and supplement drinks are available on prescription but should only be used as a second choice and with medical and dietetic supervision. They are an expensive item for GPs' budgets and their use and effectiveness needs to be carefully monitored to justify the cost.

If improving mealtime management and increasing the calorie content of foods is not successful in restoring normal growth velocity then the child should be referred to a paediatrician and on to a specialist feeding clinic.

Specialist Feeding Clinics

Children whose health may be compromised by their eating behaviour may be referred to a feeding clinic if one exists in their NHS area. Such clinics provide a coordinated multidisciplinary approach to helping families decide how to change the way they manage mealtimes and feeding children with feeding difficulties. Before referral, a child should have been seen by a doctor and any relevant investigations done.

Feeding assessments may be done by one or two trained health professionals in the home or within a specialist clinic. The combination of specialized healthcare professionals that see patients within a clinic usually includes:

- community paediatrician/paediatric gastroenterologist
- clinical psychologist
- paediatric dietitian
- speech and language therapist.

Vitamin D Deficiency and Rickets

The main source of vitamin D is not food but that made in the skin when outside in sunlight (see Chapter 1.1 page 6). Current indoor lifestyles do not always allow adequate skin synthesis even in summer for under-fives.

Although national statistics are not being collected there are reports in the literature that vitamin D deficiency and rickets in the UK are increasing (Ahmed *et al.* 2011). Deficiency not only affects growth and long-term bone health, but has also been implicated in certain forms of cancer, cardiovascular disease, tuberculosis, multiple sclerosis and type 1 and 2 diabetes.

The specific effects of vitamin D deficiency include:

- decreased calcium absorption from diet, low plasma calcium, increased plasma bone alkaline phosphatase activity (commonly measured in blood tests)
- raised parathyroid hormone concentration to mobilize calcium from bone
- rickets: swelling of rib junctions giving a characteristic lumpy appearance ('rachitic rosary'); 'bow legs' in weight-bearing children; swelling over the ends of long bones (e.g. wrist)

- enamel hypoplasia and delayed appearance of teeth
- deformity of spine (kyphoscoliosis) and pelvis in longstanding cases.

Vitamin D deficiency can only be diagnosed by a blood test and these are not done routinely. Risk factors that make vitamin D deficiency more likely include:

- Asian, African and Middle-Eastern ethnic origin
- prolonged exclusive breastfeeding with late weaning
- not taking the recommended daily supplement of vitamin D (see Chapter 5.1, page 136)
- limited options for being outside
- excess use of sunscreen which prevents cutaneous synthesis of vitamin D.

Once diagnosed, vitamin D deficiency or rickets is treated with high doses of vitamin D until symptoms resolve.

Acknowledgements

With thanks to Dr Gill Harris, Clinical Psychologist, University of Birmingham and Birmingham Children's Hospital, Birmingham.

References and further reading

Ahmed SF, Franey C, McDevitt H, *et al.* (2011) Recent trends and clinical features of childhood vitamin D deficiency presenting to a children's hospital in Glasgow. *Archives of Disease in Childhood* **96**: 694–696.

Booth IW and Aubett MA (1997) Iron deficiency in infancy and early childhood. *Archives of Disease in Childhood* **76**: 549–554.

Cooke L (2004) The development and modification of children's eating habits. *Nutrition Bulletin* **29**: 31–35.

Crowley E, Williams L, Roberts T, Jones P and Dunstan R (2008) Evidence for a role of cow's milk consumption in chronic functional constipation in children: systematic review of the literature from 1980 to 2006. *Nutrition and Dietetics* **65**: 29–33.

Davidson GP, Godwin D and Robb TA (1984) Incidence and duration of lactose malabsorption in children hospitalised with acute enteritis: study in well nourished urban population. *Journal of Paediatrics* **105**: 587–590.

Davies JH and Shaw NJ (2011) Preventable but no strategy: vitamin D deficiency in the UK. *Archives of Disease in Childhood* **96**: 614–615.

Department of Health (2009) NHS Dental Epidemiology Programme for England 2009 Oral Health Survey of 5 year old Children 2007/2008. **www.nwph.net/dentalhealth/reports/NHS_DEP_for_England_OH_Survey_5yr_2007-08_Report.pdf (accessed April 2012).**

Gibson S and Williams S (1999) Dental caries in preschool children: Associations with social class, tooth-brushing habit and consumption of sugars and sugar-containing foods. Further analysis of data from the National Diet and Nutrition Survey of children aged 1½ to 4½ years. *Caries Research* **33**(2): 101–103.

Grantham-McGregor S and Ani C (2001) A review of studies on the effect of iron deficiency on cognitive development in children. *Journal of Nutrition* **131**: 649S–666S.

Greenhalg J, Dowey AJ, Horne PJ, Fergus Lowe C, Grifffiths JH and Whittaker CJ (2009) Positive and negative peer modelling effects on young children's consumption of novel blue foods. *Appetite* **52**: 646–653.

Gregory JR, Collins DL, Davies PSW, Hughes JM and Clarke PC (1995) *National Diet and Nutrition Survey: Children aged 1½ and 4½ years*, Volume 1. Report of the Diet and Nutrition Survey. London: HMSO.

Harris G (2008) Development of taste and food preferences in children. *Current Opinion in Clinical Nutrition and Metabolic Care* **11**: 315–319.

Hinds K and Gregory JR (1995) *National Diet and Nutrition Survey: Children aged 1½ to 4½ years*, Volume 2. Report of the Dental Survey. London: HMSO.

Hoekstra JH (1998) Toddler diarrhoea: more a nutritional disorder than a disease. *Archives of Disease in Childhood* **79**: 2–5.

Houlihane JOB and Rolls CJ (1995) Morbidity from excessive intake of high-energy fluid: 'the squash drinking syndrome'. *Archives of Disease in Childhood* **72**: 141–143.

Lawson MS, Thomas M and Hardiman A (1998) Iron status of Asian children aged 2 years living in England. *Archives of Disease in Childhood* **78**(5): 420–426.

Moy RJD (2006) Prevalence, consequences and prevention of childhood nutritional iron deficiency: a child public health perspective. *Clinical and Laboratory Haematology* **28**: 291–298.

Moynihan P and Petersen PE (2004) Diet, nutrition and the prevention of dental diseases. *Public Health Nutrition* 7(1A): 201–226.

NICE (National Institute for Health and Clinical Excellence) (2010) Clinical Guideline 99. Constipation in children and young people. May 2000. **www.nice.org.uk/guidance/CG99** (accessed April 2012).

Scientific Advisory Committee on Nutrition (2007) Position statement update on vitamin D. **www.sacn.gov.uk/reports_position_statements/position_statements/update_on_vitamin_d_-_november_2007.html** (accessed April 2012).

Scottish Intercollegiate Guidance Network (2005) *Prevention and Management of Dental Decay in the Preschool Child*. Edinburgh: SIGN.

Smith MM and Lifshitz F (1994) Excess fruit juice consumption as a contributing factor in non-organic failure to thrive. *Paediatrics* **93**(3): 438–443.

Wardle J, Herrera ML, Cooke L and Gibson EL (2003) Modifying children's food preferences: the effects of exposure and reward on acceptance of an unfamiliar vegetable. *European Journal of Clinical Nutrition* **57**: 341–348.

Williams J, Wolff A, Daly A, MacDonald A, Aukett A and Booth IW (1999) Iron supplemented formula milk related to reduction in psychomotor decline in infants from inner city areas: randomised study. *British Journal of Medicine* **318**: 693–698.

Wright CM, Parkinson KN, Shipton D and Drewett RF (2007) How do toddler eating problems relate to their eating behaviour, food preferences and growth? *Pediatrics* **120**: e1069–e1075.

Resources

Infant and Toddler Forum (**www. infantandtoddlerforum.org**): Infant and Toddler Forum Factsheets: Factsheet 4.1 Common Nutritional Problems in Toddlers; Factsheet 4.4 Iron Deficiency Anaemia in Toddlers; Factsheet 3.3 Overweight and Obesity; Factsheet 2.2 How to Manage Simple Faddy Eating in Toddlers; Factsheet 2.3 Understanding and Managing Extreme Food Refusal in Toddlers; Factsheet 4.6 Constipation in Toddlers.

More J (2010) *Teach Yourself Happy Toddler Mealtimes*. London: Hodder Education.

Specialist feeding support for faltering growth and feeding difficulties

Barts and the Royal London Hospital Paediatric Feeding Clinic (**www.bartsandthelondon.nhs. uk/our-services/childrens-hospital/childrens- services/nutrition-service/**): Example of a hospital-based specialist feeding clinic.

Brighton and Hove Feeding to Thrive Service (**www. sussexcommunity.nhs.uk/downloads/sdhWeb/ information/leaflets/child_health_services/ Feeding_to_Thrive_-_August07.pdf**): Example of a community-based project.

Feeding Preschool Children in Childcare Settings

Summary

- Food intake of under-fives may change on entering nursery or childcare settings.

- Childcare settings are not required to adopt any nutritional standards but there are several

  guidance documents for them to use to develop food policies.

- Childcare settings can teach healthy eating habits to children who do not encounter a healthy diet in their home.

Opportunities and Challenges for Children Eating in Childcare Settings

When young children begin nursery or attend daycare it is an opportunity for them to encounter a wider range of foods and different ways of having foods prepared and presented. For some children this will be a positive opportunity as they will see a large peer group eating and will be able to watch and copy their behaviour and may have more control over feeding themselves than they do at home.

Toddlers who do not eat well at home may eat much better at nursery. They may have had negative experiences around eating at home and prefer the eating environment at nursery. Toddlers who eat better at nursery may include:

- those who have often been fed on their own – if they see very few people eating different foods at home they may try new foods at nursery where they see a large group of other toddlers eating different foods

- those who have experienced some of the negative actions of parents as described in Chapter 5.2; for example they may have been pressured to eat more than they wanted to.

For other children, particularly very faddy or selective eaters, being offered only unfamiliar foods in an unfamiliar environment will be a disadvantage for them. Some will eat very little and others may refuse new foods altogether. They need time to become more familiar with the new environment and the foods served. They may need to watch the other children eating a snack or a meal several times before they are prepared to try it. With time, as they become familiar with the foods served there and as they watch the other children and staff eating the foods, they will gradually gain the confidence to try the foods and then begin to learn to like them.

Feeding very selective eaters who will only eat a narrow range of foods requires a management plan agreed between the childcare setting and the parents. A food that they will eat must be offered at each meal so that they are able to join in the mealtime, sit with the other children and eat something. This might be a food the childcare setting can provide, such as bread or cooked pasta, but it may have to be food that the parents send in from home (e.g. a marmite sandwich). While eating his or her familiar food the toddler can also be offered the foods the other children are eating. However, undue pressure put on a very selective eater to eat the foods served by the childcare setting will have a negative effect.

Toddlers who eat poorly at nursery may leave feeling tired and hungry. Parents or carers need to be advised that their toddler has eaten very little so that a nutritious meal or snack can be offered immediately on arrival at home. It may be more appropriate to offer a quick snack if they are ready for a sleep and then a nutritious meal after the sleep.

Nutritious snacks for a toddler who has not eaten well at nursery include:

- slices of fruit with a small cup of milk
- ham sandwich with cherry tomatoes and a cup of water
- peanut butter and banana sandwich
- slices of apple spread with cream cheese
- pancakes spread with fruit purée and a cup of milk
- pancakes spread with chocolate spread and a cup of water
- breadsticks or crackers with cubes of cheese and celery sticks with a cup of water
- pitta bread with hummus and apple slices and a cup of water
- muffin with grapes and a small cup of milk
- crumpet spread with honey and a cup of water
- scone with butter and jam, clementine segments and a cup of milk
- yogurt or fromage frais and fruit slices
- small piece of fruit cake and a cup of milk
- small slice of pizza and a cup of water
- small bowl of breakfast cereal with banana slices and milk
- toast with peanut butter, carrot sticks and a cup of water.

Nutritional Standards for Food and Drinks Offered in Childcare Settings

There are currently no nutritional standards governing the food that is served to under-fives in childcare: a nursery or other childcare setting can serve whatever foods they choose. There are voluntary guidelines but they are not enforceable. This is a failing of our education system as a nutritious diet is very important for preschool children to:

- ensure they eat nutrient-rich foods to fulfil their high requirement for nutrients
- teach them healthy eating habits.

Some nurseries will have had expert nutritional input in developing a food and drink policy and planning their menus, however, others may not. Ideally, a working group to develop a food policy and plan menus will include:

- the catering staff
- community dietitians or nutritionists
- teaching staff
- parents.

The children should be asked about their likes and dislikes.

Menu planning for nurseries should be based on the principles of healthy eating for under-fives outlined in Chapters 1.2 and 5.1.

Poor menu planning can lead to a non-nutritious diet being offered, particularly a diet low in iron, thus exacerbating the common occurrence of iron deficiency in this age group.

Case Study

The pupils in a nursery in north-east London come from a wide variety of cultural backgrounds and parents of many children requested specific dietary restrictions. Many requests were for the children not to be given certain types of meat. Some requested no meat as the family only ate halal meat. Other parents were concerned about previous food scares and preferred their children not to have red meat. Some were from vegetarian families.

→

The nursery thought they had solved the problem by deciding to have a vegetarian menu only so that all the children could eat the same food. However, the vegetarian dishes were made up from vegetables only with cheese and eggs being included sometimes. The menu contained virtually no high-iron foods as no dishes containing pulses or nuts had been included to provide high-iron alternative foods in place of the excluded meat and fish. Consequently, the menu offered was low in iron for preschool children who have very high iron requirements.

By working with a paediatric dietitian, the nursery incorporated lentils, dhal, beans and other pulses into many of the savoury vegetarian dishes so that food with higher levels of iron and zinc was offered to the children. Chopped and ground tree nuts were incorporated into some of the desserts to further increase the nutrient content of the menu.

Nutritional guidance available for nurseries

Several agencies have developed nutritional guidance that can be used as the basis of a food policy and they can all be accessed online:

- School Food Trust: Published in June 2012 'Eat Better Start Better' Voluntary Food and Drink Guidelines for Early Years Settings in England – A Practical Guide (www.schoolfoodtrust.org.uk/parents-carers/for-parents-carers/eat-better-start-better). Nurseries and child minders can download these guidelines along with sample menus and recipes for using seasonal foods.
- Caroline Walker Trust (www.cwt.org.uk): This charity produces nutritional guidelines and staff training packs for different population groups. The publications that nurseries would find helpful are: Eating well for under-5s in childcare; Eating well for under-5s in childcare: Training materials; Eating well for under-5s: a photo resource.
- The Scottish Government (www.scotland.gov.uk/publications): In January 2006 published Nutritional Guidance for Early Years: Food Choices for Children Aged 1–5 Years in Early Education and Childcare Settings [Guidance]. These guidelines are very comprehensive, setting out exactly how often various nutritious foods should be offered to children in childcare settings. However, it is not compulsory for nurseries in Scotland to follow them.
- National Day Nurseries Association (www.ndna.org.uk): This organization has over 15 000 nurseries as members and sells two publications that they have developed with the help of a paediatric dietitian – Your Essential Guide to Nutrition, Serving Food and Oral Health and Your Essential Guide to Cooking Healthy, Tasty Food. They also offer staff training in healthy eating for toddlers.

Food for Celebrations at Nurseries

This is usually covered within the food policy if a nursery has one.

Nurseries that celebrate festivals with some traditional foods for the meal and snacks on the day of the festival offer children the opportunity to learn about the festivals that cultures other than their own celebrate.

Birthday celebrations need to be covered carefully within a food policy. If children are allowed to bring in cakes and confectionery on their birthday to share with their classmates then this can become more than an occasional treat in a large nursery group. With up to 30 young children in a group there may be a birthday every week. It would be better for the nursery to ban confectionery altogether and to offer another way of celebrating each child's birthday. For example:

- allow the birthday child to bring in non-food items such as balloons or pencils instead

- allow candles on the pudding at lunchtime for that day for the child whose birthday it is
- allow a birthday cake to be brought in but served with some fruit as the second course or pudding of the main meal.

Packed Lunches

Ideally, packed meals should include something from each of the four main food groups so that under-fives have a balanced, nutritious meal. Foods need to be easy for toddlers to eat and not require preparation by time-pressured staff.

Some ideas for children who like their foods all separate are listed in Table 5.3.1. One or two items from each food group can be put into the lunchbox.

For children who are happy to eat mixed foods, savoury items for a lunchbox could include:

- finger food pieces of pizza or quiche
- small bhajis made with lentil or chick pea flour
- sandwiches
- dips
- salads.

Sandwich fillings for sliced bread, bread rolls, bagels, pitta bread or wraps

- Cold meat such as ham, lean salami or cold roast meat with lettuce, tomato or cucumber
- Liver pâté or liver sausage
- Peanut butter with mashed banana or jam
- 1 tbsp drained tinned tuna with 1 tsp mayonnaise and 1 tsp plain yogurt
- 1 tbsp tinned sardines with a squeeze of lemon juice
- 1 tbsp of smoked fish such as smoked mackerel or smoked trout mixed with ½ tbsp of plain yogurt and ½ tbsp of mayonnaise
- Fish pâtés such as mackerel or salmon pâté
- Slices of smoked salmon
- 1 tbsp hummus mixed with ½ tbsp finely diced red pepper
- Bean spreads such as black bean spread
- Mashed avocado or guacamole or tofu
- Grated hard cheese with sliced tomatoes

Table 5.3.1 Ideas for lunchbox foods for children who like their food separate

Food groups	Food items
Group 1: Bread, rice, potatoes, pasta and other starchy foods	Bread, breadsticks, crispbreads, crackers, plain popcorn, sliced pitta bread, cooked pasta pieces, plain scones
Group 2: Fruit and vegetables	Sticks or slices of carrot, cucumber, celery, courgette Cherry tomatoes or grapes cut in half Berries (e.g. strawberries, raspberries, blueberries, blackberries) Slices of apple, pear, banana, peach, plum, apricot – these need to be wrapped to stop them going brown Orange, tangerine or clementine segments Cubes of melon Small packets of dried fruit
Group 3: Milk, cheese and yogurt	Milk to drink, cubes of cheese, pot of yogurt or fromage frais
Group 4: Meat, fish, eggs, nuts and beans	Cold sliced meat – bought or that may have been cooked the day before (e.g. roast chicken, turkey, lamb, beef or pork) Ham, pepperoni, cocktail sausages or frankfurters Fish cakes Boiled egg – whole or quarters Mini falafels
Fluids	Water, diluted fruit juice

- 1 tbsp cream cheese with ½ tsp chopped herbs such as chives or parsley
- 1 tbsp cream cheese with a scrape of marmite

Cut sandwiches made with sliced bread diagonally into four triangles so that only one side of the sandwich has a crust. Toddlers find it easier to eat the sandwich and can leave the crusts if they prefer.

Dips to go with breadsticks or vegetable sticks

- Hummus
- Cucumber, mint and yogurt dip
- Avocado dip such as guacamole
- Fish or meat pâté mixed with some extra plain yogurt or mayonnaise to make them a suitable consistency for a dip

Salads

Salads can be based on any of the following with an added mix of vegetables. You will usually need to provide a plastic fork or spoon.

- Rice
- Pasta
- Bean
- Lentil
- Potato

Pudding or second course

Fruit pieces, yogurt or fromage frais are a nutritious second course. The following cakes and biscuits all contain nutrients and can also be included as a nutritious second course, served with some fresh fruit:

- fruit cake
- carrot cake
- muffins containing fruit
- biscuits with dried fruit (e.g. Garibaldi biscuits)
- mini tarts with ground nuts (e.g. Bakewell tarts)

- cereal bars with added fruit or crushed nuts
- rice pudding.

Promoting Healthy Lifestyles and Healthy Eating Habits in Childcare Settings

When a childcare setting adopts a healthy eating policy and offers nutritious meals and snacks to the children, they will be teaching those children healthy eating habits. This will be a valuable learning experience for children who do not encounter a healthy diet in their home, such as those never offered vegetables or fruit.

In addition, other activities could be offered, such as:

- a range of interactive parental education sessions to prevent obesity
- interactive cookery demonstrations
- videos and group discussions on practical issues such as healthy eating, meal planning and local shopping for nutritious foods
- sessions to promote ideas for family activities involving physical activity, opportunities and local facilities for active play
- discussion of safety concerns that limit physical activity of young children
- encouraging more walking instead of always using the car or pushing toddlers around in a stroller.

Resources

Bedfordshire Health Authority (**www. under5healthyeatingaward.nhs.uk/**): Has an under-five healthy eating award scheme and has a series of downloadable 'Fun With Food' resources.

Caroline Walker Trust (**www.cwt.org.uk**): Resources: Eating well for under-5s in childcare; Eating well for under-5s in childcare: Training materials; Eating well for under-5s: a photo resource.

National Daycare and Nurseries Association (**www. ndna.org.uk**): Publications: *Your Essential Guide to Nutrition, Serving Food and Oral Health*; *Your Essential Guide to Cooking Healthy, Tasty Food.*

Nursery Milk (**www.nurserymilk.co.uk**): How to apply for free milk in childcare settings for under-fives.

School Food Trust (**www.schoolfoodtrust.org.uk/parents-carers/for-parents-carers/eat-better-start-better**): 'Eat Better Start Better' project resources:

Voluntary Food and Drink Guidelines for Early Years Settings in England – A Practical Guide.

Scottish Government (**www.scotland.gov.uk/publications**): *Nutritional Guidance for Early Years: Food Choices for Children Aged 1–5 Years in Early Education and Childcare Settings.*

Section 6
School Age Children

6.1 Primary School Age Children

6.2 Nutrition for Adolescents

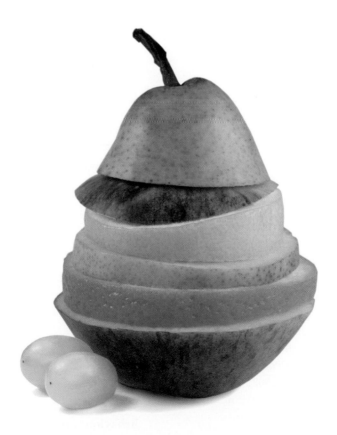

Primary School Age Children

Summary

- Children prefer familiar foods and most need to be motivated to try new foods.

- Children innately prefer sweet, salty and energy-dense foods.

- Parents and carers are responsible for food offered to primary school age children and have the power and influence to change eating habits.

- Primary school children generally satisfy their nutrient needs.

- Secondary school children make more of their own food choices and many do not satisfy their nutrient needs.

- School meals make a nutritious contribution to children's dietary intake, especially those entitled to free school meals.

- Food and nutrient-based standards for school meals are in place in England, Scotland and Wales. Northern Ireland has food-based standards.

Primary school children should be eating a diet broadly in line with a balance of the food groups in the 'eatwell plate' as discussed in Chapter 1.2.

Influences on Food Tastes and Preferences

From the age of about 5 years, children tend to eat from social cues like adults rather than regulating their energy intake according to their needs as do most infants and toddlers. This means they eat when others are eating even when they are not hungry and eat more of the foods they particularly like.

Many children continue to prefer foods with which they are familiar rather than trying new foods. They need to be motivated to taste new foods. Work in this field (Hill 2002, Cooke 2007, Brug *et al.* 2008, Scaglioni *et al.* 2008) continues to show evidence for the following factors:

- Children innately prefer sweet, salty and energy-dense foods.

- Food availability and accessibility and taste preferences are the most important determinants of children's choice and consumption of particular foods.

- As parents and carers are responsible for the foods offered to children, they have the power to influence and change children's eating habits.

- Parental control over what and how much children can eat influences food preferences but sometimes in a counterproductive way. Restricting a food such as chocolate can make it even more attractive and likely to be selected and eaten in situations where parents are not present.

- Parents are key role models – children model their own eating behaviour from their observations of their parents' eating.

- From around 7 years of age, preferences and behaviours of peer groups begin to have a stronger influence on children's food choices.

- The number of times children are exposed to a food increases the likelihood they will try the food and then learn to like it. Children eat more fruit and vegetables at schools where more fruit and vegetables are offered.

Energy and Nutrient Intakes of School Age Children

The best evidence of dietary intakes in this age group in the UK was provided by the National Diet and Nutrition Survey (NDNS) (Gregory *et al.* 2000), based on a seven-day weighed intake data obtained during 1997. A new rolling programme of national dietary surveys began in 2009 and uses a four-day reported food diary rather than weighed food intakes (Department of Health 2011). The results from a food diary are less accurate and more likely to contain under-reporting. To date, results are only available from the 870 school age children surveyed in the first two years of the rolling programme, but indications are similar to those found in the 1997 survey which surveyed twice as many. The findings include the following:

- Primary school aged children have a more nutritious diet than those 11 years and over. They also eat more fruit than older children.
- Energy intakes are below the estimated average requirement, which is probably indicative of lower physical activity levels.
- Percentages of energy derived from total fat and total carbohydrate are close to recommendations: 35 per cent and 50 per cent, respectively.
- Percentages of energy from saturated fat and non-milk extrinsic sugars (NMES) were similar throughout childhood and adolescence and exceed recommendations of 10 per cent and 11 per cent respectively. Soft drinks and confectionery were the main source of NMES.
- Protein intakes are adequate.
- Fibre intakes are low for all children when compared to the adult recommendation of 18 g/day.

- Vitamin and mineral intakes are generally adequate in primary school age children but poor in secondary school age children, particularly girls (see Table 6.2.3, Chapter 6.2, page 178).

A survey by a school meals caterer in 2005 reported that eating breakfast is at its highest in the pre-pubertal years, tending to decline, especially in girls, as adolescence approaches. Thirteen per cent of 8- to 16-year-old school children leave home in the morning having not eaten beforehand. Many buy sweets, crisps, chocolate and sweetened drinks on the way to school, but 8 per cent have nothing to eat before school (Sodexho 2005).

Portion Sizes

Energy intakes and portion sizes depend on size and gender and activity. Eating approximately within the ranges suggested in Table 6.1.1 would provide an average energy intake and nutrient sufficiency. The recommended number of servings per day from each food group is discussed in Chapter 1.2 (see Table 1.2.1, page 14).

Malnutrition in School Children

Obesity is the most common form of malnutrition in school age children in the UK. This is discussed in Chapter 7.2.

Underweight or faltering growth

Underweight children are defined as those who are below the 2nd centile line on a body mass index (BMI) centile chart. Faltering growth is usually defined as crossing 2 centile spaces downwards on a weight-for-age or height-for-age centile chart.

Both these conditions are less common in school age children than those below the age of 5 years and in school age children they are usually due to an underlying medical condition, poor appetite, family problems, concern about body image or self-imposed dietary restriction. If increasing food intake does not rectify either of these conditions

Table 6.1.1 Suggested foods from the five food groups for school age children

Group 1: Bread, rice, potatoes, pasta and other starchy foods	1–1½ slices wholegrain or white bread, muffin, roll or pancake
	Small bowl 4–9 tbsp breakfast cereal
	7–10 tbsp of hot cereals like porridge made up with milk
	4–7 tbsp of rice or pasta
	1–2 egg-sized potatoes or 3–6 tbsp of mashed potato
	2–4 crispbreads or crackers
Group 2: Fruit and vegetables	¾–1 apple, orange, pear, banana
	5–12 small berries or grapes
	3–6 tbsp freshly cooked, stewed or mashed fruit
	2–4 tbsp raw or cooked vegetables
Group 3: Milk, cheese and yogurt	150–200 mL whole cow's milk as a drink
	1–2 small pots (125 mL) yogurt or fromage frais
	3–6 tbsp grated cheese
	Cheese in a sandwich or on a piece of pizza
	100–180 mL custard or a milk pudding
Group 4: Meat, fish, eggs, nuts and pulses	3–6 tbsp ground, chopped or cubed lean meats, fish or poultry
	1 whole egg
	3–7 tbsp whole or mashed pulses (peas, beans, lentils, hummus, dhal)
	1–1½ tbsp peanut butter or 2–3 tbsp ground nuts
Group 5: Foods high in fat and sugar	1–2 digestive biscuits or 2–4 small biscuits
	1 medium slice cake
	1½ tsp butter, mayonnaise or oil
	1½ tsp jam, honey or sugar
	4–6 crisps or sweets
	1½ small fun-sized chocolate bars

The measures used are 1 tbsp = one 15 mL tablespoon and 1 tsp = one 5 mL teaspoon. These are the spoons found within a set of spoons for standard recipe measures.

then a child should be referred to a paediatrician for investigation.

Anorexia nervosa should always be considered as a cause for poor growth or weight loss. Although rare, cases have been noted in children as young as 7 years. Anorexia nervosa is a psychological eating disorder in which a person controls their food intake obsessively and reduces their intake below their needs in order to reduce their body weight. Maintaining a regular meal and snack routine and eating together as a family reduces the risk of eating disorders (Hammons and Fiese 2011).

Inappropriate dieting among children

When children choose to restrict their food intake to control weight they do not usually do this so that they meet their nutrient requirements. They often reduce their intake of nutritious foods such as milk, cheese and meat.

Girls as young as 9 years old, and some younger, indicate body dissatisfaction and a desire to be thinner. The Health Survey for England (Prescott-Clarke and Primatesta 1998) found that young children were already acting on their concerns:

- In 8–9 year olds, 9 per cent of girls and 7 per cent of boys reported that they were too heavy, and 13 per cent and 12 per cent, respectively, reported trying to lose weight.

- In 10–12 year olds, 10 per cent of both boys and girls reported that they thought they were too heavy, and 23 per cent of girls and 15 per cent of boys were trying to diet. The actual prevalence of obesity in this group was 7 per cent.

Hill (2006) found both overweight boys and girls desire weight loss and are unhappy with their body shape. He suggested this body dissatisfaction was a result of picking up on parental attitudes to weight and shape, the idealization of thinness promoted in the media and peer behaviour.

Dental caries

Children are more susceptible to dental caries than adults, although the incidence of caries in children in the UK decreased following the introduction of fluoride toothpaste in the 1970s. However, high and frequent consumption of sugar and acidic drinks contributes to (Walker 2000):

- 53 per cent of 4–18 year olds having dental decay

- 66 per cent having erosion of either their primary or permanent teeth.

When sugary food and drinks are limited to four eating occasions per day (e.g. three meals and one snack), the risk of dental caries is much lower (Moynihan and Petersen 2004).

Anaemia

Iron-deficiency anaemia is much less common in children over 5 years than in preschool children but does occur, particularly in:

- children who are vegetarian
- girls after menarche
- children with malabsorption due to an underlying disease
- children with a poor dietary intake due to dietary restriction.

Increasing the iron content of a diet is described in Chapter 5.2, page 147.

Non-haem iron uptake from eggs, nuts, pulses, cereals and vegetables can be maximized by including a good source of vitamin C with meals, such as citrus fruit, other fruits and tomatoes, and avoiding drinking tea with meals, which reduces iron absorption.

Low vitamin D levels

Blood analyses in the National Diet and Nutrition Surveys have shown that significant numbers of school children have low vitamin D levels. Sunlight on exposed skin when outside in the summer months, not diet, is the main source of vitamin D in the UK. Hence these low levels probably reflect the increased time children spend playing inside rather than outside.

The UK Department of Health does not recommend a set amount for children over 5 years of age. Other countries do set dietary recommendations of vitamin D for older children (e.g. between 5 and 10 µg/day for children in most European countries and 15 µg vitamin D for all children in the United States). The Scientific Advisory Committee on Nutrition (SACN) in the UK is currently reviewing the evidence and if they do set a recommended dietary intake then it is likely children would have to take a supplement of vitamin D as very few foods in the UK are fortified with it. This is in contrast to the United States, Canada and some Scandinavian countries, where several basic foods such as milk and orange juice are fortified with it.

School Food and Drinks

School lunches

Historically, school meals had to comply with set nutritional standards but, following the abolition of school meal standards in 1980, cheap, low-nutrient foods were often served to children as catering firms aimed to keep costs down. In 2001, England introduced school meal standards based on the food groups and changed the budget holder in many schools to the governing body rather than the Local Education Authority (LEA) in an effort to involve parents and teachers in the standards of school meals.

The food group-based standards required provision of combinations of food from all the five food groups. At least one item or a choice of two items from each food group, depending on the age group, had to be available throughout the meal service. Surveys in both primary (Nelson *et al.* 2006) and secondary (Nelson *et al.* 2004) schools showed these standards had little beneficial effect on pupils' food choices as the majority of choices were high-fat foods, chips and potatoes cooked in fat, and soft drinks.

To rectify this the School Food Trust was set up by the Government in 2005 to advise on school meal standards. This is a charity advising the Department of Education and in 2007 the Trust published nutrient-based standards for school meals and foods sold on school premises. From 2008 to 2009 the nutrient- and food-based standards became mandatory for all LEA-maintained primary,

secondary, special and boarding schools and pupil referral units in England. Scotland and Wales also have nutrient- and food-based standards. Northern Ireland has food-based standards.

The nutrient content is based on the Reference Nutrient Intakes (RNIs) for children as described in Chapter 1.1. The energy content is based on the Estimated Average Requirement (EAR) for energy for children as listed in Table 1.1.1.

In England and Wales the midday meal must provide:

- 30 per cent EAR for energy
- not less than 50 per cent energy from carbohydrate
- not more than 35 per cent energy from fat nor 11 per cent energy from saturated fat.

Minimum and maximum values of key nutrients are specified and listed in Table 6.1.2.

The figures for Scottish standards introduced in 2004 are very similar, specifying a minimum of 30–40 per cent of RNI for fibre, protein, iron, calcium, vitamin A, folate and vitamin C. These

Table 6.1.2 Energy and key nutrients that an average school lunch should provide

	Maximum or minimum amount	Primary school lunch	Secondary school lunch
Energy (kcal)		530 ± 26.5	646 ± 32.3
Protein (g)	Minimum	7.5	13.3
Carbohydrate (g)	Minimum	70.6	86.1
Non-milk extrinsic sugars (g)	Maximum	15.5	18.9
Fat (g)	Maximum	20.6	25.1
Saturated fat (g)	Maximum	6.5	7.9
Fibre (g)	Minimum	4.2	5.2
Sodium (mg)	Maximum	499	714
Vitamin A (µg)	Minimum	745	245
Vitaimn C (mg)	Minimum	10.5	14
Folate (µg)	Minimum	53	70
Calcium (mg)	Minimum	193	350
Iron (mg)	Minimum	3	5.2
Zinc (mg)	Minimum	2.5	3.3

nutrients are least likely to be consumed in sufficient amounts in Scottish diets. Maximum levels of fat, saturated fat, sugar and sodium are given for some groups of manufactured products.

Popular school meals

School children responding to The Sodexho School Meals and Lifestyle Survey in 2005 cited the following as the most popular school meals: pizza, pasta, burgers, chicken and filled jacket potatoes. Cakes, buns, doughnuts, ice cream, chocolate sponge, other sponges and yogurt were the most popular desserts.

Activity 1

Write a one-week menu for school lunches for both a primary school and a secondary school. Allocate appropriate portion sizes and use a dietary analysis programme to find out whether your menu has satisfied the average energy and nutrient requirements as set out in Table 6.1.2.

Food-based standards for all school food other than lunches

These standards apply to all food and drink provided by local authorities or school governing bodies to pupils on and off school premises, during an extended school day (up to 6 pm). They cover:

● breakfast clubs

● mid-morning break services

● vending machines

● tuck shops

● after-school snacks and meals.

Guidelines on food and drinks allowed or restricted at all school food other than lunches are described in Table 6.1.3.

School breakfasts

Many schools have begun offering school breakfasts and anecdotal claims have been made that school attendance, behaviour and performance all improve when school breakfasts are provided. However, a systematic review found that although a school breakfast is better than no breakfast, this only makes a difference in children who are malnourished. Furthermore, it was found that any improved academic performance noted may be due in part to the increased school attendance that a school breakfast encourages (Hoyland *et al.* 2009). Children say they enjoy the social side of school breakfasts.

Packed lunches

Many children bring a packed lunch rather than have school meals they dislike or that their parents either cannot afford or of which they disapprove. Packed lunches can also be of poor nutritional content: a Food Standards Agency survey of school lunchboxes in 2005 showed that 74 per cent failed to meet the food-based standards for school meals (Food Standards Agency 2005). Typically, a packed lunch comprised sandwiches, a chocolate bar, savoury snack and sweetened drink. Fresh fruit was often absent.

Ideally, lunchboxes should include foods from each of the food groups and include a drink (Table 6.1.4). A small ice pack or a frozen drink will keep a closed lunchbox cool for a few hours.

School Schemes Supporting Good Nutrition

The School Fruit and Vegetable Scheme is part of the national '5 A Day' programme designed to encourage fruit and vegetable consumption. Under the scheme, all children aged 4–6 years in LEA-maintained infant, primary and special schools are entitled to a free piece of fruit or vegetable each school day.

Subsidized school milk

The European Union provides subsidies to schools and other educational establishments so that they

Table 6.1.3 Guidelines on food and drinks allowed or restricted for all school food other than lunches

Foods encouraged	Foods restricted	Foods not allowed
Fruit and vegetables must be provided in all school food outlets. These can include fresh, dried, frozen, canned and juiced varieties	Condiments such as ketchup and mayonnaise must only be available in sachets or individual portion of not more than 10 g or 1 tsp	Confectionery such as chocolate bars, chocolate coated or flavoured biscuits, sweets and cereal bars
Nuts, seeds, vegetables and fruits with no added salt, sugar or fat	Cakes and biscuits must not be provided at times other than lunch	Snacks such as crisps
Free, fresh drinking water (still or carbonated) should be provided at all times	Starchy food cooked in fat or oil must not be provided more than three times a week across the school day	Salt must not be provided at tables or service counters
Fruit juice, vegetable juice, low-fat milk (milk with a fat content of not more than 1.8%), plain soya, rice or oat drinks enriched with calcium and plain yogurt drinks	No more than two deep-fried food items such as chips and batter-coated products can be provided in a single week across the school day	
Combinations of water (still or carbonated) and fruit and/or vegetable juice containing at least 50% juice, and may contain vitamins or minerals but no added sugar	Meat products (manufactured or homemade) are divided into four groups. A meat product from each of the four groups may be provided no more than once per fortnight across the school day	
Combinations of milk (low-fat or lactose reduced), or plain yogurt, water, fruit or vegetable juice – the milk or yogurt must be at least 50% by volume and the combined drink may contain vitamins and minerals. Less than 5% sugar or honey may be added		
Combinations of plain soya, rice or oat drink, water, fruit or vegetable juice – the soya, rice or oat drink must be at least 50% by volume, and the combined drink may contain vitamins and minerals. Less than 5% sugar or honey may be added to the soya, rice or oat component		
Combinations of milk (low-fat or lactose reduced), plain yogurt or plain soya, rice or oat drinks (with or without plain water) with cocoa. In these combinations the milk, yogurt, soya, rice or oat drink must be at least 50% by volume and the combined drink may contain vitamins and minerals. Less than 5% sugar or honey may be added to the milk, yogurt, soya, rice or oat component. No colourings are permitted		

Table 6.1.4 Suggestions for healthy packed lunchboxes

Food group	Suitable foods
Group 1: Bread, rice, potatoes, pasta and other starchy foods	Bread, bread rolls, tortilla wraps and pittas can be filled or used for sandwiches Crispbreads, crackers, oatcakes or breadsticks Pasta, rice or cooked potatoes as the base for a salad
Group 2: Fruit and vegetables	Vegetables sliced in sandwiches Combined in a salad Sticks of raw vegetables (celery, carrots, cucumber) or small tomatoes as finger foods or crunchy alternative to crisps Pieces of fruit or small packets of dried fruit Vegetable soup
Group 3: Milk, cheese and yogurt	Cheese is a popular sandwich filling Cubes, triangles, strings of cheese as finger foods Pots of yogurts, fromage frais or rice pudding make popular desserts Cartons of milk or flavoured milk as the drink
Group 4: Meat, fish, eggs, nuts and pulses	Cold meats or flaked fish can be included in sandwiches or salads Chicken drumsticks or cold sausages Falafels Nuts – if allowed in school
Foods combining more than one food group	Slices of quiche or pizza Samosas or bhajiis Vegetable soup also with lentils or other beans, meat or fish
Group 5: Foods high in fat and sugar	Small cakes or muffins (e.g. fruit cake or fruit muffins) Biscuits and cakes containing dried fruit or ground or chopped nuts Buns, scones, teabreads are a lower fat alternative Fruit juice can be included as the drink

can provide their pupils with selected milk and milk products. The aim of the scheme is to encourage consumption of milk and milk products to establish a healthy balanced diet by making them available in schools at a reduced cost to pupils. Schools choose whether they wish to sign up to this scheme and offer it. If they do, children entitled to free school meals are entitled to free milk. In England, Scotland and Northern Ireland $\frac{1}{3}$ pint of milk daily is available free to children up to the age of 5 years.

In Wales children up 7 years (in Key Stage 1) are entitled to $\frac{1}{3}$ pint milk free per day (Welsh Government 2011).

Breakfasts are now offered in many schools and have the potential to improve nutrient intakes, which is especially important for those entitled to free school meals. This can make a significant difference in the large numbers of school children who leave home without breakfast.

School-based interventions that combine the classroom curriculum, parental behaviour and school food services appear to be most effective in changing dietary habits.

Activity 2

Plan the key components to be included in a school intervention to increase the variety of foods the pupils will eat.

References and further reading

Bevelander KE, Anschütz DJ and Engels RC (2012) The effect of a fictitious peer on young children's choice of familiar v. unfamiliar low- and high-energy-dense foods. *British Journal of Nutrition* 7: 1–8.

Brug J, Tak NI, te Velde SJ, Bere E and de Bourdeaudhuij I (2008) Taste preferences, liking and other factors related to fruit and vegetable intakes among schoolchildren: results from observational studies. *British Journal of Nutrition* 99(suppl 1): S7–S14.

Cooke L (2007) The importance of exposure for healthy eating in childhood: a review. *Journal of Human Nutrition and Dietetics* **20**(4): 294–301.

Department of Health (2011) *National Diet and Nutrition Survey: Headline results from Years 1 and 2 (combined) of the rolling programme 2008/9–2009/10.* **www.dh.gov.uk/en/Publicationsandstatistics/ Publications/PublicationsStatistics/DH_128166** (accessed April 2012).

Evans CEL and Harper CE (2009) A history and review of school meal standards in the UK. *Journal of Human Nutrition and Dietetics* **22**: 89–99.

Food Standards Agency (FSA) (2005) *School Lunch Box Survey 2004.* London: FSA. **www.food.gov. uk/multimedia/pdfs/lunchbox2004report.pdf.**

Gregory J, Lowe S, Bates CJ, *et al.* (2000) *National Diet and Nutrition Survey: Young people aged 4–18 years.* London: The Stationery Office.

Hammons AJ and Fiese BH (2011) Is frequency of shared family meals related to the nutritional health of children and adolescents? *Pediatrics* **127**(6): e1565–e1574.

Hill AJ (2002) Developmental issues in attitudes to food and diet. *Proceedings of the Nutrition Society* **61**: 259–266.

Hill AJ (2006) The development of children's shape and weight concerns. In: Jaffa T and McDermott B (eds) *Eating Disorders in Children and Adolescents.* Cambridge: Cambridge University Press.

Hoyland A, Dye L and Lawton CL (2009) A systematic review of the effect of breakfast on the cognitive performance of children and adolescents. *Nutrition Research Reviews* **22**(2): 220–243.

James J, Thomas P, Cavan D and Kerr D (2004) Preventing childhood obesity by reducing consumption of carbonated drinks: cluster randomised controlled trial. *British Medical Journal* **328**: 1237–1241.

Moynihan P and Petersen PE (2004) Diet, nutrition and the prevention of dental diseases. *Public Health Nutrition* **7**(1A): 201–226.

Nelson M, Bradbury J, Poulter J, *et al.* (2004) *School Meals in Secondary Schools in England.* Research Report RR 557. London: Department for Education and Skills.

Nelson M, Nicholas J, Suleiman S, *et al.* (2006) *School Meals in Primary Schools in England.* London: Department for Education and Skills.

Prescott-Clarke P and Primatesta P (eds) (1998) *The Health of Young People 1995–1997.* London: The Stationery Office.

Scaglioni S, Salvioni M and Galimberti C (2008) Influence of parental attitudes in the development of children eating behaviour. *British Journal of Nutrition* **99**(suppl 1): S22–S25.

Sodexho (2005) *The Sodexho School Meals and Lifestyle Survey.* London: Sodexho Ltd.

Sproston K and Primatesta P (2003) *Health Survey for England 2002: The Health of Children and Young People.* London: The Stationery Office.

Walker A (2000) *National Diet and Nutrition Survey: Young people aged 4 to 18 years.* Volume 2. Report of the oral health survey. London: The Stationery Office.

Welsh Government (2011) Milk for primary school children. **http://wales.gov.uk/topics/ educationandskills/schoolshome/foodanddrink/ milkforprimaryschoolchildren/?lang=en** (accessed April 2012).

Useful Websites

British Dental Health Foundation (**www. dentalhealth.org.uk**)

British Heart Foundation (**www.bhf.org.uk**)

Caroline Walker Trust (**www.cwt.org.uk**)

Dairy Council (**www.milk.co.uk**)

Food in Schools Programme (**www.foodinschools. org**)

Health Education Trust (**www.healthedtrust.com**)

School fruit and vegetables scheme (**www.nhs.uk/ Livewell/5ADAY/Pages/Schoolscheme.aspx**)

School Meals Standards are available at: England and Wales: School Food Trust (**www.schoolfoodtrust. org.uk**), Northern Ireland (**www.niauditoffice.gov. uk/pubs/2011/nutritional_standards/8852_-_NIAO_ School_Meals_WEB.pdf**), Scotland (**www.scotland. gov.uk/library5/education/niss-00.asp**).

Subsided school milk: England: (**www.coolmilk. com/**), Wales (**http://wales.gov.uk/topics/ educationandskills/schoolshome/foodanddrink/ milkforprimaryschoolchildren/?lang=en**).

Nutrition for Adolescents

Summary

- Adolescents take more control over their food choices than younger children.

- They conform increasingly to peer pressure and less to their parents' role modelling.

- Nutritional intakes and status are poorer than in younger children.

- A diet high in fast food, sugar and soft drinks and low in milk and milk products, fruit and vegetables is mainly responsible for the nutrient deficiencies common in this age group.

- Appetite and energy intake increase during the pubertal growth spurt.

- Psychological changes and emotional difficulties at this age can lead to eating disorders.

- Committed physical training for sport requires an individual plan to cover energy needs for growth and training, competition and recovery afterwards.

- Pregnancy is usually unplanned and increases nutrient requirements.

Adolescence is a period of transition between childhood and adulthood, and involves both physical and emotional change, along with increasing independence and making more personal choices. The food choices of adolescents impact on their nutritional intake and status.

Physical Development

Sexual development occurs during adolescence and the onset of the sexual characteristics of puberty is a better marker of the stage of adolescence – and thus nutritional requirements – than age.

The pubertal growth spurt, as described in Chapter 2.1, occurs over about 3 years and is a period of rapid growth in height which occurs as a result of the synergistic effects of sex hormones and growth hormone. Adipose tissue stores also increase, with girls depositing adipose tissue at a greater rate than boys, laying down stores in the breast and hip regions. Fat deposition in boys tends to be more central.

The age at which the growth spurt begins varies enormously as it is influenced by genetics, gender, ethnicity and body weight.

In girls, it begins at the commencement of puberty, at the time breast development begins, with the greatest height increase in the year preceding menarche. On average, girls grow a further 6 cm in height after menarche which occurs around 13 years of age. The age range for menarche is 10–16.5 years, with tall, heavy girls tending to begin menstruation earlier than their smaller, leaner classmates. Vigorous exercise, such as athletics, can delay menarche because of both the physiological effects of training and the depletion of body fat.

Boys start their growth spurt on average two years later than girls and will be the shorter of the two sexes for a period of time. Growth may not cease completely at the end of adolescence and a height increase of up to 2 cm can still occur between the ages of 17 and 28 years. Boys will eventually be on average 14.5 cm taller than girls.

When growth is assessed on weight-for-age and height-for-age centile charts it is quite usual to see centile crossing for both height and weight during this growth spurt. This is because the charts show an average growth sport at an average age but there is a wide age range in timing of the growth spurt.

Emotional Changes and Food Choices

During adolescence, teenagers develop their own autonomy, often rejecting their parents' values in order to develop their own. Values relating to food and meals are no exception to this and many teenagers change their eating habits to be different from the rest of their family. They may:

- avoid family meals to avoid parental control, scrutiny and gifts of food – they may say they are not hungry or 'I'll make something for myself'
- adopt different eating patterns such as vegetarianism or diet to manage weight.

It is also a time of experimentation, with little regard for long-term consequences such as health problems in middle age. Hence they may be drawn to junk food for its taste appeal and to fall in with their peer group with no regard for nutritional consequences.

Their food choices are most likely to be based on or influenced by:

- convenience – particularly when eating outside the home
- preference
- taste
- brand name
- fashion and peer group pressure or influence
- personal ideology, such as the choice of a vegetarian diet

- a preoccupation with control of body weight – whether justified or not
- choosing less healthy foods as an act of parental defiance and peer solidarity
- following specific diets to enhance sporting prowess.

Nutritional Requirements in Adolescence

During rapid growth, energy and nutrient needs are higher, as shown in Tables 1.1.1 (page 3), 1.1.4–1.1.6 (pages 10–11). Appetite increases and parents often report boys being hungry about an hour after a large meal. If this increase in appetite is met with nutrient-dense food, then the extra energy and nutrients will be supplied. However, extra snacks are often high-energy, low-nutrient foods which may meet energy needs but not the increased need for essential nutrients.

Boys have higher energy and protein requirements than girls due to their greater gain in height and lean body mass during puberty. Undernutrition in both sexes at this time can inhibit bone development, resulting in a lower peak bone mass and lower height increase velocity, leading to stunting. Severe undernutrition can also delay puberty or halt its progression, as is seen in cases of severe anorexia nervosa.

Vitamins

Reference Nutrient Intakes (RNIs) for vitamins are generally similar to those recommended for adults except those for niacin and vitamin B6, which are slightly higher for 15–18 year olds than for adults. They are easily available in a balanced diet.

All females who could become pregnant are recommended to take a supplement of:

- 400 µg of folic acid to reduce the risk of fetal neural tube defects
- 10 µg of vitamin D to prevent hypocalcaemia in newborn infants and rickets in older infants and toddlers.

Since many pregnancies in this age group are unplanned, this advice applies to many adolescent girls but is likely to be unheeded. A folate-rich diet should therefore be recommended to all teenage girls, which would involve an increased intake of:

- yeast extract
- pulses – peas and beans
- oranges and orange juice
- green leafy vegetables (brussels sprouts, spinach and broccoli).

Minerals

The RNIs for calcium, phosphorus and iron in both genders, and magnesium in girls, are higher for adolescents than for adults. This reflects the increased needs for growth and development.

Calcium and phosphorus

Calcium and phosphorus are important for the rapid accretion of bone tissue. Sixty per cent of adult bone mass is gained during the pubertal growth spurt. Even after the growth spurt, calcification of bones continues as peak bone mass is reached at most bone sites from 16 to 30 years. Although 70–80 per cent of peak bone mass is determined by genetic factors, the remaining 20–30 per cent can be influenced by diet and exercise. In the UK, white and Asian teenagers are more susceptible to poor bone mass than other races. Adequate calcium intakes at this age may protect against osteoporosis in later life.

Low bone density and bone fractures in teenage girls are associated with a high intake of carbonated drinks (Wyshak 2000). The reason why is not clear but it may be due to the high phosphate content of carbonated drinks disturbing bone physiology along with the low-calcium diets adolescents tend towards by not having three daily servings of milk, cheese and yogurt.

Iron

Iron is a key nutrient during growth since it is a component of muscle and blood. The RNI of 11.3 mg/day set for boys 11–18 years old is higher than that for either younger or adult males. The iron requirement for girls 11–18 years old is even higher, at 14.8 mg/day to allow for menstrual losses. Achieving adequate iron stores becomes important for girls as menstrual periods become more regular and heavier as they mature.

Healthy Eating

The guidelines on healthy eating for adolescents are based on a number of daily servings from each of the five food groups in the 'eatwell plate' (see Chapter 1.2). Three large servings of milk, cheese or yogurt will ensure that calcium and phosphorus requirements are met to ensure bone deposition. Consuming two servings per day, or three for vegetarians, from the meat, fish, eggs, nuts and pulses group each day will ensure the extra iron requirement is met.

Portion sizes vary depending on size, gender and activity levels. Table 6.2.1 provides a rough guide but portions may increase during the pubertal growth spurt and for physical training.

Nutritious snacks will provide extra energy and boost nutrient intake and should be encouraged – particularly fortified foods such as breakfast cereals and bread (see Chapter 1.2). However, adolescents tend to snack outside the home and advice on healthier convenience and take-away foods with less fat, sugar and salt is appropriate. Some suggestions are provided in Table 6.2.2.

Nutritional Intakes and Status as Reported in Surveys

Despite their high requirements for nutrients, the food choices of adolescents in the UK tend to be poor compared to the food eaten by younger children.

Evidence for this comes from the National Diet and Nutrition Surveys in the UK (Gregory *et al.* 2000, Department of Health 2011) which show that many adolescents have very poor nutrient intakes of key vitamins and minerals. The current rolling programme found in the first two years that a large percentage of 11–18 year olds were not eating

Table 6.2.1 Portion sizes of foods for adolescents

Food groups	Suggested foods
Group 1: Bread, rice, potatoes, pasta and other starchy foods	2–4 slices wholegrain or white bread, muffin, roll or pancake
	Large bowl (7–9 tbsp) breakfast cereal
	Large bowl (10–16 tbsp) of hot cereals like porridge made up with milk
	5–10 tbsp of rice or pasta
	1–3 egg-sized potatoes or 3–8 tbsp of mashed potato
	2–5 crispbreads or crackers
Group 2: Fruit and vegetables	1–2 apples, oranges, pears, bananas
	6–15 small berries or grapes
	4–8 tbsp freshly cooked, stewed or mashed fruit
	4–6 tbsp raw or cooked vegetables
Group 3: Milk, cheese and yogurt	200–250 mL whole cow's milk as a drink
	2 small pots (125 mL) yogurt or fromage frais
	4–8 tbsp grated cheese
	Cheese in a sandwich or on a piece of pizza
	150–200 mL custard or a milk pudding
Group 4: Meat, fish, eggs, nuts and pulses	5–8 tbsp ground, chopped or cubed lean meats, fish or poultry
	1–2 whole eggs
	4–10 tbsp whole or mashed pulses (peas, beans, lentils, hummus, dhal)
	1–2 tbsp peanut butter or 2–4 tbsp ground nuts
Group 5: Foods high in fat and/or sugar	2–3 digestive biscuits or 2–4 small biscuits
	1 medium slice cake
	2 tsp jam, honey or sugar
	5–8 crisps or sweets
	2 small fun-sized chocolate bars

The measures used are 1 tbsp = one 15 mL tablespoon and 1 tsp = one 5 mL teaspoon. These are the spoons found within a set of spoons for standard recipe measures.

adequate amounts of certain vitamins and minerals. Only 3 per cent of a population are expected to eat less than the Lower Reference Nutrient Intake (LRNI), but the percentages of adolescents in the UK who eat less than the LRNI for several vitamins and minerals are very high (Table 6.2.3).

Fifty per cent of girls 11–18 years old had folate intakes below the RNI of 200 μg/day and 5 per cent had intakes below the LRNI. Nine per cent of girls over 11 years had a red cell folate level indicative of deficiency. The risk of low folate status is significant in this age group where unplanned pregnancies are increasingly common.

Table 6.2.2 Guidance for choosing healthier snack foods and take-away meals

Choose less	Reason	Choose instead	Reason
Fizzy drinks	High in sugar and acid which damage tooth enamel and increase risk of dental caries	Plain or flavoured milks or yogurt drinks	Good for strengthening bone and preventing fractures during sport
Diet soft drinks	High in acid which dissolves tooth enamel May decrease bone density	Plain or sparkling water	Do not damage teeth or bones and good for hydrating the skin
Crisps and other savoury snacks	High in saturated fat and salt	Sandwiches with meat, fish, egg or hummus combined with salad fillings	More protein, iron and zinc for skin repair and building muscle rather than fat
Pan-fried pizzas	High in fat	Plain oven-baked pizza bases	Less fat and a good source of nutrients depending on toppings
Doner kebab	High in fat	Shish kebab	Less fat and a better source of protein, iron and zinc
Croissants, doughnuts, sweet pastries, flapjacks	High in fat	Hot cross buns, tea bread, fruit scones, pancakes	A convenient high-energy snack and a good source of a range of nutrients
Fries with a burger	High in fat	Burger in bun with salad without the fries	Less fat and more vitamins and minerals
Fried rice/noodles or naan	High in fat	Boiled or steamed rice or chapatti	Low-fat, high-carbohydrate
Creamy and oily sauces with pasta	Sauces are high in fat	Tomato-based or vegetable sauces with pasta	Vegetables provide more vitamins and antioxidants which aid skin repair
Fried chicken and fish in batter	The batter coatings are high in fat with few nutrients	Eat the chicken and fish inside the batter and throw away the batter – or most of it	Protein, iron, zinc and B vitamins from the meat or fish are good for muscle building

Young women who do not consume fortified breakfast cereals and have low intakes of other important dietary sources of folate, such as green leafy vegetables, pulses and citrus fruits, are particularly at risk.

Food choices

The National Diet and Nutrition Surveys (NDNS) and other dietary surveys suggest that factors contributing to nutritional imbalances in this age group include the following:

- Snacking or 'grazing' is a common pattern of eating in this age group, with most adolescents eating on at least six occasions during the day.

The snacks are more likely to comprise crisps, biscuits, confectionery and carbonated drinks than fresh fruit, sandwiches or milk-based products.

- In fact, savoury snacks such as crisps, potato chips, biscuits and chocolate confectionery are among the most commonly consumed foods, with large numbers eating them every day.

- High consumption of sugar-containing foods and soft drinks provides a high intake of energy but few micronutrients.

- Fruit and vegetable consumption is poor, with many adolescents eating less than one portion a day.

Table 6.2.3 Percentage of 11- to 18-year-old boys and girls eating less than the LRNI for certain nutrients

Nutrient	Percentage eating less then the LRNI	
	Boys	Girls
Vitamin A	12	13
Riboflavin	8	17
Folate	2	5
Iron	5	43
Calcium	8	14
Magnesium	27	50
Potassium	16	31
Zinc	11	18
Selenium	22	47
Iodine	7	17

From Department of Health (2011).

LRNI, Lower Reference Nutrient Intake.

- Intake of milk-based foods was inadequate from the age of 11 years, with few drinking milk.
- High rates of dieting among teenage girls were noted. In the 1997 NDNS 16 per cent of girls aged 15–18 years old were dieting to lose weight.
- Ten per cent of 15- to 18-year-old girls said they were vegetarian in the same survey. Suitable high-iron alternatives to meat and fish such as nuts and pulses are often not included in the teenage vegetarian's diet.
- Breakfast is often not eaten which reduces nutrient intakes. A survey in 2005 found that 12 per cent of children aged 15–16 years did not eat anything before school (Sodexho 2005).
- Older boys have better nutrient intakes than girls as they eat larger quantities of food, including more biscuits, meat, fortified breakfast cereals, baked beans and potatoes.

Population differences in the dietary intakes of adolescents

- Boys appear to prefer meat and dairy products, while girls were more likely to favour fruit, low-fat products and artificially sweetened drinks, perhaps due to a desire to control body weight.
- Young people living in Scotland consumed more high-fat foods and less fruit and vegetables than those in the south of England. This impacts nutritionally and children in Scotland had lower intakes of fibre, retinol equivalents and riboflavin.
- Those from the least affluent groups had lower intakes of energy, fat and most vitamins and minerals. A greater proportion of their daily energy intake came from snacks of low nutrient density.

Nutritional status of adolescents

Blood analyses from the 1997 NDNS revealed that:

- 13 per cent of boys and 27 per cent of girls had low serum ferritin levels, indicative of low iron stores
- vitamin C, folate, riboflavin and thiamin blood levels were all low, particularly in young people in Scotland and northern England
- 8 per cent of boys and 11.5 per cent of girls had a plasma cholesterol concentration above 5.2 mmol/L
- use of salt at the table was associated with increased systolic blood pressure
- 10–25 per cent had low vitamin D plasma levels depending on the time of year measurements were made. This may reflect less time spent outside in the summer months.

Further Causes of Malnutrition

Obesity

This is discussed in Chapter 7.2.

Vegetarianism

Most dietary regimens are short lived but vegetarianism may be one way of sustaining a reduced energy intake. For some, dieting and vegetarianism are intertwined. In a US study

(Neumark-Sztainer *et al.* 1997) vegetarians were:

- twice as likely to report frequent dieting
- four times more likely to vomit for weight control
- eight times more likely to use laxatives.

In the 1997 NDNS, 10 per cent of 15- to 18-year-old girls stated that they were either vegetarian or vegan (but only 1 per cent of boys of the same age) (Gregory *et al.* 2000). This is not a problem in itself but if the diets are poorly planned and imbalanced, the result can be an inadequate intake of some micronutrients. Common pitfalls are failure to consume foods which sufficiently compensate for the loss of haem iron from the diet. In addition, alternative sources of protein and vitamin B12 are needed in a vegan diet.

Inappropriate slimming

Adolescence is the peak age for body dissatisfaction, and surveys of UK teenagers consistently show that more than 50 per cent of girls feel fat and want to lose weight. Up to 25 per cent of young adolescent girls report dieting to lose weight, their motivation driven by weight and shape dissatisfaction (Hill 2002). The Minnesota Adolescent Health Survey of 30,000 teenagers revealed that 12 per cent of girls were dieting, 30 per cent binge eating, 12 per cent vomiting and 2 per cent using laxative or diuretics (Neumark-Sztainer *et al.* 1998). The NDNS in 1997 found that 16 per cent of girls aged 15–18 years (and 3 per cent of the boys) were dieting to lose weight (Gregory *et al.* 2000). Boys are usually more concerned that they are not muscular enough.

Unsupervised and unnecessary slimming can result in low micronutrient intakes as 'the diet' often involves missing meals, particularly breakfast. Body image can be improved by encouraging physical activity, but care must be taken when discussing diet with girls who are concerned about their weight in case an over-focus on food encourages a drift towards an eating disorder. Emphasis on variety and balance rather than restriction or 'good versus bad foods' is important.

Eating disorders

A concern about body image becomes more serious if an eating disorder develops. This occurs most commonly between 15 and 25 years of age. Although eating disorders are most common in girls, studies have shown that about 10 per cent of patients with eating disorders are male.

Genetic make-up and the attitude of other family members to food may have some influence on susceptibility. It can occur in children with any cultural or racial background.

Eating disorders usually develop from a combination of many factors that make one feel unable to cope with life. This includes events, feelings or pressures such as:

- low self-esteem
- problems with friends or family relationships
- peer pressure
- the death of someone special
- problems at school, college, university or work
- high academic expectations
- lack of confidence
- sexual or emotional abuse such as being bullied
- feeling too fat.

Eating disorders have been divided into three different categories: anorexia nervosa, bulimia nervosa and eating disorder not otherwise specified.

Anorexia nervosa

Anorexia nervosa is most common in females 15–19 years but can occur in younger children. It is characterized by:

- weight loss or no weight gain during a period of growth
- intense fear of gaining weight
- distorted body image
- amenorrhoea in females – absence of at least three consecutive menstrual cycles.

Bulimia nervosa

Bulimia nervosa is characterized by:

- binge eating of abnormally large amounts of food along with a feeling of lack of control
- compensatory behaviour after the binge, including vomiting, use of laxatives, fasting or excessive exercise.

Eating disorder not otherwise specified

Eating disorder not otherwise specified is a broad diagnostic category of abnormal eating behaviours including binge eating disorder and the female athlete triad. These include aspects of anorexia and bulimia but do not meet the diagnostic criteria.

In binge eating disorders, binge eating is not followed by the compensatory behaviours.

The female athlete triad is a syndrome of sportswomen with three characteristics:

- low energy intake which may be a result of trying to lose weight for sports performance reasons, body image reasons or not understanding the energy and nutrient requirements of lifestyle and training regime
- menstrual dysfunction
- low bone mineral density which can result in bone fractures during athletic training or performance.

The long-term energy and nutrient depletion of eating disorders and the resulting malnutrition can have lasting effects on growth, sexual development and bone density. In the short term, dental erosion caused by self-induced frequent vomiting increases dental erosion.

If an eating disorder is suspected in a child then the family should be alerted and encouraged to seek professional help from a specialized treatment centre with a multidisciplinary team. Early treatment results in the most positive outcomes. When the eating disorder develops into a chronic condition, even with treatment there may be frequent relapses throughout life. In about 10 per cent of cases it causes death.

Alcohol

Alcohol intakes tend to increase during the teenage years, reaching a peak at about the age of 19. In adolescence, alcohol intake is often limited to one or two days per week and intoxication and value for money are the key aims. In the NDNS rolling survey 4 per cent of boys aged 13–15 years and 8 per cent of boys aged 13–15 years were drinking alcohol once or twice a week. UK adolescents have one of the highest levels in Europe of alcohol use, binge drinking and getting drunk.

High alcohol intakes are a cause for concern for both health and social reasons. Teenagers have less ability to metabolize alcohol than fully mature adults and are more susceptible to its adverse effects. Under the influence of alcohol they are more likely to have unsafe sex because they are less likely to use contraception, and also more likely to have sex they later regret.

Regular heavy alcohol consumption and binge drinking:

- are associated with physical problems, antisocial behaviour, violence, accidents, suicide, injuries and road traffic accidents and criminal offences
- affect school performance
- can exacerbate existing mental health problems
- may have adverse effects on health in later life.

In 2000, nearly 14 per cent of 16–19 year olds experienced dependence on alcohol (British Medical Association 2003). From a nutritional point of view, regular alcohol consumption can displace more nutrient-dense foods from the diet and, since alcohol has a high energy density but little impact on appetite, regular drinking can easily lead to over-consumption of energy.

If health advice on alcohol is over-negative it may be ignored. Emphasis is better placed on ensuring that young people:

- are aware of safe drinking limits
- know how to assess the alcoholic strength of products, particularly some of the 'designer drinks' or special brews of lagers which may have a deceptively high alcohol content.

Conditions that Increase Nutritional Requirements

Physical training for sport

Adolescents undertaking sports training at the same time as undergoing physical change and development may have very high energy requirements. Specialist input from a specialist sports dietitian can ensure that nutrient and energy requirements to support growth as well as training needs are met. If energy needs are not met, growth can be compromised.

Monthly height measurements can be used to assess when the growth spurt is taking place. Individual energy needs can be calculated using basal metabolic rate and physical activity level and adding 60–100 kcal/day to allow for extra growth (Department of Health 1991).

Adolescents undertaking sports training should aim to:

- maintain good hydration by drinking sufficient fluid
- be well hydrated before exercise and drink enough fluid during and after exercise to balance fluid losses
- eat a high-carbohydrate diet with 60–70 per cent of energy from carbohydrate
- eat sufficient protein to cover growth as well as muscle development and recovery after training or competing
- follow a balanced diet with a minimum of the daily servings of the four nutritious food groups to make sure they meet their nutrient requirements to maintain health and a strong immune system
- eat a high-carbohydrate snack or meal containing some protein within an hour of finishing training or competing – to ensure repair of muscle tissue and the replenishment of glycogen stores within muscles.

Sports beverages containing carbohydrates and electrolytes may be consumed before, during and after exercise to help maintain blood glucose concentration, provide fuel for muscles and decrease risk of dehydration and hyponatraemia. Milk is an effective recovery drink after exercise.

Pregnancy

Pregnancy and lactation during teenage years place extra nutritional requirements on girls who may not have finished growing themselves and who will not have attained their peak bone mass. Nutrient requirements have not been specified for these young mothers but a healthy balanced diet with folic acid and vitamin D supplementation is a minimum requirement. For those eating poorly, a multivitamin and mineral supplement excluding vitamin A can be recommended. As part of the Healthy Start programme, all pregnant girls under 18 are entitled to benefits regardless of their financial circumstances, including free vitamins and vouchers for milk, fruit and vegetables.

Cooking and Food Preparation Skills

Many adolescents leave home at the age of 18 or soon after, and cooking skills enable them to prepare alternatives to convenience foods for themselves. Current school curricula do not ensure they will learn to cook and many parents and carers cannot or do not teach them. Health promotion activities could usefully address this problem.

References and further reading

Aerenhouts D, Deriemaeker P, Hebbelinck M, Clarys PJ (2011) Energy and macronutrient intake in adolescent sprint athletes: a follow-up study. *Sports Science* 29(1): 73–82.

Beets MW, Swanger K, Wilcox DR and Cardinal BJ (2007) Using hands-on demonstrations to promote cooking behaviors with young adolescents: The Culinary Camp Summer Cooking Program. *Journal of Nutrition Education and Behavior* 39: 288–289.

Boutelle KN, Birkeland RW, Hannan PJ, Stat M, Story M and Neumark-Sztainer D (2007) Associations between maternal concern for healthful eating and maternal eating behaviors, home food availability, and adolescent eating behaviors. *Journal of Nutrition Education and Behavior* **39**: 248–256.

British Medical Association Board of Science and Education (2003) *Adolescent Health*. London: BMA.

Department of Health (1991) *Report No 41. Dietary Reference Values for Food Energy and Nutrients for the UK. Report of the Panel on Dietary Reference Values of the Committee on Medical Aspects of Food Policy*. London: HMSO.

Department of Health (2011) *National Diet and Nutrition Survey: Headline results from Years 1 and 2 (combined) of the rolling programme 2008/9–2009/10*. **www.dh.gov.uk/en/Publicationsandstatistics/ Publications/PublicationsStatistics/DH_128166** (accessed April 2012).

Gregory J, Lowe S, Bates CJ, *et al.* (2000) *National Diet and Nutrition Survey: Young people aged 4–18 years*. London: The Stationery Office.

Haerens L, Craeynest M, Deforche B, Maes L, Cardon G and De Bourdeaudhuij I (2008) The contribution of psychosocial and home environmental factors in explaining eating behaviours in adolescents. *European Journal of Clinical Nutrition* **62**: 51–59.

Hill AJ (2002) Developmental issues in attitudes to food and diet. *Proceedings of the Nutrition Society* **61**: 259–266.

Hill AJ (2006) The development of children's shape and weight concerns. In: Jaffa T and McDermott B (eds) *Eating Disorders in Children and Adolescents*. Cambridge: Cambridge University Press.

Lanham-New S (2011) *Sport and Exercise Nutrition*. London: Wiley-Blackwell.

Larson NI, Story M, Wall M and Neumark-Sztainer D (2006) Calcium and dairy intakes of adolescents are associated with their home environment, taste preferences, personal health beliefs, and meal patterns. *Journal of the American Dietetic Association* **106**: 1816–1824.

Larson NI, Neumark-Sztainer D and Story M (2009) Weight control behaviors and dietary intake among adolescents and young adults: longitudinal findings from Project EAT. *Journal of the American Dietetic Association* **109**: 1869–1877.

Loucks AB, Stachenfeld NS and DiPietro L (2006) The female athlete triad: do female athletes need to take special care to avoid low energy availability? *Medicine and Science in Sports and Exercise* **38**: 1694–1700.

McNaughton SA, Wattanapenpaiboon N, Wark JD and Nowson CA (2011) An energy-dense, nutrient-poor dietary pattern is inversely associated with bone health in women. *Journal of Nutrition* **141**: 1516–1523.

Matthys C, De Henauw S, Bellemans M, De Maeyer M and De Backer G (2007) Breakfast habits affect overall nutrient profiles in adolescents. *Public Health Nutrition* **10**(4): 413–421.

Miller CA and Golden NH (2010) An introduction to eating disorders: clinical presentation, epidemiology, and prognosis. *Nutrition in Clinical Practice* **25**: 110–115.

Moreno LA, Gonzalez-Gross M, Kersting M, *et al.* (2007) Assessing, understanding and modifying nutritional status, eating habits and physical activity in European adolescents: The HELENA (Healthy Lifestyle in Europe by Nutrition in Adolescence) study. *Public Health Nutrition* **11**(3): 288–299.

Nelson M, Badbury J, Poulter J, Mcgee A, Mseble S and Jarvis L (2004) *School Meals in Secondary Schools in England*. London: Department for Education and Skills.

Neumark-Sztainer D, Story M, Resnick M and Blum R (1997) Adolescent vegetarians. A behavioural profile of a school-based population in Minnesota. *Archives of Pediatric and Adolescent Medicine* **151**: 833–838.

Neumark-Sztainer D, Story M, Resnick M and Blum R (1998) Lessons learnt about adolescent nutrition from the Minnesota Adolescent Health Survey. *Journal of the American Dietetic Association* **98**: 1449–1456.

Pearson N, Biddle SJ and Gorely T (2008) Family correlates of fruit and vegetable consumption in children and adolescents: a systematic review. *Public Health Nutrition* **12**(2): 267–283.

Robinson-O'Brien R, Perry CL, Wall MM, Story M and Neumark-Sztainer D (2009) Adolescent and young adult vegetarianism: better dietary intake and weight outcomes but increased risk of disordered eating behaviors. *Journal of the American Dietetic Association* **109**(4): 648–655.

Rodriguez NR, DiMarco NM, Langley S, American Dietetic Association, Dietetians of Canada, American College of Sports Medicine (2009) Position of the American Dietetic Association, Dietitians of Canada, and the American College of Sports Medicine: Nutrition and athletic performance. *Journal of the American Dietetic Association* **109**(3): 509–527.

Sjöberg A, Hallberg L, Höglund D and Hulthén L (2003) Meal pattern, food choice, nutrient intake and lifestyle factors in The Göteborg Adolescence Study. *European Journal of Clinical Nutrition* **57**(12): 1569–1578.

Sodexho Ltd. (2005) *The Sodexho School Meals and Lifestyle Survey*. London: Sodexho Ltd.

Stevenson C, Doherty G, Barnett J, Muldoon OT and Trew K (2007) Adolescents' views of food and eating: Identifying barriers to healthy eating. *Journal of Adolescence* **30**: 417–434.

Vicari RM, Bramlet D, Olivera B, *et al.* (2007) Atherosclerosis and teen eating study. *Journal of Clinical Lipidology* **1**: 194–197.

Vue H and Reicks M (2007) Individual and environmental influences on intake of calcium-rich food and beverages by young adolescent girls. *Journal of Nutrition Education and Behaviour* **39**: 264–272.

Wyshak G (2000) Teenaged girls, carbonated beverage consumption, and bone fractures. *Archives of Pediatric and Adolescent Medicine* **154**(6): 610–613.

Resources

Eating Disorders Association (**www.b-eat.co.uk/**)

Healthy Start Programme (**www.healthystart.nhs.uk**)

Section 7
Nutrition for Chronic Conditions

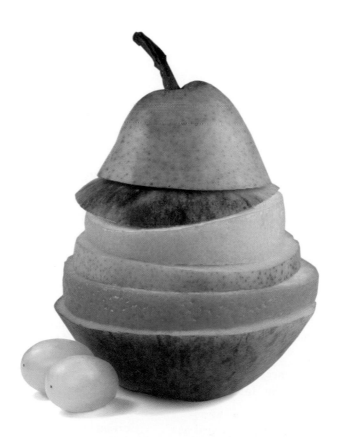

Food Hypersensitivity – Food Allergies and Intolerances

Summary

- Food hypersensitivity can be either an allergic reaction involving the immune system or an intolerance that is an adverse reaction to food not involving the immune system.

- Symptoms of food allergy that appear rapidly involve the production of immunoglobulin E (IgE). A slower onset of symptoms at least two hours after eating the food may not involve IgE.

- Common foods that children in the UK have adverse reactions to are milk, eggs, fish, peanuts and other tree nuts.

- Food hypersensitivity is less common than parents report and is diagnosed by one or more of the following: clinical history, skin prick tests, blood tests, food challenge or trial exclusion diet.

- European law requires that the following foods must be listed in the ingredients list on the label if they are present in a food: milk, cereals containing gluten, eggs, fish, shellfish, peanuts or ground nuts, tree nuts, soybeans, celery, mustard, sesame seeds, lupin, sulphur dioxide and sulphites.

The number of children who are allergic or intolerant to foods may be rising and the increase depends on the country they live in and the foods involved. For example, peanut allergy may be increasing in some countries and milk allergy increasing in other countries. This changing pattern is difficult to explain but may be due to factors such as:

- exposure to a wider range of chemicals in the environment, many of which have only been introduced in the last 50 or so years

- exposure to a less diverse range of microorganisms due to lifestyle factors, including how clean homes are kept

- improving public health measures including immunizations that prevent infections in infants and toddlers

- the changes in food and drinks consumed as they are more likely to be processed with a long shelflife and less likely to be fresh from a local producer.

Food Hypersensitivity

Although most people use the term 'food allergy' loosely to cover all unpleasant reactions to food, the current clinical classification is based on the type of adverse response to food (Johansson *et al.* 2004). 'Food hypersensitivity' is the umbrella term used to cover all the different types of physiological reactions to foods (Figure 7.1.1). Food allergy triggers the immune system to respond to a food protein, whereas the term 'food intolerance' is used when the immune system is not involved and the reactions may be triggered by chemicals in a food that are either naturally occurring or have been added in the processing of that food.

Current management of food hypersensitivity is to exclude the food causing the problem, but the degree of avoidance needed is very individual. It is important to monitor the condition so that foods are not excluded for longer than is necessary.

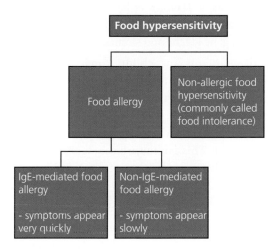

Figure 7.1.1 Classification of adverse reactions to food

Food allergy

The foods that are most likely to cause an allergic reaction vary from country to country. In the UK they are:

- cow's milk – more likely in infancy
- eggs
- peanuts, also called ground nuts
- tree nuts – almonds, hazelnuts, walnuts, cashew nuts, pecan nuts, brazil nuts, pistachio nuts, macadamia nuts and Queensland nuts
- fish
- shellfish – prawn, shrimp, crab, lobster and crayfish
- wheat
- soya
- sesame
- kiwi fruit.

When an infant or child is allergic to a food, a protein in that food triggers their immune system to respond in a variety of ways. It may be a rapid, mainly severe response or a slower, less severe response depending on whether the antibody immunoglobulin E (IgE) is released by the immune system or not. Not all allergic reactions involve the production of IgE.

IgE-mediated food allergy

In infants and children who do make the specific antibody IgE to a food, a protein in the food reacts with the IgE and one or more of the following symptoms will appear within two hours of eating the food:

- diarrhoea
- asthma/wheeze
- breathing difficulties
- eczema gets worse
- hives (blotchy red rash) or urticaria
- itching
- pallor
- rashes
- redness – particularly a red facial flush in infants and young children
- swelling of lips, tongue, face
- vomiting
- anaphylaxis.

Anaphylaxis is the most serious reaction and includes breathing problems, and a rapid drop in blood pressure. Children who suffer in this way need immediate medical attention. Death from fatal allergic reaction to food is rare: around 1 in 800 000 per year. Children with asthma have the highest risk.

Parents of children at risk of anaphylaxis need to be taught how to use an adrenaline auto-injector (e.g. Epipen or Anapen). The adrenaline reverses the reaction. Two adrenaline auto-injectors need to be with the child at all times so that it can be accessed rapidly and used in an emergency.

The Anaphylaxis Campaign provides useful information for food allergy sufferers with anaphylaxis (www.anaphylaxis.org.uk).

Non IgE-mediated food allergy

When immune cells other than IgE are involved in the reaction to a protein in the food, the symptoms appear more slowly – usually a few hours after eating the food. The typical symptoms are:

- abdominal pain or colic, bloating and wind
- constipation
- diarrhoea
- eczema – a gradual increase in the number and size of the sites being affected
- reflux
- vomiting a few hours after meal
- wheeze.

Non-allergic food hypersensitivity or food intolerance

When a child has a food intolerance, the immune system does not respond to the food but an unpleasant reaction to food still occurs. The symptoms usually appear a few hours or even days after eating the food and they are rarely life-threatening. Foods which children can be intolerant to include:

- citrus fruits: these fruits sometimes contain high levels of benzoic acid which can cause a harmless flare reaction around the mouth
- fruits and vegetables containing salicylates or histamines can cause reactions similar to food allergy such as hives and skin rashes, even facial swelling in some toddlers. The foods with the highest levels that are most likely to cause such a reaction are strawberries, tomatoes, blueberries and blackberries.

Foods containing biogenic amines can cause headache, nausea and giddiness. They include:

- cheese, especially if matured
- fermented foods such as blue cheese, sauerkraut, fermented soya products
- yeast extracts
- fish, especially if stale or pickled
- microbial contaminated foods
- chocolate

- some fruits, especially citrus fruits, bananas and avocado pears
- foods containing monosodium glutamate (MSG) as a flavour enhancer. Some foods contain large amounts of MSG and it may cause flushing, headache and stomach ache
- milk – infants and children may sometimes become intolerant to lactose, which is the sugar in milk, for a short time following a bout of viral gastroenteritis. During this time they lack the enzyme lactase and consequently do not digest the lactose. This can cause loose stools and wind but usually resolves within a few weeks.

Additives

Whether additives in food such as artificial colours and preservatives cause reactions is currently unclear and needs further investigation. The Food Standards Agency advises that any foods, drinks or medicines containing the following should not be given to infants and children:

Colours:	
Tartrazine	E102
Ponceau 4R	E124
Sunset yellow	E110
Carmosine	E122
Quinoline yellow	E104
Allura red AC	E129
Preservative:	
Sodium benzoate	E211

How Common Are Food Allergies?

Many parents suspect their child has a food allergy but it is only clinically diagnosed in about 10 per cent of these children. The symptoms listed above may be caused by other environmental substances rather than food, such as dust mites. For example, fewer than half of the infants and children with eczema have this skin condition because of a reaction to food. Food allergy is more likely in children with severe and widespread eczema.

Between 2 and 4 per cent of children 1–3 years old are affected but most grow out of it by about 3 years of age (Zuberbier *et al.* 2004, Venter *et al.* 2008). Those with slow onset symptoms are more likely to outgrow their food allergies than those who experience rapid appearance of symptoms. In general (Venter and Arshad 2011):

● 80–90 per cent of infants will outgrow their milk allergy by 3 years

● 50 per cent of infants will outgrow their egg allergy by 3 years

● 20 per cent of children may outgrow their peanut allergy.

Only about 2 in 100 toddlers remain allergic to one or more foods as they get older. Children should therefore be retested with a food challenge at an appropriate age to check if they have grown out of it.

Diagnosing Food Allergies and Intolerances

There is no simple diagnostic test for food allergy or food intolerance. A detailed history is an important part of the diagnosis, and the National Institute for Health and Clinical Excellence (NICE) recommends the following points are included (NICE 2011):

● individual and family history of atopic disease – eczema, asthma, allergic rhinitis and also food allergy – in parents or siblings

● any personal history of atopic disease especially eczema

● the suspected allergen

● details of any foods that are avoided and why

● presenting symptoms and other symptoms that may be associated with food allergy, including age of first onset, speed of onset, duration, severity and frequency, reproducibility of symptoms on repeated exposure and what food and how much exposure to it causes a reaction

● feeding history (e.g. weaning)

● details of any previous treatment or exclusions and the response.

A paediatrician or allergy clinic can organize additional investigations that may be helpful, including:

● specific IgE testing

● skin prick tests (SPT)

● patch tests

● endoscopy and biopsy.

There is no clinical or scientific evidence to support the use of various other tests including hair analysis, kinesiology and bioresonance (NICE 2011). However, many alternative therapists use them.

Specific IgE tests measure the level of food-specific IgE levels in the blood and are highly predictive of foods causing allergic reactions. However, a child with a high food-specific IgE level will not always have an adverse reaction to that food.

A positive skin prick test causes redness and swelling of the skin. The size of the skin wheal formed is graded. They are:

● rarely negative in someone with true IgE-mediated allergic reactions

● almost always negative in non-IgE-mediated reactions.

However, a positive blood or skin test can be seen in the absence of food allergy. The positive blood or skin response merely means that the child is making IgE to the proteins in that food. There is no need to avoid a food that a child is regularly eating without symptoms even if the SPT or blood test to that food is positive.

If the child has a history of a reaction to a food, however, and the SPT or blood test is positive, that would mean a clinical allergy in most cases and the food needs to be avoided. A food challenge may be needed for a definitive diagnosis in some cases.

If the SPT or blood test is positive and the child has never knowingly eaten the food, a food challenge will be needed to rule out food allergy.

Food Challenges

Food challenges are the most definitive part of diagnosis but are not always necessary if the clinical history is convincing. They will either:

- detect a specific food which causes symptoms and needs to be excluded from the diet; or
- confirm that a specific food is not responsible for symptoms and does not need to be restricted.

They are also used to determine if and when a child has outgrown their food allergy.

The gold standard test is the placebo-controlled double blind food challenge. In clinical practice, however, open challenges are usually performed. A paediatric or allergy specialist dietitian needs to be involved as the food suspected to be the cause of symptoms must be consumed by the child and the response monitored.

Challenges must be carried out in appropriately staffed and equipped settings because of the risk of a severe reaction. For children with any level of specific IgE or any size SPT to the food or who have developed symptoms to a food less than two hours after eating it in the past, the food challenge should be done in hospital where the necessary medication can be administered to reverse any severe symptoms.

Food challenges can usually be carried out at home in children with no specific IgE levels to a food or negative SPT and a history of only slow onset symptoms (NICE 2011).

A food challenge for non-severe, slower onset symptoms of non-IgE-mediated food allergy and non-allergic food hypersensitivity usually involves:

1. recording the symptoms and foods eaten while on a normal diet for one or two weeks

2. recording the symptoms and foods eaten while on a diet excluding the suspected food – usually for one or two weeks

3. recording the symptoms and foods eaten for a further period of time with the suspected food eaten to see if the symptoms reappear if they have disappeared in step 2.

Expert advice is needed from a dietitian to cut out a suspected food completely as parents and children may not be aware of all the foods that can contain traces of a suspected food.

Grading the severity of the symptoms to be recorded helps make the parent or carer recording the symptoms more objective. For example, diarrhoea can be graded as follows:

Severity of symptoms	Diarrhoea
0	Formed stool
1	Slightly loose stool
2	Very loose stool
3	Liquid stool

During the period of investigation the parent/carer records the timings of all the food and drinks consumed by the infant or child along with the time of any symptoms and the grade of severity. For example:

Time	Food and drinks consumed	Symptoms
7:30	Small bowl Cheerios with full-fat milk + banana slices	
	1 cup milk	
8:30		Diarrhoea – 2
10:30	120 mL cup of apple juice diluted 50% with water	
	1 digestive biscuit	
12:00	2 tbsp pasta	
	1 tbsp meat sauce	
	3 carrot sticks	
	2 cauliflower florets	
	1 flavoured fromage frais	
	6 grapes	
	120 mL cup of water	
13:00		Diarrhoea – 1

The dietitian can then assess the diary and discuss with the parents whether the suspect food is likely to be causing the adverse reaction or not.

Managing Diagnosed Food Hypersensitivity

Once an allergy or intolerance to a food is diagnosed, the current management is to avoid the culprit food or foods.

The extent to which the food needs to be avoided will vary from child to child. Some infants and children with IgE-mediated food allergies need to completely avoid the food – even in trace amounts. Others may be able to tolerate small amounts of the food they are allergic or intolerant to.

All children with food allergy should be under the care of a paediatrician or GP. Children with severe food allergies may need an adrenaline auto-injector prescribed for them (Figure 7.1.2).

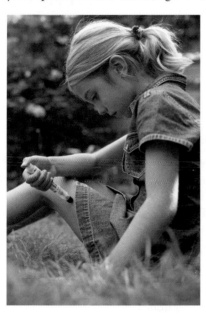

Figure 7.1.2 An adrenaline auto-injector pen

All children should know which foods they need to avoid and should be encouraged to tell others about their food allergy or intolerance.

Clothes, stickers, t-shirts, watches and jewellery that alert people to food allergy are available from certain websites (e.g. www.kidsaware.co.uk, www.medicalert.co.uk, www.sostalisman.com).

Recent research suggests that, in the future, treatment for food allergy may change to exposing children to small quantities of the suspected food and increasing that quantity over time to induce tolerance of that food (Fisher *et al.* 2011). This is still very much in the experimental phase.

Coeliac Disease

This disease is not a food allergy or a food intolerance but is an autoimmune disease. Infants and children with this condition cannot tolerate the protein gluten which is found in the three cereals: wheat, rye and barley. All food and drinks made from these three cereals need to be eliminated from the diet. Some children may also need to avoid oats if they are also sensitive to a protein in oats which is similar to gluten. Often oats are contaminated with traces of wheat, rye or barley and so children may be advised to avoid oats along with wheat, rye and barley as a matter of course.

Coeliac disease is discussed further in Chapter 7.3.

Treating Food Hypersensitivity with an Exclusion Diet

Children may be hypersensitive to more than one food. Exclusion diets which exclude the food or foods the child is hypersensitive to can lead to a nutritional inadequacy and therefore all children should see a paediatric or allergy specialist dietitian for nutritional assessment and advice.

An excluded food can often be substituted with other foods from the same food group (see Chapter 1.2). However, if the food suspected of causing a reaction is milk then that whole food group must be excluded. A dietitian can recommend suitable alternative milks which may be prescribable by a doctor.

The responsibilities of a dietitian managing any exclusion diet are to advise:

- which foods a child can eat and which foods he or she will have to avoid
- which family foods to use in place of excluded foods
- how to check food labels for food ingredients that must be avoided
- on any food products or milks a child may be entitled to have prescribed

- on supplements that may be required to ensure nutritional adequacy
- where to buy certain foods
- which organizations can give extra advice and support
- on menu planning and recipe modification
- a nursery or school about the special diet the child needs.

Avoiding certain foods becomes more complicated when processed foods are used. The ingredients in commercial foods may also contain traces of foods that need to be avoided and this may not always be obvious. Some manufacturers and supermarkets provide lists of foods free from certain foods but the ingredients list should always be checked as recipes of processed foods are often modified.

Useful advice for parents and children is summarized in Table 7.1.1.

Cutting out eggs

Many foods (e.g. cakes, some biscuits, some ice cream, mayonnaise, quiche, pancakes and some pasta) contain eggs as an ingredient. Often eggs are used to glaze baked goods.

Some children may be able to eat very small quantities of egg in cooked foods such as cakes as cooking denatures some of the protein, making it less likely to cause a reaction (Lemon-Mule *et al.* 2008).

Cutting out peanuts and tree nuts

Peanuts are from a different biological family to tree nuts and children may not be allergic to both peanuts and tree nuts. However, whatever the nut allergy it is prudent to avoid both types of nuts as they are often processed in the same factories, which can lead to cross-contamination of tree nuts with traces of peanuts or vice versa.

Cutting out sesame

Many foods contain sesame or tahini: particularly hummus, halvah and many Turkish, Greek, Chinese and Japanese foods. Sesame can also be present in bread, biscuits, salad dressings and sauces.

Cutting out milk

Because this involves the elimination of a whole food group, a child needs to have a substitute food to provide the same nutrients that milk, cheese and yogurt provide.

Most infants and children who are allergic to cow's milk will also be allergic to goat, buffalo, camel and sheep milk so these cannot be used instead. Hydrolysed infant formulas are prescribable for infants. Soya formula milk is not considered appropriate for infants less than 6 months of age (see Chapter 4.1, page 94). Soya or oat milk which is fortified with extra calcium and vitamins is often the substitute milk for children over 12 months.

Rice milk is not recommended for children under 5 years as it may contain small amounts of arsenic.

Cutting out wheat

Cutting out wheat is very difficult as many foods are based on wheat flour. This includes bread, pasta, couscous and almost all biscuits and cakes. Wheat flour is often used as an ingredient for thickening sauces and wheat rusks are added to sausages and other processed meats.

There are a variety of pastas, breads and crispbreads based on flours made from other cereals or foods, such as maize, polenta, rye, oats, chick peas, gram, lentil, bean, potato, rice, millet, arrowroot and buckwheat. Labels need to be checked carefully to make sure they are 100 per cent wheat free as some may contain a small percentage of wheat flour, making them unsuitable. For example, rye bread may be made from 90 per cent rye flour and 10 per cent wheat flour and oat flapjacks often contain some wheat flour.

Cutting out soya

Soya flour is used along with wheat flour in many foods – most breads have some soya flour in them.

Table 7.1.1 Foods to avoid and suggested alternatives

Food to be excluded by the child	Foods and ingredients to avoid	Foods to replace the excluded food
Milk	Butter, casein, cheese, cow/sheep/goat's milk, evaporated or condensed milk, cream, yogurt, fromage frais, cheese, ice cream, curd, ghee, lactoglobulin, lactose, milk solids, whey, yogurt, milk proteins	GP can prescribe a replacement milk for infants. Children can use a prescribed replacement milk or calcium-enriched soya or oat milks, soya-based yogurts and desserts and tofu
Egg	Albumin, dried egg, egg powder, egg protein, egg white and yolk, frozen egg, globulin, lecithin (E322), livetin, ovalbumin, ovoglobulin, ovomucin, ovovitellin, pasteurized egg, vitellin	Meat, fish, nuts and pulses
Wheat	Bran, breadcrumbs, bulgar wheat, cereal filler, couscous, durum wheat, farina, flour, rusk, semolina, starch, vegetable protein, wheatgerm and wheatgerm oil	Rice, potatoes, wheat-free breads, pasta and flours, sago, tapioca, quinoa and millet, buckwheat
Foods containing gluten	Bran, breadcrumbs, bulgar wheat, cereal filler, couscous, durum wheat, farina, flour, rusk, semolina, starch, vegetable protein, wheatgerm and wheatgerm oil, rye, barley and oats, spelt	Rice, potatoes, corn, maize, sago, tapioca, quinoa, millet and gluten-free cereals, breads and flour Gluten-free products can be prescribed by a GP for children diagnosed with coeliac disease
Fish or shellfish	Anchovy, Worcestershire sauce, aspic, caviar, fish stock and fish sauce	Meat, eggs, nuts and pulses To replace the omega 3 fats in fish: walnuts and walnut oil, rapeseed oil
Peanuts – also known as ground nuts	Peanuts, ground nuts, peanut oil which could also be called arachis oil or hypogeaia, peanut flour, peanut protein. It is best to avoid all other nuts as well as they may be contaminated with small amounts of peanuts	Meat, fish, eggs and pulses
Other nuts which are called tree nuts	Almonds, hazelnuts, walnuts, cashews, pecan nuts, Brazil nuts, pistachio nuts, macadamia nuts and Queensland nuts (You do not need to avoid coconut, pine nuts, nutmeg and butternut squash) Pesto often contains cashew nuts	Meat, fish, eggs and pulses
Soya	Hydrolysed vegetable protein, soya lecithin, soya sauce, miso, soya albumin, soya beans, soya flour, soya milk, soya nuts, soya oil, soya proteins, soya sprouts, tempeh, texturized vegetable protein, tofu	Meat, fish, eggs and nuts
Sesame	Sesame seeds, sesame oil, tahini, aqualibra drinks	–

Naan breads, breakfast muffins and pancakes are usually soya free.

Food Labels

Parents, carers and older children need to check food labels very carefully by reading the list of ingredients to check for anything that needs to be avoided – even when the food product is well used. Sometimes the manufacturer may change the recipe slightly and include new ingredients. The label will not always be modified to say 'new' or 'improved'.

European legislation now requires that all pre-packed food must be clearly labelled if it contains any of the following foods:

- cereals containing gluten (i.e. wheat, rye, barley, oats, spelt, kamut or their hybridized strains)
- eggs
- fish
- shellfish
- peanuts or ground nuts
- soybeans
- milk and lactose
- nuts
- celery
- mustard
- sesame seeds
- sulphur dioxide and sulphites
- lupin
- molluscs.

These foods must be included in the ingredients list if they are included in the food.

However, foods sold loose, in small packages and bottles and catering packages are exempt from this guidance and will not usually display this information. Because of this risk the guidance on foods sold loose is under review and some changes should be seen in the UK in the next few years.

'Free-from' foods and lists

Some supermarkets and manufacturers also produce 'free-from' lists on which all their own-brand products are listed according to their suitability for various diets. Clients can telephone customer care lines to request a list of 'free-from' foods for the food allergy or intolerance that a child has. This does not replace checking the food labels prior to purchase or offering to the child as the recipe may have changed since the 'free-from' list was last updated.

Adapting Family Foods for a Food Allergy or Intolerance

Many recipes can be adapted but there are now recipe books for particular food allergies in all good bookshops. Dietitians or others with a food allergy may be able to provide some well-tested recipes.

To prevent cross-contamination of foods that need to be avoided by a child:

- cooking utensils must be washed thoroughly
- special care taken when washing chopping boards or work surfaces
- hands must be washed thoroughly before preparing special foods for the food-allergic child
- oil for cooking different foods must not be re-used
- the same spoon must not be used when dishing up different foods.

Eating Outside the Home

Eating outside the home presents several challenges, especially if a child has an IgE-mediated allergy. It is best to avoid foods if the full list of ingredients is not known rather than taking risks.

In the United States it has become common for people to carry a 'chef card' that outlines the foods that a child must avoid. The card can be presented to the chef or manager and serves as a reminder of the food allergy. However, chefs often have a poor understanding of food allergies (Bailey *et al.* 2011).

At nursery and school

Teaching staff and carers need written information about a child's food allergy or intolerance that includes what to avoid and which foods can be offered in their place. It is important that nursery staff understand:

- how to check food labels
- how to ascertain ingredients in catering packs even if it means that the company should be contacted

- what degree of food avoidance is required for each food
- any other allergic conditions
- dealing with milk – severe allergic reactions.

Travel to non-English-speaking countries

When travelling abroad to foreign countries, families who do not speak the local language will need accurate translations of the key foods and ingredients that a child needs to avoid. Various websites provide a series of translation sheets for various allergies (www.allergyaction.co.uk, www.allergyuk.org, www.kidsaware.co.uk, www.yellowcross.co.uk).

Activity

Devise a one-day menu for a 2-year-old child who is allergic to wheat, milk, fish and soya protein.

Acknowledgements

With thanks to Dr Carina Venter, Specialist Allergy Dietitian, Isle of Wight.

References

Allen KJ, Davidson GP, Day AS, *et al.* (2009) Management of cow's milk protein allergy in infants and young children: an expert panel perspective. *Journal of Paediatric and Child Health* **45**(9): 481–486.

Bailey S, Albardiaz R, Frew AJ and Smith H (2011) Restaurant staff's knowledge of anaphylaxis and dietary care of people with allergies. *Clinical and Experimental Allergy* **41**(5): 713–717.

Boyce JA, Assa'ad A, Burks AW, *et al.* (2010) Guidelines for the diagnosis and management of food allergy in the United States: report of the NIAID-sponsored expert panel. *Journal of Allergy and Clinical Immunology* **126**(6 suppl): S1–58.

Du Toit G and Lack G (2011) Can food allergy be prevented? The current evidence. *Pediatric Clinics of North America* **58**(2): 481–509, xii.

Du Toit G, Meyer R, Shah N, *et al.* (2010) Identifying and managing cow's milk protein allergy. *Archives of Disease in Childhood Education and Practice Edition* **95**(5): 134–144.

Fiocchi A, Brozek J, Schunemann H, *et al.* (2010) World Allergy Organization (WAO) Diagnosis and Rationale for Action against Cow's Milk Allergy (DRACMA) Guidelines. *Pediatric Allergy and Immunology* **21**(suppl 21): 1–125.

Fisher HR, du Toit G and Lack G (2011) Specific oral tolerance induction in food allergic children: is oral desensitisation more effective than allergen avoidance?: a meta-analysis of published RCTs. *Archives of Disease in Childhood* **96**(3): 259–264.

Greer FR, Sicherer SH and Burks AW (2008) Effects of early nutritional interventions on the development of atopic disease in infants and children: the role of maternal dietary restriction, breastfeeding, timing of introduction of complementary foods, and hydrolyzed formulas. *Pediatrics* **121**(1): 183–191.

Host A, Halken S, Muraro A, *et al.* (2008) Dietary prevention of allergic diseases in infants and small children. *Pediatric Allergy and Immunology* **19**(1): 1–4.

Johansson SG, Bieber T, Dahl R, *et al.* (2004) Revised nomenclature for allergy for global use: Report of the Nomenclature Review Committee of the World Allergy Organization, October 2003. *Journal of Allergy and Clinical Immunology* **113**(5): 832–836.

Lemon-Mule H, Sampson HA, Sicherer SH, Shreffler WG, Noone S and Nowak-Wegrzyn A (2008) Immunologic changes in children with egg allergy ingesting extensively heated egg. *Journal of Allergy and Clinical Immunology* **122**(5): 977–983.

NICE (National Institute for Health and Clinical Excellence) (2007) Atopic eczema in children. Management of atopic eczema in children from birth up to the age of 12 years. **www.nice.org.uk/nicemedia/live/11901/38559/38559.pdf** (accessed April 2012).

NICE (2011) Clinical Guidance 116. Diagnosis and assessment of food allergy in children and young people in primary care and community settings. **http://guidance.nice.org.uk/CG116/Guidance** (accessed April 2012).

Nowak-Wegrzyn A, Assa'ad AH, Bahna SL, Bock SA, Sicherer SH and Teuber SS (2009) Work Group report: oral food challenge testing. *Journal of Allergy and Clinical Immunology* **123**(6 suppl): S365–S383.

Royal College Paediatrics and Child Health (2011) Allergy Care Pathways for Children: Food allergy. **www.rcpch.ac.uk/sites/default/files/2011_RCPCH-CarePathway-FoodAllergy_v6_(16.26).pdf.pdf** (accessed April 2012).

Sicherer SH and Burks AW (2008) Maternal and infant diets for prevention of allergic diseases: understanding menu changes in 2008. *Journal of Allergy and Clinical Immunology* **122**(1): 29–33.

Venter C and Arshad SH (2011) Epidemiology of food allergy. *Pediatric Clinics of North America* **58**(2): 327–349.

Venter C and Meyer R (2010) Session 1: Allergic disease: The challenges of managing food hypersensitivity. *Proceedings of the Nutrition Society* **69**(1): 11–24.

Venter C, Pereira B, Voigt K, *et al.* (2008) Prevalence and cumulative incidence of food hyper sensitivity in the first 3 years of life. *Allergy* **63**(3): 354–359.

Venter C, Vlieg-Boerstra BJ and Carling A (2009) The diagnosis of food hypersensitivity. In: Skypala I and Venter C (eds) *Food Hypersensitivity: Diagnosing and managing food allergies and intolerances.* Oxford: Blackwell, p. 85.

Wright T (2001) *Food Allergies – enjoying life with a severe food allergy.* London: Class Publishing Ltd.

Wright T (2009) In: Skypala I and Venter C (eds) *Food Hypersensitivity: Diagnosing and managing food allergies and intolerances.* Oxford: Blackwell, pp. 265–277.

Zuberbier T, Edenharter G, Worm M, *et al.* (2004) Prevalence of adverse reactions to food in Germany – a population study. *Allergy* **59**(3): 338–345.

Resources

The Anaphylaxis Campaign (**www.anaphylaxis.org.uk**)

Childhood Obesity

Summary

- Overweight and obesity are measured by body mass index (BMI) which is calculated by dividing a person's weight in kilograms by the square of their height in metres.

- BMI varies throughout childhood, decreasing from about 1 year to 5–6 years and then slowly increasing throughout the rest of childhood.

- BMI-for-age centile charts are used to classify children as overweight or obese – above the 91st centile is considered overweight and above the 98th centile is classified as obese.

- Organic causes of obesity are very rare and family lifestyle is the most common cause of childhood obesity.

- Families first need to acknowledge that their child is overweight or obese and be motivated to address this through lifestyle changes if interventions are to be successful.

- Lifestyle changes are very difficult for families to make and they may need considerable support to achieve change.

Definitions of Overweight and Obesity in Children

In children, overweight and obesity are defined by body mass index (BMI) centile. As discussed in Chapter 2.1, BMI is a measure of weight relative to height and is calculated by dividing the weight in kilograms by the square of the height in metres:

$$BMI = \frac{weight\ in\ kg}{(height\ in\ m)^2}$$

BMI varies throughout childhood and this variation is slightly different between boys and girls. Hence there are gender-specific BMI-for-age centile charts.

Other characteristics to note about BMI values are that they:

- increase during infancy
- decrease from 1 year or when the toddler becomes increasingly mobile until about 5–6

years of age – the average BMI at one year is 17.5, falling to about 15.5 at 5–6 years of age

- steadily increase from about 6 years of age until adulthood.

BMI is only considered accurate as a measure of whether a child is a normal or abnormal weight for their height from about 2 years of age.

Clinical definitions of overweight and obesity in the UK

Once a child's weight and height have been measured accurately on calibrated equipment the BMI is calculated and then plotted on a BMI-for-age centile chart. In a clinical setting a child is:

- overweight if they are between the 91st and 98th centile lines
- obese if they are on or above the 98th centile line.

Table 7.2.1 Percentage of children classified as obese in National Child Measurement Programme

Age	Percentage of children classified as obese			
	2006/07	2007/08	2009/10	2010/11
Reception (4–5 year olds)	9.9	9.6	9.8	9.4
Year 6 (10–11 year olds)	17.5	18.3	18.7	19

Other definitions of overweight and obesity

To date, UK Government statistics use the 85th BMI centile as the cut-off for overweight and the 95th BMI centile as the cut-off for obesity. As these 2 centile lines are not marked in the BMI charts in clinical use, they are not used in clinical practice.

Definitions used in other countries vary and the International Task Force on Obesity set cut-offs that are similar to those used clinically in the UK but not exactly the same.

Assessing overweight or obesity

Studies have shown that neither healthcare professionals nor parents can reliably assess, just by eye, whether a child is overweight or obese. The assessment must be carried out more objectively, using the BMI centile.

Waist circumference centile charts can be used to estimate truncal fat stores and the consequent risks to health. Waist circumference has increased at a greater rate than BMI over the last few decades.

Where an adolescent is in relation to their pubertal growth spurt should be taken into consideration as full height may not have been reached.

Prevalence of Childhood Obesity in the UK

The prevalence of childhood overweight and obesity has been increasing in developed countries over the last few decades. In the UK rates have risen from around 8 per cent in 1974 to around 30 per cent in 2010.

The National Child Measurement Programme in UK schools measures children when they enter Reception, age 4–5 years, and again in their final year of primary school – Year 6, age 10–11 years. About 93 per cent of children take part, as they are able to opt out. The figures (Table 7.2.1) may be a slight underestimate as parents of obese children are more likely to request that their children are not measured.

The latest figures also showed that obesity levels were highest in London and lowest in the southern home counties. Obesity is also more prevalent in deprived areas and urban environments and lower socio-economic groups (Jotangia *et al.* 2006).

Figures from the Health Survey for England 2010 show similar figures but are over a wider age range (Table 7.2.2).

Table 7.2.2 Percentage of children classified as overweight or obese in Health Survey for England 2010

Age range	Percentage of children	
	Overweight	Obese
2–4 years	15	11
5–10 years	13	17
11–15 years	15	18

Factors Associated with Childhood Obesity

Eating patterns, activity levels, ethnicity, genetics, low socio-economic status and environment all play a part in the development of obesity. Evidence is emerging that genetic differences may make some children more susceptible to obesity in an obesogenic environment (Bouchard 2009).

The vast majority of overweight and obesity is caused by a higher energy intake (amount of calories consumed in food and drinks) than energy expenditure (amount of energy used in growth, development and activity). The excess energy intake is stored as extra adipose tissue which contributes to the physical and metabolic changes seen in obesity.

Medical causes of obesity in children are extremely rare and include:

- endocrine disorders often signalled by short stature such as hypothyroidism, Cushing's syndrome and growth hormone deficiency
- single-gene defects (e.g. leptin deficiency and melanocortin 4 receptor (MC4R) deficiency)
- chromosomal disorders, such as Prader–Willi syndrome, Bardet Biedl syndrome, Alstrom syndrome and Cohen syndrome.

Excess weight gain in preschool children is of particular concern. A Dutch study found poor lifestyle patterns at 5 years were associated with later childhood obesity (Gubbels et al. 2011). A UK study found that most of the excess weight in 9-year-old children had been gained as excess weight before 5 years of age (Gardner et al. 2009).

As part of the Avon Longitudinal Study of Parents and Children (ALSPAC), also known as the 'Children of the 90s' study, Reilly et al. (2005) identified the following risk factors for childhood obesity at age 7 years irrespective of whether the child was overweight at 3 years or not:

- parental obesity of one or both parents
- high birthweight
- rapid weight gain in the first year – crossing upwards across weight for age centile lines after 8 weeks of age
- catch-up growth between birth and 2 years
- an early adiposity rebound at 3–4 years of age when the BMI does not continue to decrease as expected on BMI centile charts
- sedentary behaviour: more than eight hours watching TV per week at 3 years

- less than 10½ hours sleep/24 hours at 3 years – normally 3 year olds sleep for about 12 hours in every 24 hours.

Parental obesity

Having one obese parent increases the risk, and if that parent is the mother the risk is higher. The highest risk is in children with two obese parents (Dorosty et al. 2000, Reilly et al. 2005). This could be due to a combination of factors: genetic, social or environmental.

Weight gain in infancy

Whether breastfeeding in early infancy plays a role in preventing obesity in childhood or not remains controversial. Formula-fed infants lose less weight in the first few days after birth and their overall growth pattern is different to that of exclusively breastfed babies. As discussed in Chapter 4.1 it is easier to overfeed a baby by bottlefeeding than by breastfeeding. However, there are many lifestyle factors throughout the toddler years and early childhood, in addition to the mode of milk feeding during infancy, that may contribute to the development of obesity (Hediger et al. 2001, Clifford 2003). Rapid weight gain in the first 3 months in infancy is also related to low socio-economic status (Wijlaars et al. 2011), which is in turn associated with a higher risk of obesity.

Adiposity rebound

'Adiposity rebound' is the term given to the time when BMI begins to increase after falling to a low point at around 5–6 years. Children with an early adiposity rebound (i.e. whose BMI begins to increase earlier than 5–6 years) are at higher risk of obesity.

Consequences of Obesity

The health risks associated with obesity in childhood are:

- increased severity of asthma and other respiratory disease
- lower levels of fitness

- social discrimination, such as bullying, victimization and social exclusion that can lead to low self-esteem, lower quality of life and lower academic achievement
- orthopaedic and musculoskeletal problems
- increased risk of insulin resistance and type 2 diabetes
- higher incidence of atherosclerosis
- increased risk of cardiovascular disease
- non-alcoholic fatty liver disease
- kidney disease
- several cancers.

Obese adolescents may also develop one or more of the following:

- sleep apnoea
- hypertension and dyslipidaemia – found in 80 per cent
- type 2 diabetes
- gallstones
- encopresis
- steato-hepatitis
- gastro-oesophageal reflux.

An overweight child has a 40–70 per cent chance of becoming an obese adult. The older an overweight child is, the more likely they will remain overweight or obese as an adult.

Preventing Obesity

Preschool and primary school children are dependent on parents and carers for their food and opportunities for physical activity, so it is the parents and carers who must take responsibility for a healthy family lifestyle. A recent systematic review found the following factors should be included in interventions (Bond *et al.* 2011):

- cultural sensitivity
- sustained moderate to vigorous exercise
- active engagement of the parents in the programme and as role models of healthy living
- active engagement of the children in nutrition education.

Secondary school children make more of their own lifestyle decisions and the responsibility for preventing obesity is a shared responsibility between themselves and their parents and carers. However, the lifestyle habits and preferences of secondary school children, particularly around food and physical activity, will have been largely learned by parental role modelling when they were younger. Environmental factors and marketing will also influence lifestyle choices of adolescents.

Food and drinks

Adopting the principles of nutritious balanced diets as discussed in Chapter 1.2 is a key part of obesity prevention. Although most infants and preschool children tend to regulate their energy intakes to their needs, some young children do not regulate their energy intake well and some derive considerable pleasure from sweet, high-energy foods. From 5 years children tend to eat to social cues and easily override their feelings of satiety. Portion control becomes important for children who do not regulate their intake according to their feelings of satiety.

However, providing food is an emotional issue for parents and many show their love through giving food. Research has found that more parents are concerned about their young children being underweight than overweight (Pagnini *et al.* 2007). Some parents:

- coerce children to finish up larger portions than the child wants to eat
- give high-energy, low-nutrient foods as treats, rewards or for comfort.

Small amounts of foods high in fat and sugar are acceptable but children often eat these foods to excess – particularly sweetened drinks and high-fat snack foods such as crisps. The rise in obesity is parallel to the increase in consumption of sweetened drinks by children. Restricting these foods and drinks in today's environment requires discipline, as children naturally prefer energy-dense foods (Cooke 2004).

Family meals and planned snacks are preferable to allowing unplanned snacking and grazing throughout the day as unplanned snacks tend to include higher energy, lower nutrient foods than planned meals and snacks.

Physical activity

Physical activity accounts for about 25–35 per cent of children's energy expenditure (Ball *et al.* 2001).

When toddlers and preschool children are encouraged and given the opportunities for active play they will develop coordination and skills that will allow them to enjoy sport as they get older. Most preschool children do not need encouragement for active play but opportunities depend on their housing situation and the local environment.

As children get older they may need more motivation to take part in physical activity.

The Department of Health (2011) now recommends that:

- children under 5 years are physically active for at least three hours each day. Short periods of activity can be spread out over the day
- children 5–18 years should engage in moderate to vigorous intensity physical activity for at least 60 minutes and up to several hours every day
- vigorous intensity activities, including those that strengthen muscle and bone, should be incorporated at least three days a week.

Studies show that physical activity tends to decrease in girls after the age of 10–12 years, whereas boys remain more active although activity levels are lower in those aged 15–18 than in 11–14 year olds. Girls aged 15–18 years are the least active. Few adolescents achieve the recommended 60 minutes or more of physical activity of at least moderate intensity. In 2004 a study found that among 15 year olds only 29 per cent of girls and 48 per cent of boys in England and 18 per cent of girls and 40 per cent of boys in Wales achieved this on five occasions per week (Currie *et al.* 2004). Adolescents cite greater embarrassment and self-consciousness about their bodies – along with lack of time – as barriers to physical activity.

The role of physical activity in obesity prevention remains controversial, as a recent UK study reports that when children become overweight they reduce their activity and that inactivity is less implicated in causing obesity than a high energy intake through foods (Metcalf *et al.* 2011).

Some suggested activities that can contribute towards the recommended 60 minutes of daily activity include:

Moderate-intensity activities:

- Brisk walking
- Swimming
- Cycling
- Dancing
- Playground games
- Gymnastics
- Trampolining
- Horse riding
- Most sports including rounders, cricket, football, rugby, tennis

Vigorous-intensity activities that enhance strength:

- Climbing
- Skipping
- Jumping
- Resistance exercises

Limiting sedentary behaviour

The same Department of Health guidelines recommend that all children and young people should minimize the amount of time spent being sedentary (sitting) for extended periods. In the United States and elsewhere watching television is not recommended for the under-twos, and for those aged 3 and over the American Academy of Pediatrics recommends no more than two hours per day in sedentary behaviours such as TV viewing. A recent literature review found that video games and computers do not represent such a high risk compared to watching TV (Rey-López *et al.* 2008).

Many toddlers and young children spend a lot of time being babysat by a TV/DVD/video when parents are busy doing chores.

Getting enough sleep

Several studies have reported an association between inadequate sleep and obesity (Chaput *et al.* 2011). The mechanism by which less sleep might affect growth and predispose young children towards obesity is not clear but it may be via hormonal influences on growth.

Changing lifestyles in families with children at risk of obesity

Initiatives to improve lifestyles in families at risk of obesity need to be undertaken sensitively and should involve support for parents to improve their parenting skills. Preschool children learn by copying, so parents need to adopt healthy lifestyle patterns themselves. Home visits during pregnancy and infancy may be a time when parents are receptive to advice on healthy eating for young children (Bull *et al.* 2004).

Changing eating habits is usually difficult but particularly so for parents who:

- do not understand the principles of healthy eating
- do not have the cooking skills necessary to prepare simple home-cooked food and instead rely on convenience foods which are usually higher in energy, fat, sugar and salt
- do not have set mealtimes either as a family or for their children so that frequent snacking forms part of their eating pattern.

Childcare settings

NICE guidance (2006) recommends that all nurseries and childcare facilities should:

- minimize sedentary activities during play time, and provide regular opportunities for enjoyable active play and structured physical activity sessions
- implement Government guidance on food procurement and healthy catering
- ensure that children eat regular, healthy meals in a pleasant, sociable environment free from

other distractions (such as television). Children should be supervised at mealtimes and, if possible, staff should eat with children.

Activity 1

Make a list of obesity-prevention measures to be included in obesity-prevention programmes for families with children.

Treating Obesity

Most NHS Trusts have a locally agreed protocol for treating childhood obesity. Scottish guidance recommends that children with a BMI over the 99.6th centile should be referred to a paediatrician for investigation.

In pre-pubertal obese and overweight children, weight loss may not be required but weight gain should be slowed or stopped temporarily through lifestyle changes so that BMI declines as the child grows taller. Older children who have already been through their pubertal growth spurt and very obese pre-pubertal children will require weight loss to reduce their BMI. Bariatric surgery is available in some areas for post-pubertal children who have tried lifestyle change.

The most effective way of managing overweight and obesity in children remains uncertain as the evidence base is limited (Ross *et al.* 2010). Successful interventions include a combination of:

- change in dietary habits to reduce energy intake but maintain a balanced, nutritious diet
- increase in physical activity
- decreasing sedentary behaviour
- ensuring adequate sleep for growth
- family-based behavioural therapy.

Engaging parents

Most parents do not recognize that their children are overweight or obese so healthcare professionals need to be sensitive when discussing the issue. Parents could be asked how they feel about their child's weight as a way of beginning a discussion. A measurement of the child's weight and height/length could then be offered. Showing a parent how the BMI of their overweight/obese child relates to the normal range by using the BMI centile chart is a good way to continue the discussion.

Unless parents acknowledge that there is a problem and are ready to change their lifestyle there is little that can be achieved for an overweight or obese preschool or primary school child.

Supporting parents to make lifestyle changes

Lifestyle changes for the whole family are preferable to just targeting the behaviour of the overweight or obese child on their own. When lifestyle changes become a normal part of their family life they are more likely to be maintained long term. Each family will probably have a preference for either:

- a single family intervention or
- a multi-family group programme although accessibility to group programmes may be limited.

In most cases the cause of the obesity will be multifactorial and a single solution will not suit every family. Parents are likely to be aware of factors but they may involve emotional issues, making change seem more difficult (Pagnini *et al.* 2007).

Discussion points to explore with a family with an overweight or obese child:

Weight change – what are the aims for this child/family?

Adolescent growth spurt – has this occurred yet and how does this affect weight change goals?

Planned meal and planned snack routine rather than allowing grazing on food and drinks

Snacks – changes towards low energy, higher nutrient planned snacks

Portion sizes eaten by child – are they appropriate or do they need to be reduced?

Speed of eating – children who eat quickly tend to eat larger quantities of food

Child's enjoyment of food vs. enjoyment of non-food activities

Family attitude to food and food as rewards, treats or for comfort

Family activities that can be introduced to replace food and drink-based activities

Current family lifestyle balance between physical activities and sedentary activities

Overweight child's aspirations to try new non-food-related activities

Increasing children's self-esteem around non-weight-related activities or skills. Praise from parents when achievements are made is important.

Once contributing factors have been identified, families can explore which of these factors they feel they may be able to change. The barriers to making changes may be considerable for some families because of:

- the family lifestyle
- lack of knowledge of what a nutritions balanced diet is
- lack of cooking skills or facilities to prepare lower energy foods
- housing and facilities in the local environment
- limited finances.

There will be pros and cons, and solutions may not always be clear cut. For instance, excess sedentary behaviour and lack of physical activity could be a major factor for a family living in a cramped flat in a high-rise building with no access to a playground or garden. Taking a young child to play outside would impact on the time a busy mother might have to prepare ideal foods. A carefully structured assessment of need will enable healthcare professionals to support parents in balancing needs and priorities.

NICE (2006) guidelines noted that for a programme to be considered a behavioural intervention for children it must incorporate the following aspects:

- stimulus control
- self-monitoring
- goal setting
- rewards for reaching goals
- problem solving.

Although not strictly defined as behavioural techniques, giving praise and encouraging parents to role-model desired behaviours are also recommended.

Stimulus control

This involves removing inconsistencies in the family environment. Parents can limit the availability of foods and triggers that lead to overeating, for example:

- ideally, not bringing high-calorie, low-nutrient foods into the house at all
- buying an individual packet rather than multi-packs of snack foods or biscuits that must be stored somewhere in the house
- not going to 'all you can eat for £x' style restaurants
- having set mealtimes, preferably with all the family eating together
- having readily available healthy snacks to use in between meals.

Goal setting

Families can agree simple goals for behaviour change and what benefits they will achieve. Three or less goals are ideal. They should not lead to conflict between family members and should be SMART (Table 7.2.3).

When these changes have been made and sustained, the family can be encouraged to consider another set of lifestyle changes.

Self-monitoring

By keeping records of the goals and the achievements the family can review them. When goals are not achieved, it can be an opportunity to re-evaluate motivation and the complexity or effort required to achieve that goal.

Reward systems

Children are more willing to repeat behaviours that are rewarded. The degree of the reward should match the magnitude of the effort required by the child to achieve that goal. A star chart can be used to work towards a larger reward in several stages. If a goal is not achieved then the reward agreed for it should not be given; however, earned rewards should not be withdrawn to punish poor behaviour. Rewards should not be food or drinks. More suitable non-food rewards include playing games with children, reading books to them, taking them on a swimming trip or other outing.

Problem solving

Through reviewing how difficult lifestyle changes are to make, problems can be identified and possible solutions explored.

Other solutions

Drug therapy and bariatric surgery are sometimes considered for older adolescents who are morbidly obese but not for those who:

Table 7.2.3 Making goals SMART

Aspect of goal	Good examples	Poor examples
Specific	Have sugar-free squash in place of ordinary squash	Choose healthy drinks
Measurable	Have one packet of crisps each week	Eat fewer crisps
Achievable	Walk to school twice next week	Walk to school every day from now on
Relevant	Reduce the number of sweets I eat	No candyfloss at the funfair
Time-limited	Play football with Dad in the park once this weekend	Play more football in the park with Dad this year

- are pregnant
- have an eating disorder
- have failed to adopt healthy living principles.

Support for parents who are not ready to make lifestyle changes

Parents need to understand that obesity is a clinical condition with health implications rather than just a question of how someone looks. Discuss the benefits of making changes to physical activity and eating patterns and give them details of someone they can contact when they are ready to consider making changes.

Activity 2

Decide on a lifestyle change you would like to make yourself. Set yourself a goal making it adhere to all the SMART aspects of a goal. List the challenges and barriers to making those changes and any problem solving required to overcome those barriers.

Acknowledgements

With thanks to Dr Paul Chadwick, Clinical Psychologist, CRUK Health Behaviour Research Centre, University College London; Dr Helen Croker, Clinical Research Dietitian, CRUK Health Behaviour Research Centre, University College London and Julie Lanigan, Research Dietitian, Institute of Child Health, University College London.

References and further reading

Ball EJ, O'Connor J, Abbot R, *et al.* (2001) Total energy expenditure, body fatness and physical activity in children aged 6–9 y. *American Journal of Clinical Nutrition* 74: 524–528.

Bond M, Wyatt K, Lloyd J and Taylor R (2011) Systematic review of the effectiveness of weight management schemes for the under fives. *Obesity Review* 12(4): 242–253.

Bouchard C (2009) Childhood obesity: are genetic factors involved? *American Journal of Clinical Nutrition* 89(suppl): 1494S–501S.

Bull J, McCormick G, Swann C and Mulvihill C (2004) Ante- and post-natal home-visiting programmes: a review of reviews: Evidence Briefing. Health Development Agency. **www.nice.org.uk/nicemedia/documents/home_visiting_summary.pdf** (accessed April 2012).

Chaput JP, Lambert M, Gray-Donald K, *et al.* (2011) Short sleep duration is independently associated with overweight and obesity in Quebec children. *Canadian Journal of Public Health* 102(5): 369–374.

Clifford TJ (2003) Breastfeeding and obesity. *British Medical Journal* 327: 879–880.

Cole TJ (2004) Children grow and horses race: is the adiposity rebound a critical period for later obesity? *BMC Pediatrics* 4: 6.

Cole TJ, Bellizzi MC, Flegal KM and Dietz WH (2000) Establishing a standard definition for child overweight and obesity worldwide: international survey. *British Medical Journal* 320: 1240–1253.

Cooke L (2004) The development and modification of children's eating habits. *Nutrition Bulletin* 29: 31–35.

Currie C, Roberts C, Morgan A, *et al.* (2004) *Young People's Health in Context. Health behaviour in school-aged children (HSBC) Study: International Report from the 2001/2002 Survey.* Health Policy for Children and Adolescents, No. 4. Copenhagen: World Health Organization, 2004.

Department of Health (2011) *UK Physical Activity Guidelines.* **www.dh.gov.uk/en/Publicationsandstatistics/Publications/PublicationsPolicyAndGuidance/DH_127931** (accessed April 2012).

Dorosty AR, Emmett PM, Cowin IS and Reilly JJ (2000) ALSPAC Study Team. Factors associated with early adiposity rebound. *Pediatrics* 105: 1115–1118.

Gardner DS, Hosking J, Metcalf BS, Jeffery AN, Voss LD and Wilkin TJ (2009) Contribution of early weight gain to childhood overweight and metabolic health: a longitudinal study (EarlyBird 36). *Pediatrics* 123(1): e67–73.

Gidding SS, Dennison BA, Birch LL, *et al.* (2006) American Heart Association Dietary recommendations for children and adolescents: a guide for practitioners. *Pediatrics* 117(2): 544–559.

Gubbels JS, Kremers SP, Goldbohm RA, Stafleu A and Thijs C (2011) Energy balance-related behavioural patterns in 5-year-old children and the longitudinal association with weight status development in early childhood. *Public Health and Nutrition* **29**: 1–9.

Hediger ML, Overpeck MD, Kuczmarski RJ and Ruan WJ (2001) Association between infant breastfeeding and overweight in young children. *Journal of the American Medical Association* **285**: 2453–2460.

Jotangia D, Moody A, Stamatakis E and Wardle H (2006) *Revised: Health Survey for England 2005: Obesity among children under 11*. London: National Statistics, pp. 1–23.

Lagou V, Manios Y, Moran CN, *et al.* (2007) Developmental changes in adiposity in toddlers and preschoolers in the GENESIS study and associations with the ACE I/D polymorphism. *International Journal of Obesity* **31**: 1052–1060.

Metcalf BS, Hosking J, Jeffery AN, Voss LD, Henley W and Wilkin TJ (2011) Fatness leads to inactivity, but inactivity does not lead to fatness: a longitudinal study in children (EarlyBird45). *Archives of Disease in Childhood* **96**: 942–947.

Monasta L, Batty GD, Macaluso A, *et al.* (2011) Interventions for the prevention of overweight and obesity in preschool children: a systematic review of randomized controlled trials. *Obesity Reviews* **12**: e107–e118.

NICE (National Institute for Health and Clinical Excellence) (2006) Clinical Guideline 43. Obesity guidance on the prevention, identification, assessment and management of overweight and obesity in adults and children. **www.nice.org.uk/nicemedia/pdf/CG43NICEGuideline.pdf** (accessed April 2012).

Pagnini DL, Wilkenfeld RL, King LA, Booth ML and Booth SL (2007) Mothers of pre-school children talk about childhood overweight and obesity: The Weight of Opinion study. *Journal of Paediatrics and Child Health* **43**(12): 806–810.

Reilly JJ (2010) Assessment of obesity in children and adolescents: synthesis of recent systematic reviews and clinical guidelines. *Journal of Human Nutrition and Diet* **23**(3): 205–211.

Reilly JJ, Armstrong J, Dorosty AR, *et al.* (2005) Early life risk factors for obesity in childhood: cohort study. *British Medical Journal* **330**: 1357–1359.

Rey-López JP, Vicente-Rodríguez G, Biosca M and Moreno LA (2008) Sedentary behaviour and obesity development in children and adolescents. *Nutrition and Metabolism Cardiovascular Disease* **18**(3): 242–251.

Ross MM, Kolbash S, Cohen GM and Skelton JA (2010) Multidisciplinary treatment of pediatric obesity: nutrition evaluation and management. *Nutrition in Clinical Practice* **25**(4): 327–334.

Scottish Intercollegiate Guidelines Network (SIGN) (2010) Guideline 115. Management of obesity. **www.sign.ac.uk/guidelines/fulltext/115/index.html** (accessed April 2012).

Stewart L, Reilly JJ and Hughes AR (2009) Evidence-based behavioral treatment of obesity in children and adolescents. *Child and Adolescent Psychiatric Clinics of North America* **18**(1): 189–198.

Waters E, de Silva-Sanigorski A, Hall BJ, *et al.* (2011) Interventions for preventing obesity in children. *Cochrane Database Systematic Reviews* **12**: CD001871.

Wijlaars LP, Johnson L, van Jaarsveld CH and Wardle J (2011) Socioeconomic status and weight gain in early infancy. *International Journal of Obesity (London)* **35**(7): 963–970.

Resources

British Dietetic Association Teenage Weight Wise (**www.teenweightwise.com**).

Hunt C and Rudolf M (2008) *Tackling Obesity with HENRY*. London: Community Practitioners' and Health Visitors' Association.

Infant and Toddler Forum (**www.infantandtoddlerforum.org**): Factsheet 3.3 Overweight and Obesity.

National Obesity Observatory (**www.noo.org.uk**)

Nutrition for Children with Chronic Diseases and Syndromes

Summary

- Various medical conditions require dietary modification and a paediatric dietitian can advise on how to make these while ensuring nutritional adequacy to support health and normal growth.

- Nutritional support is required for several conditions and may be delivered using higher energy family foods or prescribable sterile nutritional supplements.

- Some or all of a child's nutritional requirements may be provided by tube feeding when they are unable to consume their energy and nutrient requirements orally.

- Pumps and plastics for home enteral tube feeding can be delivered directly to the home or a holiday destination.

- Children with coeliac disease need to eat a gluten-free diet and are entitled to a monthly allowance of gluten-free products on prescription.

- Children with cystic fibrosis usually need a diet higher in energy and certain nutrients and usually take pancreatic enzymes with each meal and snack.

- Children with cancer may need nutritional support when their appetite is decreased.

- Children with insulin-dependent diabetes need to control the carbohydrate content of their diet and the distribution of the carbohydrate throughout each day.

Medical Conditions Requiring Dietary Modifications

Several medical conditions in infants and children require a modified nutritional intake to treat or ameliorate either the condition itself or the consequences of some medical treatments. Table 7.3.1 lists the dietary modifications required for several medical conditions, the more common of which are discussed in further detail in the rest of this chapter. For a comprehensive guide to the treatment for all paediatric conditions requiring dietary modification, students and practitioners should use the 4th edition of *Clinical Paediatric Dietetics* edited by Vanessa Shaw and published by Wiley (Shaw 2013).

Considerations when Advising and Supporting Parents and Carers

When an infant or child is diagnosed with a medical condition, it can be very traumatic for the family and they may need time to come to terms with the diagnosis before they can embark on a programme of learning about the extra responsibility of following the dietary modifications required of them. Parents may have to deal with guilt feelings, particularly if their child's condition was genetically inherited.

Individualized advice from a paediatric dietitian with experience of the medical condition is needed for any dietary modification. The aims of dietary treatment are to meet the nutritional and energy

Table 7.3.1 Medical conditions and the main dietary modifications

Medical condition	Dietary modifications
Autistic spectrum disorders including attention deficit hyperactivity disorder (ADHD) and Asperger's syndrome	Extra nutrient supplementation to address any nutritional deficiencies in children with very selective eating Parents can be supported when they wish to trial various dietary modifications to ascertain if this will improve symptoms in their child
Burns	Increased energy, protein nutrient or fluid requirements depending on the extent of the injury, mobility and albumin levels Early enteral feeding in children with major burns Increased intake of prebiotics and probiotics in those with diarrhoea
Cancer	Varies according to symptoms. Frequently nutritional support to address poor growth or a poor appetite as a result of cahexia or drug treatments
Carbohydrate intolerances	Avoidance or limited intake of the sugar causing the intolerance. The sugar may be lactose, sucrose, glucose, fructose or galactose
Coeliac disease	A gluten-free diet avoiding the protein gluten found in wheat, rye and barley. Some children may also need to avoid the protein avenin in oats
Congential heart disease	Increased energy requirements and/or energy to be provided in smaller volumes of food or fluid
Cystic fibrosis (CF)	Increased energy, protein and nutrient requirements to address malabsorption. Nutritional support is frequently needed to promote growth and an adequate BMI About 90 per cent of children with cystic fibrosis take oral pancreatic enzyme treatments to improve their digestion and absorption of protein, fat and some vitamins
Diabetes – type 1	Controlled carbohydrate intakes to coordinate with insulin treatment
Epilepsy	When patients do not respond to medication, a ketogenic diet, which is very high in fat and low in carbohydrate, may be tried
Fat malabsorption	Reduced fat intake or a modified fat intake
HIV and AIDS	Healthy eating to optimize immune system as even with undetectable viral loads, these children are more vulnerable to infection Nutritional support when appetite is reduced or growth faltering Limited saturated fat intake if cholesterol levels are raised
Inherited metabolic disorders	Can affect metabolism of protein, fat or carbohydrate. Varies with the disorder – likely to be the restricted intake of one or more nutrients (e.g. specific amino acids)
Inflammatory bowel diseases: Crohn's disease	Varies according to symptoms of intestinal inflammation, nausea, poor appetite, malabsorption and malnutrition Some centres use periods of a specified formula feed in place of all food to induce remission of symptoms followed by a diet excluding any foods that induce symptoms in that particular child
Kidney disease	Nutritional support to address poor appetite and malnutrition. High-energy diet with modified fluid, protein, phosphate, sodium, potassium, calcium intakes may be required depending on the severity and type of disease and mode of renal replacement
Liver disease	Nutritional support to address malnutrition and poor appetite. High-energy diet using specialized feeds, modified fat to address fat malabsorption, addition of branched chain amino acids and fat-soluble vitamins depending on the severity and type of disease

Table 7.3.1 Medical conditions and the main dietary modifications (*Continued*)

Neurological impairment, e.g. cerebral palsy and Down's syndrome	Food texture modifications or nutritional support to address feeding difficulties resulting from impaired oral motor functions such as poor chewing and swallowing Decreased energy requirements if there is limited mobility Portion control where there is a tendency towards obesity as in Down's syndrome Increased energy requirements when there are frequent unwanted movements or congenital heart defects
Poorly functioning or non-functioning gastrointestinal tract (intestinal failure)	Parenteral nutrition Minimal enteral (trophic) feeding to maintain brush border integrity of the gastrointestinal tract may be appropriate
Phenylketonuria	Controlled low intake of the amino acid phenylalanine
Physical disabilities	Food texture modifications to address feeding difficulties Decreased energy requirements if there is limited mobility
Prader–Willi syndrome	Nutritional support for faltering growth in the first 2 years followed by controlled energy intake to prevent or minimize obesity

requirements for each child. This can sometimes be achieved using family foods and extra nutrient supplementation using over-the-counter supplements found in supermarkets and pharmacies. However, for more complex dietary needs, specialist dietary products are prescribable for specific conditions (listed in British National Formulary Appendix 7: Borderline Substances).

When giving individualized advice to families, the paediatric dietitian needs to consider:

- family routines and food and drink preferences
- family budget for food, drinks and supplements
- family's knowledge of food and cooking skills
- how well the parents and child understand the dietary treatment aims
- the facilities available to the family for managing the dietary modifications.

The impact of dietary modifications on family lifestyle and the quality of life of the child or whole family should not be underestimated. Some modifications may make it difficult or even prevent the child from eating at school or at friends' homes or going away on holidays or school trips, for example.

Non-compliance with dietary treatment may occur for several reasons:

- young children may refuse foods if they do not like the taste, texture or appearance

- older children may refuse to follow the dietary modifications in social settings rather than appear different to their peer group
- adolescents may refuse to comply with both dietary and medical treatments to assert their independence
- children may realize that by refusing to comply they are able to manipulate their parents or carers.

Nutritional Support for Children with an Inadequate Appetite to Satisfy their Energy and Nutrient Requirements

Malnutrition develops when children are unable to eat sufficient quantities of food and drink to satisfy their energy and nutrient requirements in the long term. This may begin to impact on health and growth if it is not addressed. The main causes of an inadequate oral intake are:

- decreased appetite due to the medical conditions and/or treatments
- malabsorption increases the energy and nutrition requirements above that for healthy children
- increased nutrient requirements due to altered metabolism, chronic illness, fever or a high level of physical activity.

The options available to increase energy and nutrient intakes are:

- more energy-dense foods and drinks so that more energy is taken within the same volume of food/drink
- prescribable high-energy drinks or sip feeds to supplement or replace oral intake
- supplementary tube feeding by bolus during the daytime or by pump during the day or overnight
- 100 per cent of energy and nutrient requirements via tube feeding.

Increasing the energy density of the normal diet by adding extra carbohydrate and/or fat

Advice needs to be tailored to foods normally eaten and may include:

- adding extra sugar or sweet syrups to breakfast cereals, puddings, drinks and other sweet foods
- stirring extra cream or powdered milk into milk drinks and puddings
- frying foods rather than grilling or baking them
- adding extra oil or butter to vegetables, pasta, rice, sauces and gravies
- adding a prescribable supplement containing carbohydrate and/or fat. These are much less sweet than sugar and should not greatly alter the taste of the food/drink. Suitable products include: Maxijul, Polycal, Vitajoule (carbohydrate), Calogen (fat) and Duocal (combined carbohydrate and fat).

Prescribable high-energy drinks or sip feeds

Several companies make a wide variety of these prescribable products which are either milk-based or juice-style drinks. A wide variety of flavours are available and it is a matter of trial and error to find which flavours each individual child will drink. They come in a variety of sizes but usually 200–250 mL bottles or cartons for drinking. One such drink per day may be adequate or a child may need to try and drink two or three. When they are drunk at the end of a meal or snack they are less likely to reduce the appetite for normal foods.

As they are an expensive item for a GP's budget, care should be taken to review the prescription frequently to make sure they are not being wasted by being thrown away once a child has begun to refuse them through taste boredom.

Tube feeding using prescribable feeds

When children are not able to eat or drink as much as they need to maintain a normal growth rate, feeding via a tube may be recommended. Tube feeding may provide:

- some of their nutrient requirements to supplement a limited oral intake
- all their energy and nutrient requirements where no oral intake is possible
- specialized formulas for various disease states that may be unpalatable to the child who refuses to take them orally.

Tube feeding can be either continuous or bolus feeding:

- In continuous feeding the food is supplied over a long period of time via a pump. The flow rate can be adjusted. This is usual for overnight feeding when a child is in bed. For daytime tube feeding a child can wear a small back pack containing a small portable pump. The child can carry on with most daily activities while being tube fed this way.
- Bolus feeding can also use a pump or can be administered using gravity for the feed to drain down the tube.

Children who may need to be tube fed for some time are those who:

- are critically ill and require ventilation
- have severe developmental delay
- have malformations around the mouth
- have faltering growth.

The routes of tube feeding can be via:

- a nasogastric tube or much less commonly an orogastric tube
- a nasojejunal tube when the stomach needs to be bypassed
- a tube connected to a gastrostomy or jejunostomy button – used for longer term feeding.

Nasogastric tube feeding

This route is used when a child initially requires tube feeding or requires it for a short time. A thin tube is passed through the child's nose down into the stomach so that liquids can be slowly pumped into the stomach. The tube is usually held in place by being taped to the child's cheek. They are easily pulled out and can be repassed quite easily if the child is cooperative.

Orogastric tube feeding

In orogastric tube feeding the tube is passed via the mouth down into the stomach.

Gastrostomy feeding

If tube feeding continues to be necessary for a longer period of time (about 6 weeks or more) a gastrostomy is formed which requires a minor surgical procedure: a short tube is passed directly through the child's skin and stomach wall and into the stomach. It is held in position with a plastic clamp or a button with a small inflatable balloon that sits inside the stomach. The feeding tube can then be connected directly to the gastrostomy device without having to go via the nose/mouth. When this form of feeding is no longer needed, the gastrostomy device can be removed and the small hole in the skin and stomach wall will close over and heal. A tiny scar may be the only indication that this route of feeding was ever used.

Jejunostomy feeding is either via a nasojejunostomy tube or a jejunostomy button. Jejunostomy feeding must be slow and continuous using a pump so that the jejunum does not receive large volumes of feed over a short period of time; this can result in malabsorption. Bolus feeding is not appropriate when the natural reservoir of the stomach is bypassed. The pump flow rate will depend on what the child can tolerate.

Feeds available for tube feeding

Several companies make a variety of sterile tube feeds that are 'ready to feed'. They can provide either complete nutrition or partial nutrition. Standard feeds have an energy content of 1 kcal/mL and are designed for different age groups to provide adequate energy, nutrients and fibre within a suitable fluid load for that age range: 0–1 year, 1–6 years and 7–12 years. Children over 12 years are usually given feeds formulated for adults.

Non-standard feeds include those providing complete nutrition:

- in lower volumes
- with lower or higher energy content
- with varying levels of fibre
- with varying fat content such as different combinations of long and medium chain triglycerides
- with varying protein type such as complete protein, hydrolysed protein or simple amino acids.

Although there is a choice of brands, commonly an NHS Hospital Trust will have a contract with one of the companies and use their products exclusively, where possible, at a lower cost. Feeds for children at home are prescribed by their GP usually on the advice of a paediatric dietitian or paediatrician.

Selecting a feed and feeding regimen

A paediatric dietitian can assess a child's nutritional needs and advise on the type of feed and feeding regimen that meets their nutritional requirements. The assessment will include an estimation of their:

- energy requirements, taking into account mobility, activity level, body temperature and the need for catch-up growth or energy restrictions to address obesity

● fluid requirements

● nutrient and fibre requirements.

Requirements are usually based on a child's weight so, as the child grows, requirements and the feeding regime need to be regularly reassessed and recalculated.

Considerations when initiating tube feeding

If a child has not been eating for some time a feed may need to be started slowly and increased over several days according to how the child tolerates an increased flow rate or increased energy density. Stomach pain, vomiting and diarrhoea are all indications that the child is not tolerating the feed. However, these symptoms need to be interpreted according to the clinical condition of the child.

The gradual introduction of feed over several days will also protect against the risk of 'refeeding syndrome' in those children who have had very little nutrition for some time.

Support for home tube feeding

When infants and children are tube fed at home parents and carers need to be trained in:

● operating the pump using appropriate flow rates or bolus volumes

● frequency and method of changing the plastic tubes (giving sets and reservoirs)

● appropriate flushing of tubes before and after feeding episodes

● cleaning the gastrostomy site

● clearing blocked tubes.

Companies making the feeds all have home delivery services to deliver both the sterile plastic tubes (giving sets and reservoirs) and the feeds either to a local pharmacy or directly to the home. They can usually arrange deliveries to holiday accommodation as well. They also have 24-hour helplines to answer carers' queries and offer support to cope with any problems.

Parenteral feeding for critically ill children with very poor gut function

This is an expensive treatment and usually only used in hospital. The child is fed directly into a vein with a combination of sterile solutions prepared by a pharmacy. The solutions must be calculated carefully and prescribed for each child. Together these solutions provide fat, carbohydrate, protein, vitamins and minerals. Occasionally a child can be fed at home by this method but parents require considerable support and training to do this safely and effectively.

Common Medical Conditions Requiring Dietary Modifications

Autistic spectrum disorders, including attention deficit hyperactivity disorder (ADHD) and Asperger's syndrome

Some children with these disorders only eat a narrow range of foods. This selective eating may be related to either over- or under-sensory perception with tastes, smells, texture and temperature of foods as well as the visual appearance of food. Diaries of foods normally eaten can be assessed by a paediatric dietitian for nutritional adequacy and a supplement recommended for any deficiencies.

Parents often wish to try a variety of dietary modifications for which there is varying anecdotal evidence of symptom improvement in some children. A dietitian can support parents to do this safely so that there is no nutritional risk to the children. Such dietary interventions requested include:

● supplements of zinc, iron, magnesium, omega 3 fatty acids (eicosapentaenoic acid (EPA) in particular), vitamin A, methyl sulphonyl methane/magnesium sulphate, folinic acid, betaine and/or methylcobalamine

● excluding phenolic compounds, salicylates, aspartame, monosodium glutamate (MSG), artificial colours or benzoates

- casein and gluten-free diet
- ketogenic diet – very high-fat and low-carbohydrate.

To assess the effectiveness of any dietary intervention for a particular child, an objective record of symptoms must be kept during a baseline period of the regular diet, the intervention period and then a return to the regular diet as described for open food challenges (see Chapter 7.1, page 190).

Before embarking on an exclusion diet with a child who eats very selectively it is advisable to assess whether excluding any key foods they normally eat will compromise their energy or nutrient intake, as once foods have been excluded for a while the child may refuse to begin eating them again.

Cancer

Children with cancer may have a reduced appetite due to:

- pain
- repeated infections when the immune system is compromised due to chemotherapy and radiotherapy
- nausea and vomiting caused by chemotherapy and radiotherapy
- diarrhoea because of antibiotic treatments or because of cancer treatments
- changes to their taste buds making food less enjoyable.

Children eating poorly can become malnourished quite quickly, which will further lower their immune system and they may begin to lose weight.

Considerations for nutritional support

- Small frequent snack-style meals about 5 or 6 times each day may be preferable to 3 big meals and 2–3 small snacks.
- If the child has a sore mouth, very soft foods may be preferable.
- If nausea occurs, cold food may be preferred to hot food.

- Increasing energy intake using extra oil, butter and cream may not be suitable when a child is feeling nauseous. It may be better to try the prescribable high-calorie/high-nutrient drinks.
- Overnight tube feeding is often recommended as it can help to maintain growth, boost the immune system and prevent weight loss.

Coeliac disease

In children with this autoimmune disease, the protein gluten causes the production of destructive antibodies which damage the tissue of the small intestine, causing malabsorption of food.

Gluten is found in the three cereals: wheat, rye and barley. All food and drinks made from these cereals need to be eliminated from the diet of a child with coeliac disease. Some children may need to avoid oats as well as they may be sensitive to a similar protein, avenin, in oats. Sometimes oats are contaminated with traces of wheat, rye or barley.

Children with undiagnosed coeliac disease or who are not following their diet may have any of the following symptoms:

- weight loss
- poor growth
- diarrhoea
- nausea
- wind
- tiredness
- constipation
- anaemia
- mouth ulcers
- headaches
- hair loss
- skin problems.

Foods that should be included or eliminated in a gluten-free diet are listed in Table 7.3.2.

Parents and children need to check the labels on food packaging of all commercial foods for their

Table 7.3.2 Foods to include or eliminate in a gluten-free diet

Food groups	Foods allowed	Foods to eliminate	Special gluten-free foods available
Group 1: Starchy foods: bread, rice, potatoes, pasta and other starchy foods	Rice, potatoes, yam, millet, sago, tapioca, quinoa Flours made from arrowroot, buckwheat, chick peas (gram flour), corn, lentil, maize and rice Some brands of corn flakes and rice krispies	Any foods made from wheat, rye, barley, spelt or oats. This includes a large range of commercial bread, pasta, couscous, semolina, crackers, breakfast cereals, pizza bases, buns, pancakes	Gluten-free flours, cereals, breads, crackers and crispbreads. Some are prescribable
Group 2: Fruit and vegetables	Fresh, frozen, tinned and dried fruits and vegetables	Vegetable soups thickened with wheat flour	
Group 3: Milk, cheese and yogurt	Breast milk, infant formulas, follow-on milks, cow's milk, goat's milk, toddler milks, yogurts, cheese, milk puddings, calcium-enriched soya milks, tofu	Milk puddings that are thickened with wheat flour	
Group 4: Meat, fish, eggs, nuts and pulses	Meat, fish, eggs, nuts and pulses (lentils, dhal, chick peas, hummus, kidney beans and other similar starchy beans)	Any foods coated in flour, batter or breadcrumbs	Chick pea, lentil and gram flour
Group 5: Foods high in fat and/or sugar	Cream, butter, margarines, cooking and salad oils, jam, honey, syrup, crisps, most soft drinks	Biscuits, cakes, foods with pastry Most commercial sauces are thickened with wheat flour Ready meals will often contain flour Some drinks contain barley	Gluten-free biscuits, cakes and pastry
Fluids	Water, milk, diluted fruit juices		

suitability. Although foods are often marked as 'gluten free' on the label, the ingredients list needs to be checked for any of the following ingredients, which contain gluten or avenin: wheat, farina, flour, rusk, semolina, starch, vegetable protein, wheatgerm and wheatgerm oil, rye, barley, barley malt, oats and spelt.

Coeliac UK (www.coeliac.org.uk) is the charity that offers support and advice to families with coeliac disease. Each year they update their Food and Drink Directory, which lists all the gluten-free commercial foods available in the UK.

Prescribable gluten-free foods
There are many specialist food companies that make gluten-free food products, and children with coeliac disease are entitled to a certain quantity on prescription from their GP.

The prescribable foods are all allocated a unit:

Food	No. of units
400 g bread	1
100–250 g rolls/baguettes	½
250–400 g rolls/baguettes	1
500 g bread mix/flour mix	2
100 g savoury biscuits/crackers	½
200 g savoury biscuits/crackers/crispbreads	1
250 g pasta	1
500 g pasta	2
2 ×110–180 g pizza bases	1

Table 7.3.3 Entitlement of age groups to gluten-free foods on prescription

Age (years)	Units of gluten-free food per month	Example of monthly prescription
1–3	10	6 × 400 g bread (or 3 × 500 g mix suitable for making bread) 2 × 500 g pasta
4–6	11	6 × 400 g bread (or 3 × 500 g mix suitable for making bread) 2 × 500 g pasta 1 (2 × 110–180 g) pizza bases
7–10	13	8 × 400 g bread (or 4 × 500 g mix suitable for making bread) 2 × 500 g pasta 1 (2 × 110–180 g) pizza bases
11–14	15	8 × 400 g bread (or 4 × 500 g mix suitable for making bread) 3 × 500 g pasta 1 (2 × 110–180 g) pizza bases
15–18	18	8 × 400 g bread (or 4 × 500 g mix suitable for making bread) 4 × 500 g pasta 2 (2 × 110–180 g) pizza bases

The number of prescribable units children are entitled to increases with their age, as shown in Table 7.3.3.

Cystic fibrosis

Cystic fibrosis is a genetic disorder which is inherited from both parents. It is relatively common in white populations and less so in Asian, African and Middle Eastern families. Several of the glands in the body do not function very well and this causes lung disease, malabsorption of food and very salty sweat. Cystic fibrosis is usually diagnosed by measuring the amount of salt in a child's sweat.

Symptoms of the disease vary considerably between children and some may have more respiratory problems while others have more problems with malabsorption of food, particularly the fat in food.

The problems of malabsorption are due to a poor production of enzymes from the pancreas which are needed to digest foods in the small intestine so that they can be absorbed into the body. To improve the absorption of their food, about 90 per cent of children with cystic fibrosis are prescribed pancreatic enzyme supplements to be swallowed along with meals and snacks. The amount recommended varies from child to child depending on their symptoms. A vitamin and

mineral supplement is also prescribed as the fat-soluble vitamins A, D, E and K are usually poorly absorbed.

Infants and children with cystic fibrosis generally need a higher energy intake than normal healthy children. To achieve this, children with cystic fibrosis need to eat more food with a higher energy content. They are encouraged to eat foods containing high amounts of fat and sugar in addition to a balanced diet of foods from the four main foods groups described in Chapter 1.2.

Unfortunately cystic fibrosis infants and children often have a poor appetite, especially if they are often ill with respiratory illnesses. Some may have reflux which can cause pain on eating. Poor appetites often cause considerable stress for parents, who are very keen for their children to eat well to prevent more illness. Parents of toddlers with cystic fibrosis report more feeding problems than do parents of healthy toddlers.

Parents and older children usually plan the child's diet with a dietitian and he or she will advise on how many capsules of pancreatic enzymes to take with each meal and snack.

Children whose growth is inadequate may be prescribed high-calorie drinks as supplements. From time to time their calorie intake may be supplemented by tube feeding. Overnight tube feeding is commonly used, particularly in teenagers.

Diabetes

There are two types of diabetes:

- *Type 1 diabetes* is an autoimmune disease in which the cells in the pancreas that produce the hormone insulin are destroyed. It affects about 25 000 children in the UK and can be diagnosed at any age. It is treated with insulin.

- *Type 2 diabetes* develops when the cells in the body become resistant to insulin. It affects around 400 children in the UK, usually arising in obese teenage children. It may be controlled initially just by diet or hyperglycaemic agents but insulin treatment may be instigated as the disease progresses.

Without enough insulin or with insulin resistance, glucose in the blood will not pass into the body's cells to provide a source of energy. The glucose remains in the blood, resulting in hyperglycaemia. When this occurs before children are diagnosed they may lose weight and complain of excessive thirst. Ketones may be smelt in the breath as they are released when cells break down fat as a source of energy in the absence of glucose.

Type 1 diabetes

There are several options for giving the insulin and the medical team will discuss and agree what is the best regimen for each child. Insulin may be given via:

- a number of injections throughout each day. This may be a set regimen or calculated at several points during the day after measuring the blood glucose levels with a finger prick test.

- a small insulin pump. A fine tube from the pump is inserted under the skin. The pump is set to automatically provide around half of the daily dose of insulin as a low continuous basal dose. The child then controls the pump to give a calculated bolus dose just prior to each meal or snack.

A balanced, nutritious diet based on the five food groups as described in Chapter 1.2 is the basis of a diabetic diet for diabetic children. The diet and eating routine for each individual child is planned in consultation with a dietitian around the energy and carbohydrate needed by that child depending on:

- their age and appetite
- activity levels
- growth rate.

NICE guidelines (NICE 2011) recommend that the energy content of the diet is:

- >50 per cent carbohydrate
- 10–15 per cent protein
- 30–35 per cent fat.

Carbohydrate is digested in the small intestine into sugars that are absorbed into the blood and transported as glucose. The amounts and timing of the carbohydrate eaten should balance the effects of the insulin administered or vice versa so that blood glucose levels remain relatively close to the normal range.

When physically active for any length of time without extra carbohydrate, blood glucose levels can fall as exercise increases the non-insulin-dependent uptake of glucose by cells as well as insulin sensitivity. Hence before extra physical activity children should eat some extra carbohydrate as rapidly absorbable sugary food (e.g. confectionery or chocolate snack bars). With experience, children and parents learn to estimate how much should be eaten to avoid hypoglycaemia during sustained physical activity.

When advising on a diabetic diet parents and older children need to understand or be taught:

- how much carbohydrate is to be consumed
- how to distribute it through the day and load it at times just before the child is going to be particularly physically active
- how to calculate how much carbohydrate has been ingested when the whole meal or snack is not consumed.

Often, a list of foods each containing 10 g carbohydrate is used to help work out how much food will provide the appropriate amount of carbohydrate. These food portions are called '10 g carbohydrate exchanges' and examples are listed in Table 7.3.4. The range is from about 13–18 exchanges of 10 g carbohydrate each day for a toddler to 35–40 exchanges for a very active teenager going through their adolescent growth spurt.

Commercial foods state the amount of carbohydrate on the label and this can be used to work out how much carbohydrate is in a portion of food that the child eats.

Sweet puddings, confectionery and other sugary foods do not have to be cut out altogether. The overall sugar intake can be about 10 per cent of total energy as for normal healthy eating. This

Table 7.3.4 Ten-gram carbohydrate exchanges

Food items		Quantity providing 10 g carbohydrate
Bread	Wholemeal or white slices	½ large slice or 1 small slice
	Rolls or baps	½ roll
Breakfast cereals	Porridge	7 tbsp
	Weetabix	1 biscuit
	Corn flakes/Cheerios	5 tbsp
Rice and pasta	Cooked brown or white rice	3 tbsp
	Cooked pasta shapes	3 tbsp
	Spaghetti	10 long strands
	Tinned spaghetti	$\frac{1}{3}$ small tin
Potatoes	Boiled potatoes	1 small
	Baked potatoes	1 medium
	Chips	5 thick cut
Beans	Baked beans in tomato sauce	5 tbsp
	Dried uncooked beans	2 tbsp
Fruit	Apple	1 medium
	Pear	1 medium
	Banana	1 medium
	Grapes	10
	Orange	1 medium
	Satsumas/clementines	2 small
	Dried fruit	1 tbsp
Yogurt and ice cream	Natural yogurt	1 carton
	Fruit sweetened yogurt	½ carton
	Ice cream	1 scoop
Biscuits	Oatcakes	1 large
	Crackers	2
	Crispbreads – wholewheat or rye	2
	Digestive	1
Drinks	Milk	2 glasses of 100 mL
	Unsweetened pure fruit juice	2 glasses of 50 mL pure juice diluted with 50 mL water

1 tbsp = one 15 mL tablespoon.

is about 20 per cent of the carbohydrate allowance. Sugary foods are better given at the end of meals rather than as snacks as at the end of a meal the sugar will be absorbed more slowly and therefore less likely to make the blood glucose levels rise quickly.

Special diabetic foods are not necessary and are better avoided. Sorbitol, which is a sweetener, is often used in special diabetic foods and can cause diarrhoea.

A routine of meals and snacks is important so that similar amounts of carbohydrate are offered at each meal and snack. A young child having 15 carbohydrate exchanges each day may have them distributed through the day like this:

Breakfast	3
Mid-morning snack	2
Midday meal	3
Mid-afternoon snack	2
Evening meal	3
Snack before bed	2
Total for the day	15

An example one-day menu for such a child is shown in Table 7.3.5.

Glycaemic index

The glycaemic index of the meals and snacks eaten is a measure of how quickly blood glucose levels rise after eating that meal or snack. Sugary foods,

Table 7.3.5 Sample one-day menu for a young child with diabetes allowed 15 carbohydrate exchanges

Meal or snack		Number of carbohydrate exchanges	Total number of carbohydrate exchanges for each meal or snack
Breakfast	2 Weetabix	2	3
	100 mL milk	½	
	½ banana sliced	½	
Mid-morning snack	½ apple sliced	½	2
	1 digestive biscuit	1	
	100 mL milk to drink	½	
Midday meal	1 large slice toast with butter	2	3
	2½ tbsp baked beans	½	
	Cucumber and carrot sticks		
	5 grapes	½	
Mid-afternoon snack	1½ digestive biscuits	1½	2
	1 satsuma	½	
	Water to drink		
Evening meal	3 tbsp cooked pasta	1	3
	Bolognaise sauce		
	Broccoli florets		
	1 carton fruit yogurt	1	
	5 strawberries	½	
	50 mL fruit juice diluted with water	½	
Snack before bed	1 large slice toast with butter	2	2

such as sweets and confectionery, have a very high glycaemic index as the blood sugar rises high very quickly when these are eaten on their own. To keep the glycaemic index of a meal or snack low so that the blood sugar rises slowly a balanced diet as described in Chapter 1.2 should be offered, including foods with fibre at each meal:

- Include fruit with breakfast and at least one fruit and one vegetable with the other two meals.
- Offer a mixture of white and some wholemeal varieties of bread and cereals (e.g. wholemeal bread and porridge).

Hypoglycaemia

Hypoglycaemia (low blood glucose levels) may occur when:

- a child has not had enough carbohydrate to eat – he or she may be late for a meal or a snack or may have refused to eat
- a child has had extra exercise without eating extra carbohydrate or reducing the insulin dose
- too much insulin has been given or it may have been given at the wrong time
- food may not have been absorbed because the child has diarrhoea or has vomited
- alcohol has been consumed – one effect of alcohol consumption is to lower blood glucose levels.

During hypoglycaemia blood glucose levels become too low for the brain to function properly and a child will not always be able to indicate that they need more glucose to correct the hypoglycaemia.

General symptoms of hypoglycaemia are:

- pallor
- mood swings
- irritability
- headache
- hunger
- fatigue
- becoming uncooperative
- becoming confused
- finally losing consciousness and fitting.

Young children may not be able to describe any of these early symptoms but parents, teachers or carers might notice a child becoming confused or uncooperative. A young child might say he feels funny or has shaky or wobbly legs. The older child may be able to clearly recognize their early signs of hypoglycaemia.

To treat hypoglycaemia a child needs to be given some carbohydrate that will be rapidly absorbed to restore the blood glucose levels to within the normal range. Carbohydrate that is rapidly absorbed will be glucose or sugar or a sugary food or drink.

Examples are:

- glucose tablets or sweets to suck
- about 50 mL of a glucose drink or non-diet squash or
- 2–3 teaspoons of jam or honey or syrup.

If a child becomes confused or uncooperative it may be preferable to squeeze a glucose gel into the mouth or rub it on the gums. The glucose will be absorbed rapidly to raise blood glucose levels out of the danger zone. Glucose gels are available over the counter from pharmacies and can be prescribed. A store can be kept handy for hypoglycaemic emergencies.

If hypoglycaemia happens frequently then it is time to reassess the child's insulin regimen and carbohydrate intake. The solution may be either to increase the daily carbohydrate intake or reduce the insulin regimen.

Coping with food refusal in children with diabetes

As discussed in Chapter 5.1, toddlers and young children may at times refuse to eat or they may eat much less of a food than expected, particularly if they are going through a phase of food refusal. Food refusal can cause more anxiety for parents of diabetic toddlers who are concerned about hypoglycaemia. If parents begin to offer alternative foods, a child soon learns to manipulate the parent through food refusal. Force feeding should never be used and parents can try to minimize their anxiety, relying on the child becoming hungry as their blood glucose level falls. One solution is to inject insulin after meals and snacks, rather than before, calculated on how much carbohydrate has been consumed.

Adolescents may also refuse to follow their usual routine, refusing both insulin treatment and/or dietary routines for a period – just to test out the necessity of it. Some may be tempted to reduce insulin intake as a means of losing weight.

Type 2 diabetes

Dietary treatment in children with type 2 diabetes is also a nutritious, balanced, low glycaemic index diet with carbohydrate spread out evenly throughout the day. Obese children should also aim for a negative energy balance so that they lose weight because the progression of their disease will be slower in the absence of obesity.

Inflammatory bowel diseases – Crohn's disease

The intestinal inflammation in Crohn's disease is believed to be caused by an immune reaction against the bacteria living in the bowel. The normal food residues passing through the gastrointestinal tract are thought to be the energy source for these bacteria. Hence, to induce remission from the inflammation some centres change patients to a synthetic liquid diet free of all food residues for 6–8 weeks. Other centres use steroid treatment instead of a change in diet, and evidence for which is the preferable treatment is debatable (Zachos *et al.* 2007, Critch *et al.* 2012).

The synthetic liquid diet has one of the following as a protein source:

- single amino acids – an elemental feed
- short chains of amino acids – an oligopeptide or hydrolysed protein feed
- whole protein from a single source (e.g. casein).

The choice of feed is made by the medical team and at present evidence does not favour one over the others (Critch *et al.* 2012). A paediatric dietitian must ensure that the quantity of whichever feed is consumed will provide adequate energy and nutrients for the child. With the onset of the disease, often these children have a reduced appetite and may have already lost weight. Growth faltering may also be present.

The feeds are usually drunk orally but can be taken via a tube if children do not like the taste or cannot manage the required volume orally. Once the inflammation has resolved – usually after about 6–8 weeks – normal foods are introduced one by one. Any food that causes symptoms is stopped and introduction of other foods continues. The final diet is then made up of foods that do not cause symptoms. If there are any nutritional deficits then a dietitian can advise on a suitable supplement to correct the deficiency.

Neurological disabilities – cerebral palsy, Down's syndrome, muscular dystrophy and degenerative disorders

When motor function is affected in children with a neurological disability poor nutritional intake can result. The more severe the disability, the more limited the oral intake and the more likely malnutrition will arise.

Impairment of oral motor function can limit the ability to suck, drink, bite, chew, seal the lips, use the tongue effectively and swallow. Symptoms include:

- weak sucking in infants
- poor progression through food textures during weaning
- coughing, choking and gagging on foods
- vomiting
- frequent respiratory infections from aspiration of food into the lungs.

Gastrointestinal muscle tone may also be impaired, resulting in limited absorption of nutrients and/or gastro-oesophageal reflux.

Feeding takes longer and usually requires a parent or carer's dedicated time as well. A multidisciplinary assessment is important:

- *Speech and language therapist* can assess biting and chewing skills and safety of swallow.

Video-fluoroscopy of swallowed liquid and solids may be used to ascertain whether food/drink is spilling into the air passages and lungs causing coughing, wheezing and chest infections.

- *Occupational therapist* can advise on the most appropriate seating for mealtimes and on any eating aids that will help.
- *Physiotherapist* can advise on an ideal position for oral feeding.
- *Dietitian* can assess their nutritional intake with the current regimen and suggest improvements.
- *Paediatrician* can treat any gastro-oesophageal reflux, oesophagitis, slow gastric emptying or constipation.

Thickening liquids may help with control of swallowing liquids. However, if oral feeding is not considered safe then tube feeding directly into the stomach must be commenced. Most children will require nutritional support and tube feeding to provide partial or total nutritional intake.

Ideally, all children with neurological disabilities should have regular assessments of their:

- energy and nutrient requirements – both increase as children grow and care needs to be taken during the adolescent growth spurt when nutritional needs increase markedly to support this rapid growth rate. Overall energy requirements may be lower than the norm in children with limited mobility or higher than the norm in children who make frequent involuntary movements
- actual nutritional intake and challenges to achieving their nutritional needs – this may change with time
- weight and growth – this may require the use of specialist anthropological measuring equipment depending on the child's posture and muscle tone. It may be necessary to track growth through limb measurements or sitting height rather than standing height.

Cerebral palsy

Most children with cerebral palsy have feeding difficulties and many of these children need to be tube fed to support their limited oral intake.

Down's syndrome

Children with Down's syndrome often have:

- reduced muscle tone leading to minor feeding difficulties
- congenital heart defects which may increase their energy requirement
- gastrointestinal problems such as constipation and gastro-oesophageal reflux.

When assessing their needs, growth must be plotted on specialist Down's syndrome charts because short stature is a component of the syndrome.

Activity 1

Plan a one-day menu for a diabetic diet for a 12-year-old girl, with 50 per cent of her energy requirements as carbohydrate spread evenly over three meals and two snacks. Add in an extra 20 g of rapidly absorbed carbohydrate for volley ball practice after school.

Activity 2

Write a letter to a school outlining the needs and menu suggestions for a newly diagnosed 7-year-old boy with coeliac disease who wishes to continue eating school meals with his friends rather than take in a packed lunch and have to sit in another room.

Activity 3

Design a feeding regimen using a feed that provides 1 kcal/mL for a 5-year-old girl with cancer. She has lost weight and now weighs 14 kg and needs 40 per cent of her energy and nutrient requirements as an overnight feed. She is in bed from 7 pm to 6.30 am. Her parents go to bed at 11 pm.

Acknowledgements

With thanks to Vanessa Shaw, Head of Dietetics, Great Ormond Street Hospital for Children NHS Trust, London.

References and further reading

Brown AC, Rampertab SD and Mullin GE (2011) Existing dietary guidelines for Crohn's disease and ulcerative colitis. *Expert Review of Gastro enterology and Hepatology* **5**(3): 411–425.

Critch J, Day AS, Otley A, King-Moore C, Teitelbaum JE and Shashidhar H; on Behalf of the NASPGHAN IBD Committee (2012) Use of enteral nutrition for the control of intestinal inflammation in pediatric Crohn's disease. *Journal of Pediatric Gastroenterology and Nutrition* **54**(2): 298–305.

Eilander A, Hundscheid DC, Osendarp SJ, Transler C and Zock PL (2007) Effects of n-3 long chain polyunsaturated fatty acid supplementation on visual and cognitive development throughout childhood: a review of human studies. *Prostaglandins, Leukotrienes and Essential Fatty Acids* **76**(4): 189–203.

ESPGHAN Committee on Nutrition, Agostoni C, Braegger C, Decsi T, *et al.* (2011) Supplementation of N-3 LCPUFA to the diet of children older than 2 years: a commentary by the ESPGHAN Committee on Nutrition. *Journal of Pediatric Gastroenterology and Nutrition* **53**(1): 2–10.

NICE (National Institute for Health and Clinical Excellence) (2009) *Clinical Guidance 86. Recognition and Assessment of Coeliac Disease.* London: NICE.

NICE (2011) *Clinical Guidance 15. Type 1 Diabetes: Diagnosis and management of type 1 diabetes in children, young people and adults.* London: NICE.

Shaw V (2013) *Clinical Paediatric Dietetics*, 4th edn. London: Wiley.

Zachos M, Tondeur M and Griffiths AM (2007) Enteral nutritional therapy for induction of remission in Crohn's disease. *Cochrane Database of Systematic Reviews* **1**: CD000542.

Resources

Cerebral palsy (**www.scope.org.uk/cerebral-palsy-charity**)

Children with Diabetes (**www.childrenwithdiabetes.com**)

Children's HIV Association (**www.chiva.org.uk**)

Coeliac UK (**www.coeliac.org.uk, www.coeliac.co.uk**)

Crohn's disease (**www.crohns.org.uk**)

Down's Syndrome Association (**www.downs-syndrome.org.uk**)

Juvenille Diabetes Research Foundation (**www.jdrf.org.uk**)

Scottish Government (2011) Healthy Eating in Schools: Supplementary guidance on diet and nutrition for children and young people with additional support needs. **http://dera.ioe.ac.uk/2636/1/0114781.pdf**

Glossary

Allergen – A substance that causes an immune response.

Allergy – A hypersensitivity reaction initiated by specific immunological mechanisms.

Amino acids – A group of compounds that proteins are made of. Essential amino acids are those that we cannot make ourselves and therefore we must eat them in food. Non-essential amino acids are those that we can make for ourselves if our diets are adequate.

Anaphylaxis – Severe difficulty breathing and heart malfunction due to a fall in blood pressure, usually as a result of a serious allergic reaction. It can result in death but if adrenaline is administered the body is quickly restored to normal.

Apnoea – A transient absence of spontaneous respiration. It may occur during sleep in very obese children.

Asperger's syndrome – One of several autism spectrum disorders (ASD) characterized by difficulties in social interaction and by restricted and stereotyped interests and activities.

Atopy – A characteristic making one susceptible to develop immediate allergic reactions to substances such as pollen, food, dander and insect venoms and manifested by hay fever, asthma, food allergies, eczema or similar allergic conditions.

Autism – Autistic spectrum disorders (ASD) are a spectrum of psychological conditions characterized by widespread abnormalities of social interactions and communication, as well as severely restricted interests and highly repetitive behaviour.

Autoimmune disease – A disease in which the body produces antibodies that attack its own tissues.

Body mass index (BMI) – An index calculated by dividing body weight in kilograms by the height in metres squared.

Coeliac disease – An autoimmune disease in which the protein gluten causes the production of destructive antibodies which damage the tissue of the small intestine causing malabsorption of food.

Corrected age – The age of a child born preterm minus the weeks the baby was born early.

Cushing's syndrome – Disorder caused by excessive levels of the hormone cortisol which causes rapid weight gain, particularly of the trunk and face.

Dehydration – Condition that results from excessive loss of body water. This may occur due to a high temperature and excessive sweating or it may be due to normal water losses through skin, breathing, passing water and stools coupled with an inadequate intake of water.

Dyslipidaemia – An excess of lipids in the blood, usually the lipids cholesterol and triglycerides.

Estimated date of delivery (EDD) – For a premature baby this is the date they were expected to be born if they had remained in the womb for a normal-length pregnancy of 40 weeks gestation.

Encopresis – Involuntary faecal soiling of underwear in children who are already toilet trained.

Endocrine disorders – Abnormalities of hormone secretion or action.

Food allergy – An abnormal or exaggerated immunological response to specific food proteins.

Gag on food – Food is not successfully swallowed and comes back into the mouth.

Gastro-oesophageal reflux – The contents of the stomach flow backwards: back up out of the stomach into the oesophagus.

Glucose – A form of sugar. Sugar in the blood is always in the form of glucose.

Gluten – A protein found in wheat, rye and barley. Oats contain a very similar protein.

Growth hormone – A hormone secreted by the pituitary gland which stimulates growth and cell reproduction.

Halal – Means 'lawful' and relates to meat which is acceptable to Muslims. Animals must be ritually slaughtered to provide meat that is Halal.

Hypoglycaemia – Blood sugar levels are lower than the normal range for blood sugar.

Hypothyroidism – Insufficient production of thyroid hormone by the thyroid gland.

Hyperglycaemia – Blood sugar levels are higher than the normal range for blood sugar.

Hypersensitivity – Objectively reproducible symptoms or signs initiated by exposure to a defined stimulus at a dose tolerated by normal persons.

Hypertension – Raised blood pressure.

Infant – A child under 12 months of age.

Kangaroo care – The practice of securing a very young or preterm infant against the mother's skin, usually on her chest between her breasts to maximize body contact. The benefits include reduced morbidity and mortality.

Kosher – This means that animals and birds have been slaughtered by the Jewish method, carried out by a trained and authorized person.

Leptin – A hormone secreted by adipose tissue that plays a key role in regulating energy intake and energy expenditure, including the regulation of appetite and metabolism.

Non-milk extrinsic sugars – Sugars in food that are the most harmful to teeth – sucrose, glucose and fructose not within the intact cells of fruit (e.g. fructose from processed fruit such as fruit juices).

Oesophagus – The part of the digestive canal that food and drinks pass through between the throat down to the stomach.

Personal Child Health Record (PCHR) – A record of a child's growth, development and uptake of preventive health services (e.g. immunizations), designed to enhance communication between parents and health professionals.

Pesticide – Chemicals including herbicides, insecticides and fungicides used to kill pests.

Phytochemicals – Compounds that occur naturally in plants (phyto means 'plant' in Greek), which may have biological significance but are not established as essential nutrients. They are responsible for some colour and smell, such as the deep purple of blueberries and smell of garlic. In the diet they play a role in the immune system and provide long-term protection against cancer and heart disease. They include the brightly coloured pigments in fruits and vegetables and are also called flavanoids, flavanols or isoflavones.

Phyto-oestrogens – Plant chemicals that behave the same way in the body as the hormone oestrogen.

Prader–Willi syndrome – A condition caused by a chromosomal abnormality. Babies are floppy at birth and go on to develop obesity due to an excessive appetite and overeating. Other characteristics are small hands and feet, mental retardation, poor emotional and social development and immature development of sexual organs and other sexual characteristics.

Prebiotics – Fibre that encourages the growth of good bacteria in the intestine.

Preterm babies – Babies born before 37 weeks gestation.

Probiotics – Bacteria present in fermented food that colonize the intestinal tract and improve the intestinal microbial balance. Examples are bifidobacteria and lactobacilli.

Protein – A complex molecule consisting of a particular sequence of chains of amino acids. Proteins are essential constituents of all living things.

Pulses – A group of foods that includes lentils, peas and starchy beans but excludes green beans. Examples of starchy beans are chick peas, black eye beans, baked beans, white and red kidney beans, flageolet beans.

Reflux – See gastro-oesophageal reflux.

Retch – Make an involuntary effort to vomit.

Stool – Evacuated faecal matter passed through the anus.

Supine – Lying on the back.

Teratogenesis – The development of physical defects in the embryo.

Term babies – Babies born after 37 weeks gestation.

Answers to Activities

Chapter 1.3

Activity 3

Your answer may include:

- lack of understanding why change is needed
- lack of confidence in the advice given by health professionals
- communication difficulties with language barriers and sometimes issues with literacy
- senior members of the family being held in great respect and their views on diet having considerable influence, which negatively affects compliance with guidance given by health professionals
- negative prior experience of receiving inappropriate and insensitive guidance ignoring cultural and religious beliefs.

Activity 4

Your answer may include:

- access to food and shops
- prices of food in accessible shops and markets
- budgeting strategies
- patterns of food choice
- social and cultural acceptability
- other pressures for allocation of money (e.g. rent, heating, lighting, clothes/shoes for the children)
- food preferences within the household
- concerns for food waste
- lack of education on benefits of healthy diet
- social support available for families (e.g. Healthy Start Scheme).

Activity 5

Your answer may include these items:

Nutritious choices	Lower nutrient foods that should be limited to very small amounts occasionally
Bread	Fortified sugar-coated breakfast cereals
Breakfast cereals – fortified but not sugar coated	Fizzy drinks
Cheese	Fruit juices
Yogurt	Fruit smoothies
Fromage frais	Chocolate
Fish fingers	Sweets and confectionery
Frozen vegetables	Biscuits Cakes Fast food sold with little or no vegetables Ice cream Crisps and other packet snacks Cereal bars

Activity 6

Your answer may include:

- reduced energy expenditure as it displaces more active pastimes
- exposure to food advertising that negatively affects nutritious food choices
- misleading food advertising confuses the understanding of healthy eating.

Activity 7

Your answer could include:

- what parents/carers already 'know' about food (carers are more likely to accept, integrate and act on nutrition information that corresponds with their existing knowledge)
- established food patterns and customs and the extent to which they are followed in the household
- hierarchy within the family
- social pressures and socio-economic factors
- multicultural competencies of health professionals giving the advice, such as using the correct terminology
- access to appropriate foods in the local area
- availability of different foods.

Activity 8

Your answer may include:

- eat with their children as often as possible
- eat the foods they would like their children to eat
- make positive comments about the foods they want their children to eat
- plan a daily routine of 3 meals and 2–3 nutritious snacks
- always offer nutritious foods at meals and snacks
- set boundaries around food, drinks, meals and snacks and stick to them.

Activity 9

Your answer should include ideas involving:

- parental time and attention
- books and toys
- non-food-related activities.

Activity 10

Your answer may include:

- no strong role models for children to copy positive eating behaviours

- children adopt antisocial mealtime behaviours
- children do not learn to like the food their parents eat.

Chapter 3.1

Activity 1

(a) An underweight woman: balanced eating plan with increased energy intake with the aim of weight gain and increased nutritional stores, exercise levels, alcohol intake, caffeine intake.

(b) An overweight couple: balanced eating plan with decreased energy to reduce weight to a healthy BMI for both man and woman, exercise levels, alcohol intake, caffeine intake.

(c) A couple both of normal weight: balanced eating plan to improve nutritional status, alcohol intake, exercise levels, caffeine intake, zinc supplements, hazards in the working environment.

Activity 2

Answer to include:

- reduce weight to BMI 18.5–25 at least 3–4 months prior to conception
- reduce HbA1c to below 6.1 per cent, and not try to conceive if HbA1c is above 10 per cent
- follow a nutritions balanced diet with a supplement of 5 mg folic acid and 10 µg vitamin D.

Chapter 3.2

Activity 1

Answer should include:

- nutritions balanced diet
- vitamin supplementation of folic acid and vitamin D
- three servings of milk, cheese and yogurt per day
- encourage high-iron foods
- register for the benefits of the Healthy Start scheme.

Activity 2

Your menu should include:

● food group 1: bread, rice, potatoes, pasta and other starchy foods – the base for each meal and some snacks using mainly wholegrain varieties

● food group 2: fruit and vegetables – one or more of these at each meal and some snacks

● food group 3: milk and dairy foods – 2–3 servings of milk, cheese, yogurt using low-fat varieties

● food group 4: meat, fish, eggs, beans and nuts – 2 or 3 servings

● food group 5: foods and drinks high in fat and/ or sugar – small quantities

● fluid intake: 6–8 drinks.

Activity 3

Answer should include:

● reheat all food thoroughly so it is piping hot right through

● cook thoroughly all meat and eggs, and foods containing them

● avoid unpasteurized milk and milk products

● avoid pâté and mould-ripened soft cheese

● wear gloves when gardening, dealing with soil or cat litter trays

● wash fruit and vegetables thoroughly to remove any soil

● wash hands after contact with pets

● limit foods containing vitamin A

● limit oily fish to two servings per week.

Chapter 4.4

Activity 1

	Requirements per kg	Requirements for infant of 1.8 kg	300 mL mature breast milk	300 mL preterm formula: Nutriprem 1
Fluids (mL)	135–200	243–360	300	300
Energy (kcal)	110–135	198–243	207	240
Protein (g)	3.5–4.0	6.3–7.2	3.9	7.8
Sodium (g)	69–115	124.2–207	45	210
Potassium (mg)	66–132	119–238	174	246
Calcium (mg)	120–140	216–252	102	282
Phosphorous (mg)	60–90	108–162	45	186
Magnesium (mg)	8–15	14.4–27	9	24
Iron (µg)	2000–3000	3600–5400	2100	4800
Vitamin A (µgRE)	400–1000	720–1800	186	1083
Vitamin D (IU)	800–1000 /day	800–1000	–	360
Vitamin E (mg)	2.2–11	3.96–19.8	1.02	10.5
Vitamin K (µg)	4.4–28	7.92–50.4	–	18
Thiamin (µg)	140–300	252–540	80	420
Riboflavin (µg)	200–400	360–720	90	600

Activity 2

Baby was born 13 weeks, or 3 months, early before the EDD (estimated date of delivery), so 5–8 months after the date of birth is 2 (5 minus 3) to 5 (8 minus 3) months past the EDD.

Chapter 5.1

Activity

High-iron foods:

	Day 1	Day 2	Day 3
Breakfast	Egg	Baked beans	Muesli with added ground almonds
Midday meal	Chick pea	Dhal	Lentils
Evening meal	Tofu	Egg	Hummus

High-vitamin C foods:

	Day 1	Day 2	Day 3
Breakfast	Small glass diluted orange juice	Small glass diluted orange juice	Strawberries
Midday meal	Strawberries	Mango slices	Tomato in bolognaise sauce
Evening meal	Cherry tomatoes	Pepper slices	Kiwi fruit

Chapter 6.1

Activity 2

Your answer may include:

- developing familiarity with foods by holding cooking sessions, tasting sessions involving teachers making positive comments about the food, and classroom activities such as counting, colouring in, drawing, painting, stories, word searches, quizzes, weighing out foods as part of maths lessons and games.

- involving the pupils, parents and staff in planning menus and foods available in other catering outlets

- getting the teachers to eat with the children, eat the same food and make positive comments about the foods

- developing taught curriculum to contain the concepts of nutrients and components in food in relation to health.

Chapter 7.2

Activity 1

Your answer may include a range of components, including demonstrations, videos and group discussions rather than focusing on parental education alone. For example:

- planning more nutritious meals and snacks that can be substituted for the high-fat and high-sugar foods that they may normally offer

- interactive cookery demonstrations

- cook-and-eat sessions for parents to improve their cooking skills and their knowledge of healthy eating, and to empower parents to provide healthier family meals

- exploring children's activities that can be substituted for watching TV or DVDs

- increasing daily family physical activity by encouraging more walking instead of always using the car or pushing preschool children around in a stroller

- engaging in local facilities with opportunities for active play and sports.

Appendix 1: Function and Food Sources of Nutrients

Nutrient	Function in the body	Food sources
Protein – usually provides about 15% of energy	Provides structure for all the cells in the body. Enzymes and carrier molecules are made of protein It can be broken down to provide energy if necessary	The main sources are milk, yogurt, cheese, meat, fish, eggs, nuts chopped and ground or as butter Other sources are pulses such as dhal, lentils, baked beans, hummus and other starchy beans: chick peas, butter beans and red kidney beans Breakfast cereals and foods containing flour such as bread, chapatti and pasta also provide some protein
Carbohydrate – should provide about 50% of the energy (calories) There are three types: 1. 'simple' sugars, such as lactose in milk, fructose in fruit and added sugar – sucrose and glucose 2. starch 3. fibre is made up of carbohydrate complexes that are not absorbed in the intestine	Starch and sugar provide energy (calories)	Potatoes, yam, breakfast cereals, couscous, rice and any foods containing flour such as bread, chapatti, pasta, biscuits and cakes Fruit contains the sugar fructose Milk contains the sugar lactose Sweetened foods contain the sugars sucrose and glucose
Fibre – also called 'non-starch polysaccharides' Fibre includes: 1. non-digestible carbohydrates, mostly derived from plant material, that are fermented in the colon 2. prebiotics	Fibre keeps the gastro intestinal tract functioning normally. Too little will cause constipation but too much can cause diarrhoea and could slow growth Prebiotics feed the bacteria in the colon that are important in the normal functioning of the intestines	Fruits, vegetables, cereals and foods made from flours White flour and breads contain some fibre while wholemeal or wholegrain contain more Wholegrain cereals such as porridge, Ready Brek and Weetabix contain more fibre than more processed cereals Prebiotics are a type of fibre found in onions, leeks, garlic and bananas
Fat – should provide about 35% of the energy (kcal) It is made up of: 1. fatty acids that are: saturated, monounsaturated or polyunsaturated, including omega 3 and omega 6 2. complex fats (e.g. cholesterol and phospholipids)	Provides energy and carries some vitamins around the body All cells have fats in their structure All the fatty acids needed can be synthesised by the human body except the omega 3 and omega 6 fatty acids, which we need to have in our food. Brain, nerves and skin contain very high amounts of omega 3 and omega 6 fats	Oils and fats used in cooking foods Butter, margarine and other spreads for bread Cream and cheese Cakes, biscuits and ice cream Small amounts in whole milk and yogurt, egg yolks and lean meat Toddlers need a good balance of omega 3 and omega 6 fats. There are usually plenty of omega 6 fats in the diet Oily fish are good sources of omega 3 long-chain fats, DHA (docosahexaenoic acid) and EPA (eicosapentaenoic acid) Rapeseed oil and walnut oil are good sources of omega 3 ALA (alpha-linolenic acid). Most pure vegetable oil in the UK is made from rapeseed Olive and soya oils have a good balance of omega 3 and omega 6

Water	For maintaining normal hydration; blood pressure and fluid balance	Most water comes from drinks: milk, fruit juices and diluted squashes are all about 90% water Soups, sauces, fruit and vegetables have high water contents. Drier foods contain less
Vitamins		
Vitamin A (retinol and carotene)	Ensures normal growth and development, strengthens the immune system; important for healthy intestines and skin and good vision	Full fat cow's milk Egg yolks Butter and other fats spreads (margarines) Orange, red and dark green fruit and vegetables such as carrots, red peppers, tomatoes, sweet potato, pumpkin, apricots, mangoes, cantaloupe melons, broccoli Oily fish Liver and liver pâté has very high levels so only give it to your toddler once per week at the most
B vitamins: thiamine, folate, niacin, riboflavin, pyridoxine, biotin, pantothenic acid, vitamin B12	Growth and development of healthy nervous system Involved in the processes that convert food into energy	Liver pâté and yeast extracts such as Marmite are the only foods that contain all the B vitamins Most breakfast cereals are fortified with extra B vitamins Other good sources are meat, milk, yogurt, cheese, fish, eggs, seeds, bread and vegetables
Vitamin C (ascorbic acid)	Helps absorb iron from non-meat sources Is part of the immune system and protects cells from damage Maintains blood vessels, cartilage, muscle and bone	Most fruit and vegetables contain some The richest sources are blackcurrants, kiwi fruit, citrus fruits, tomatoes, peppers and strawberries Potato, sweet potatoes and mangoes are also good sources Certain fruit juices such as blackcurrant and orange have higher levels than other fruit juices
Vitamin D	Needed to absorb calcium into the body. Also regulates calcium levels, ensures bone growth and is part of the immune system	Most vitamin D is made in the skin when toddlers are outside during the summer months i.e. April–September in the UK The few food sources are oily fish and foods fortified with vitamin D which include margarine, some yogurts and fromage frais, one or two breakfast cereals and growing up formula milks
Vitamin E	Antioxidant that protects cell structures throughout the body	In a wide variety of foods Rich sources are vegetable oils and margarine, avocados, almonds, meat, fish and eggs

(Continued)

(Continued)

Nutrient	Function in the body	Food sources
Vitamin K	Blood clotting	Mainly produced by bacteria in the large bowel. Food sources are green leafy vegetables and broccoli
Minerals		
Calcium	Needed for growing bones and teeth Needed for muscle contractions, for the structure and functioning of all cells and the working of nerves	Richest sources are milk, cheese, yogurt and fortified soya milk White bread is fortified with calcium Ground almonds Canned fish with bones such as sardines
Copper	Making energy and protein	In small amounts in most foods
Fluoride	Strengthens tooth enamel and makes it resistant to attack by the bacteria that cause tooth decay	A smear of fluoride toothpaste on toothbrush when cleaning teeth twice a day provides enough It is in tap water in some areas of the UK where tap water is fluoridated or the water naturally contains adequate levels of fluoride. However, large areas of the UK have water that contains very, very little fluoride
Iodine	Part of the hormone thyroxine, which helps convert food into energy and is needed for mental and physical development	Fish, milk, yogurt and eggs
Iron	Necessary for carrying oxygen around the body in the blood and needed for growing muscles, energy metabolism and the immune system	Best sources are red meat (beef, lamb and pork) and dark poultry meat (e.g. chicken legs and thighs). White meat such as chicken breast has less Other sources are: fortified breakfast cereals, ground or chopped nuts (see below for caution with peanuts and whole nuts), dhal, lentils, hummus, popadums made with lentil flour, bhajis and Bombay mix made with chick pea flour Smaller amounts are in fruit and vegetables
Magnesium	Helps in bone development, making protein and converting food into energy	Best sources are wholegrain breakfast cereals, milk and yogurt Also in meat, egg, dhal, lentils, hummus, potatoes and some vegetables
Phosphorus	Building bone growth and using energy	Richest source is milk and it is present in most other foods
Potassium	Important for fluid balance, muscle contraction and nerve conduction	Milk, vegetables and potatoes Bananas, dried apricots, prunes, dates and kiwi fruit are also good sources
Selenium	Antioxidant and necessary for the production of the thyroid hormone thyroxine	Bread, meat, fish, nuts, eggs and other foods made from flour

Sodium	Regulation of fluid balance and blood pressure	Salt is the main source of sodium and salt is used in making bacon, ham, cheese and bread Salt is added to most ready meals, sauces, soups, snacks and other processed foods Sodium is also found naturally in small quantities in most fresh foods particularly meat, fish, eggs, milk and yogurt Foods with added salt such as crisps and processed foods should be kept to a minimum
Zinc	Helps wounds heal and is involved in the function of many enzymes and hormones	Best sources are meat, fish, shellfish and eggs Other good sources are milk, wholegrain breakfast cereals, such as porridge, Shredded Wheat, Weetabix, and bread Some in potatoes, dhal, lentils, hummus and leafy vegetables
Other bioactive substances		
Phytochemicals in plants that provide long-term protection against cancer and heart disease Also called flavanoids, flavanols and isoflavones (e.g. lycopene, lutein and quercetin)	Among other things, they act as antioxidants protecting all cells from damage and they are an important part of the immune system	Fruits, vegetables, spices, herbs, nuts and foods made from cereals – particularly those that are brightly coloured Cocoa and chocolate
Probiotics are bacteria in food that will colonize the intestine and provide health benefits	Increase the number of beneficial bacteria in the intestine and consequently reduce the effects of harmful bacteria that may cause infection	Live yogurt

Appendix 2: Growth Charts

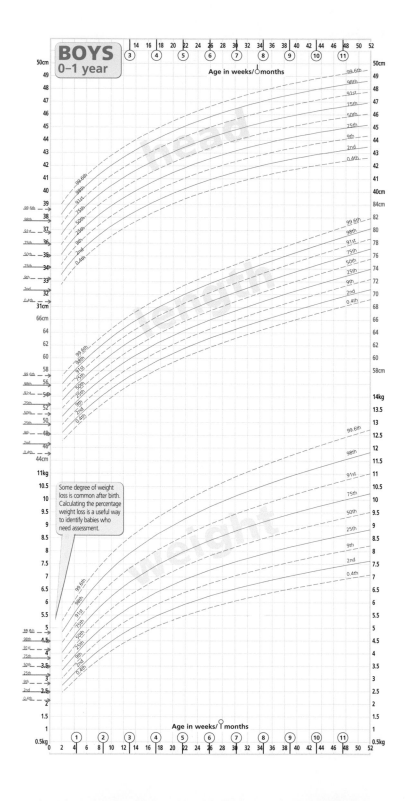

BOYS
0–1 year

Age in weeks/ months

Some degree of weight loss is common after birth. Calculating the percentage weight loss is a useful way to identify babies who need assessment.

Age in weeks/ months

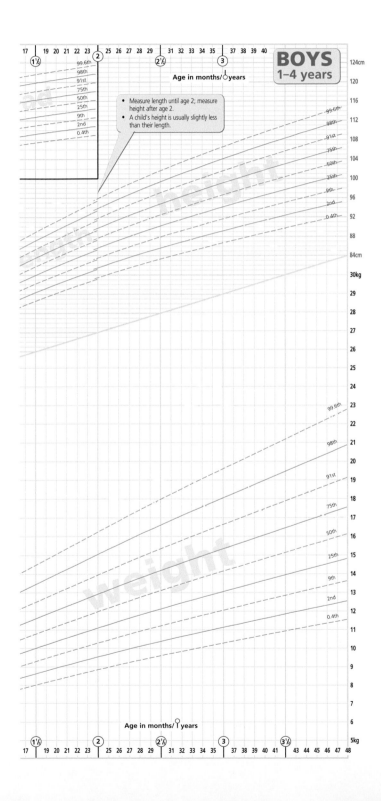

BOYS
1–4 years

- Measure length until age 2; measure height after age 2.
- A child's height is usually slightly less than their length.

Age in months/years

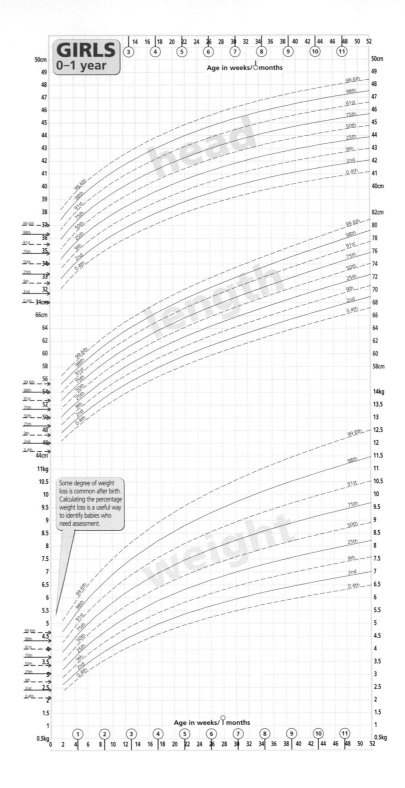

GIRLS
0–1 year

Age in weeks/months

Some degree of weight loss is common after birth. Calculating the percentage weight loss is a useful way to identify babies who need assessment.

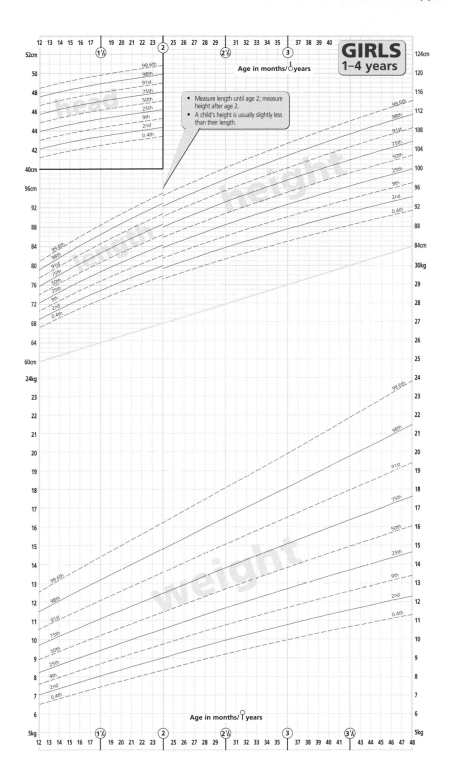

GIRLS
1–4 years

Age in months/years

- Measure length until age 2; measure height after age 2.
- A child's height is usually slightly less than their length.

Age in months/years

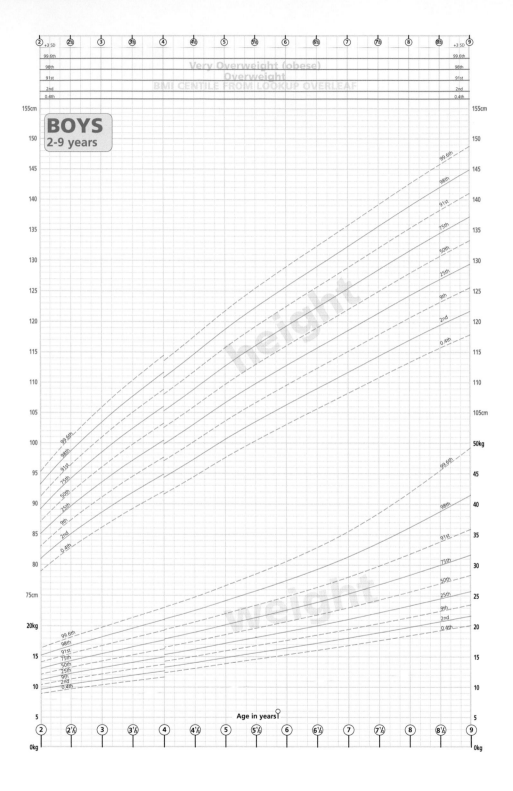

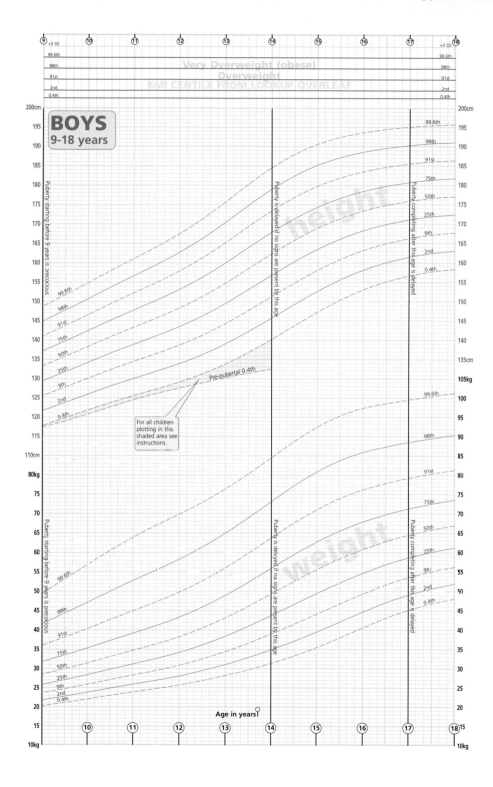

BOYS
9-18 years

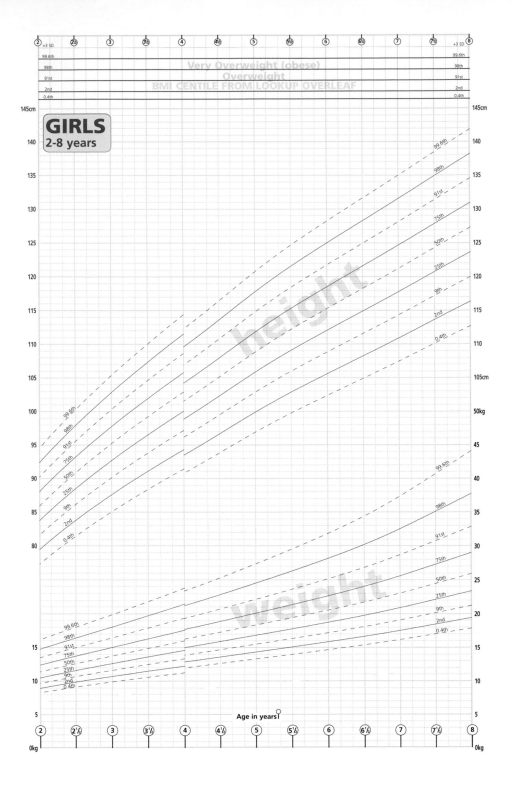

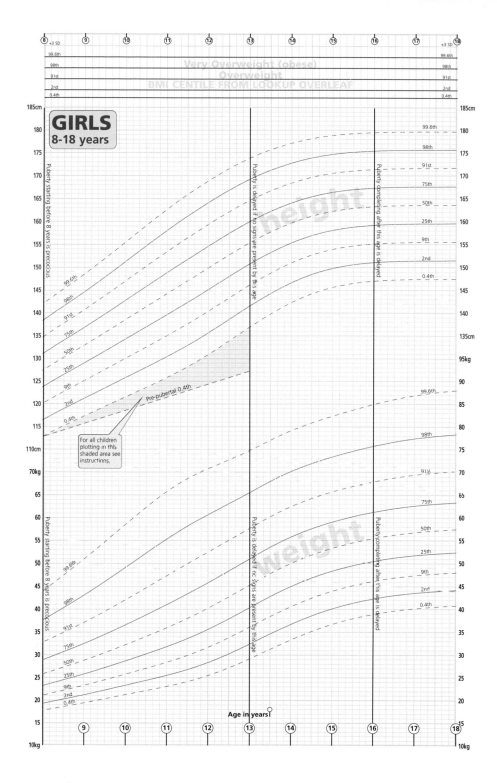

GIRLS
8-18 years

Very Overweight (obese)
Overweight
BMI CENTILE FROM LOOKUP OVERLEAF

Pre-pubertal 0.4th

For all children plotting in this shaded area see instructions.

weight

Weight

Age in years

Appendix 3: BMI and Waist Circumference Charts

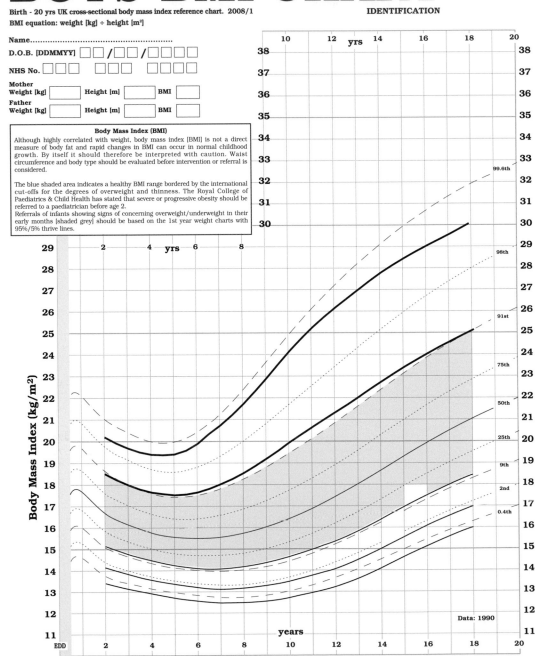

BOYS BMI CHART

Birth - 20 yrs UK cross-sectional body mass index reference chart. 2008/1

BMI equation: weight [kg] ÷ height [m²]

IDENTIFICATION

Name...

D.O.B. [DDMMYY] □□ / □□ / □□□□

NHS No. □□□   □□□   □□□□

Mother
Weight [kg] □   Height [m] □   BMI □

Father
Weight [kg] □   Height [m] □   BMI □

Body Mass Index (BMI)

Although highly correlated with weight, body mass index [BMI] is not a direct measure of body fat and rapid changes in BMI can occur in normal childhood growth. By itself it should therefore be interpreted with caution. Waist circumference and body type should be evaluated before intervention or referral is considered.

The blue shaded area indicates a healthy BMI range bordered by the international cut-offs for the degrees of overweight and thinness. The Royal College of Paediatrics & Child Health has stated that severe or progressive obesity should be referred to a paediatrician before age 2.
Referrals of infants showing signs of concerning overweight/underweight in their early months [shaded grey] should be based on the 1st year weight charts with 95%/5% thrive lines.

Data: 1990

Body mass index reference curves for the UK, 1990 (Cole TJ, Freeman JV, Preece MA) *Arch Dis Child* 1995; **73**: 25-9
Establishing a standard definition for child overweight and obesity: international survey (Cole TJ, Bellizzi MC, Flegal KM, Dietz WH) *BMJ 2000*; **320**: 1240-3
Body mass index cut-offs to define thinness in children and adolescents: international survey (Cole TJ, Flegal KM, Nicholls D, Jackson AA) *BMJ 2007*; **335**: 194-7

Manufacture 21 May 12   BMIBI

BOYS WAIST CIRCUMFERENCE

D.O.B. [DDMMYY] ☐☐ / ☐☐ / ☐☐☐☐

Because a high BMI by itself may not be a guarantor of obesity/overweight, a high waist centile added to a high BMI centile will confirm fatness more conclusively. The shaded area represents a healthy waist range.

Measuring the Waist

The waist is defined as the mid-way point between the lowest rib cage and the iliac crest and should be measured, preferably, with a special tension tape [see illustrations below].

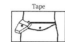
Tape

When measuring his waist, the boy should ideally be wearing only underclothes. Ask him to stand with his feet together and weight evenly distributed with his arms relaxed. Ask him to breathe normally and take the waist measurement at the end of a normal expiration.

The waist can also be identified by asking him to bend to one side. Measurement is taken at the point of flexure.

If he is wearing a shirt or vest, deduct 1cm before recording and plotting the waist measurement.

There is no consensus about how to define paediatric obesity using waist measurement. For clinical use the 99.6th or 98th centiles are suggested cut-offs for obesity and the 91st centile for overweight, like the BMI [see chart overleaf].

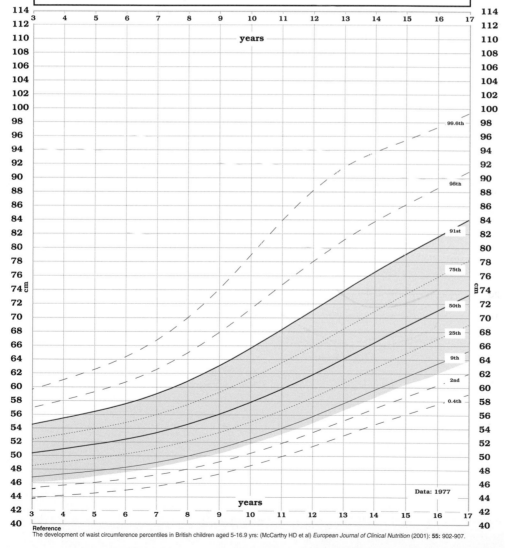

Reference
The development of waist circumference percentiles in British children aged 5-16.9 yrs: (McCarthy HD et al) *European Journal of Clinical Nutrition* (2001): **55:** 902-907.

GIRLS BMI CHART

Birth - 20 yrs UK cross-sectional body mass index reference chart. 2008/1

BMI equation: weight [kg] ÷ height [m²]

IDENTIFICATION

Name...

D.O.B. [DDMMYY] ☐☐ / ☐☐ / ☐☐☐☐

NHS No. ☐☐☐ ☐☐☐ ☐☐☐☐

Mother
Weight [kg] ☐   Height [m] ☐   BMI ☐

Father
Weight [kg] ☐   Height [m] ☐   BMI ☐

Body Mass Index (BMI)

Although highly correlated with weight, body mass index [BMI] is not a direct measure of body fat and rapid changes in BMI can occur in normal childhood growth. By itself it should therefore be interpreted with caution. Waist circumference and body type should be evaluated before intervention or referral is considered.

The red shaded area indicates a healthy BMI range bordered by the international cut-offs for the degrees of overweight and thinness. The Royal College of Paediatrics & Child Health has stated that severe or progressive obesity should be referred to a paediatrician before age 2.

Referrals of infants showing signs of concerning overweight/underweight in their early months [shaded grey] should be based on the 1st year weight charts with 95%/5% thrive lines.

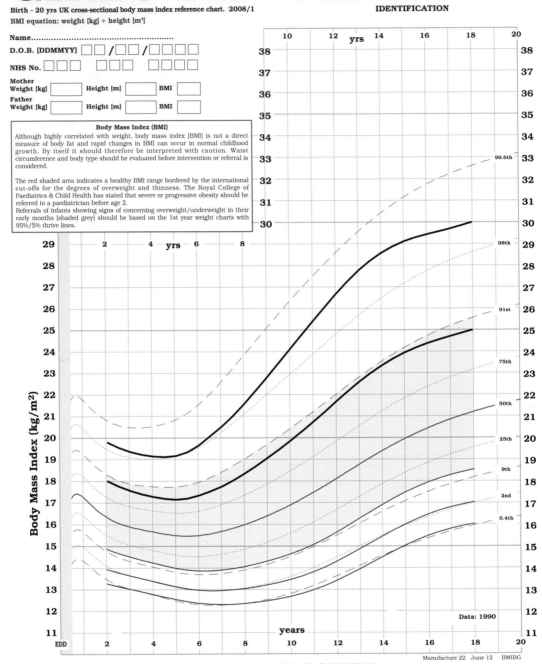

Data: 1990

Manufacture 22   June 12   BMIBG

Body mass index reference curves for the UK, 1990 (Cole TJ, Freeman JV, Preece MA) *Arch Dis Child* 1995; **73:** 25-9
Establishing a standard definition for child overweight and obesity: international survey (Cole TJ, Bellizzi MC, Flegal KM, Dietz WH) *BMJ 2000;* **320:** 1240-3
Body mass index cut-offs to define thinness in children and adolescents: international survey (Cole TJ, Flegal KM, Nicholls D, Jackson AA) *BMJ 2007;* **335:** 194-7

GIRLS WAIST CIRCUMFERENCE

D.O.B. [DDMMYY] ☐☐ / ☐☐ / ☐☐☐☐

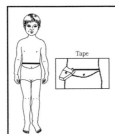

Tape

Because a high BMI by itself may not be a guarantor of obesity/overweight, a high waist centile added to a high BMI centile will confirm fatness more conclusively. The shaded area represents a healthy waist range.

Measuring the Waist

The waist is defined as the mid-way point between the lowest rib cage and the iliac crest and should be measured, preferably, with a special tension tape [see illustrations below].

When measuring her waist, the girl should ideally be wearing only underclothes. Ask her to stand with her feet together and weight evenly distributed with her arms relaxed. Ask her to breathe normally and take the waist measurement at the end of a normal expiration.

The waist can also be identified by asking her to bend to one side. Measurement is taken at the point of flexure.

If she is wearing a shirt or vest, deduct 1cm before recording and plotting the waist measurement.

There is no consensus about how to define paediatric obesity using waist measurement. For clinical use the 99.6th or 98th centiles are suggested cut-offs for obesity and the 91st centile for overweight, like the BMI [see chart overleaf].

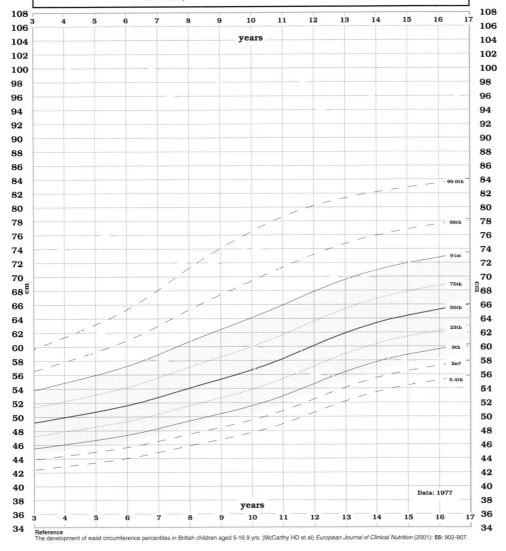

Data: 1977

Reference
The development of waist circumference percentiles in British children aged 5-16.9 yrs: (McCarthy HD et al) *European Journal of Clinical Nutrition* (2001): **55**: 902-907.

Index